VOICES OF MENTAL HEALTH

Other books by Martin Halliwell

Romantic Science and the Experience of Self (1999; 2016)
Modernism and Morality (2001)
republished as *Transatlantic Modernism* (2006)
Critical Humanisms: Humanist/Anti-Humanist Dialogues (2003)
(with Andy Mousley)
Images of Idiocy: The Idiot Figure in Modern Fiction and Film (2004)
The Constant Dialogue: Reinhold Niebuhr and American Intellectual Culture (2005)
American Culture in the 1950s (2007)
American Thought and Culture in the 21st Century (2008)
(edited with Catherine Morley)
Beyond and Before: Progressive Rock since the 1960s (2011)
(with Paul Hegarty)
Therapeutic Revolutions: Medicine, Psychiatry, and American Culture, 1945–1970 (2013)
William James and the Transatlantic Conversation (2014)
(edited with Joel Rasmussen)
Neil Young: American Traveller (2015)
Reframing 1968: American Politics, Protest and Identity (forthcoming)
(edited with Nick Witham)

VOICES OF MENTAL HEALTH

Medicine, Politics, and American Culture, 1970–2000

MARTIN HALLIWELL

RUTGERS UNIVERSITY PRESS
New Brunswick, Camden, and Newark, New Jersey, and London

Library of Congress Cataloging-in-Publication Data

Names: Halliwell, Martin, author.
Title: Voices of mental health : medicine, politics, and American culture, 1970-2000 / Martin Halliwell.
Description: New Brunswick, New Jersey : Rutgers University Press, [2017] | Includes bibliographical references and index.
Identifiers: LCCN 2016053289 | ISBN 9780813576787 (hardcover : alk. paper) | ISBN 9780813576794 (e-book (epub)) | ISBN 9780813576800 (e-book (web pdf))
Subjects: | MESH: Mental Disorders—history | Mental Disorders—therapy | Health Policy—history | Mental Health Services—economics | Psychiatry in Literature | Motion Pictures as Topic | History, 20th Century | United States
Classification: LCC RC455 | NLM WM 11 AA1 | DDC 362.196/89–dc23
LC record available at https://lccn.loc.gov/2016053289

A British Cataloging-in-Publication record for this book is available from the British Library.

∞ The paper used in this publication meets the requirements of the American National Standard for Information Sciences—Permanence of Paper for Printed Library Materials, ANSI Z39.48–1992.

www.rutgersuniversitypress.org

Manufactured in the United States of America

Contents

Illustrations

Preface

I began this book during winter 2012–13 at a time when two high-profile cinema releases profiled stories of individuals who are forced to confront uncomfortable medical interventions and intractable life issues. The first of these, *Silver Linings Playbook*, sees discharged mental health patient Patrick Solitano (Bradley Cooper) struggling to reintegrate into suburban Philadelphia after being institutionalized in a Baltimore psychiatric facility following the disintegration of his marriage. Avoiding prescription drugs when he can, Pat tries to adopt a positive "silver lining" attitude to life, but only hours after his trial discharge he feels hemmed in by his overprotective mother, his aloof father, fearful former colleagues, and an unsympathetic local policeman. He devises the mantra "excelsior" in an attempt to banish negativity but discovers that life does not deliver happy endings—that is, until he meets Tiffany Maxwell (Jennifer Lawrence), who has been taking similar medication. An unlikely therapeutic relationship develops between the pair as Tiffany slowly comes to terms with the untimely death of her husband and Pat broadens his perspective from his all-consuming desire to mend his broken marriage. Based on Matthew Quick's 2008 novel, the film focuses on Tiffany's intervention in Pat's story, through which she helps him to confront the messiness of life and realize that recovery is an ongoing process of adjustment.

The second film, Steven Soderbergh's *Side Effects*, explores the relationship between psychiatry and the pharmaceutical industry by focusing on a very different central character, Emily Taylor (Rooney Mara). Whereas *Silver Linings Playbook* has a comic edge, *Side Effects* hinges on a dark neo-noir plot in which none of the characters seem wholly innocent. Referencing a powerful literary account of depression—William Styron's 1989 memoir *Darkness Visible* (a text I discuss in chapter 8)—Emily is overwhelmed with depressive feelings when her husband returns from a stint in jail for insider trading, and she attempts suicide by slamming her car into the wall of a parking garage. Surviving the crash, Emily is placed on new medication, Ablixa, with its promise to "take back tomorrow." The drug appears to dull her anxiety but also triggers sleep-walking, during one episode of which she stabs her husband with a kitchen knife. The second half of *Side Effects* focuses on the extent to which Emily is guilty of murder (she is eventually plea-bargained into a local hospital) and the backlash against her psychiatrist, Jonathan Banks (Jude Law), for prescribing an untested drug. Whereas *Silver Linings Playbook* retains a largely realistic frame, *Side Effects* weaves depression and anxiety into a conspiracy involving Emily and another psychiatrist (Catherine Zeta Jones) who is making money from the sale of Ablixa. Hints of Emily's duplicity and Banks's professional misconduct complicate the malpractice case, resulting in a story in which viewers, like the patient and doctor, must find their way through a fog of uncertainty.

Neither film offers a straightforward critique of medical practices, nor do they see formal therapy or medication as simple solutions for bipolar disorder and chronic depression. Both characters have seemingly supportive doctors, yet Pat and Emily appear to be searching for an inner personal voice that has been muted by their drug treatment and distorted by their medical and social interactions. As a romantic comedy, *Silver Linings Playbook* offers a more optimistic therapeutic arc than the cynical *Side Effects*, but the twin focus on the patient's voice and the need to establish a coherent narrative links the two films.

These were just two of a group of cinematic releases in winter 2012–13 that address mental health issues; the group includes the subtle depictions of President Lincoln's famous melancholy in Steven Spielberg's *Lincoln*, the pain of cultural dislocation in Terence Malick's trancelike *To the Wonder*, and the damaging effects of obsession and torture in Kathryn Bigalow's *Zero Dark Thirty*. This third film echoes the opening episodes of the first season of the Showtime TV series *Homeland* (2011), in which CIA agent Carrie Mathison's bipolar disorder both sharpens and distorts her suspicions about the motives of returning U.S. marine Nicholas Brody, who has been held captive in Iraq for eight years, has secretly converted to Islam, and suffers postconflict trauma on returning to family life in the suburbs of Washington, DC. These examples cross borders of genre, gender, and geography and push us to think about how so many stories that deal with mental health pose questions about the veracity of who speaks and with what degree of knowledge and insight.

To pursue these questions, *Voices of Mental Health* focuses on health conditions that rose to public attention in the late twentieth century and that captured the interest of physicians, policy makers, the media, and cultural practitioners. Just as the voices in this book are diverse and plural, so the book takes the topic of mental health to encompass a spectrum of experiences and behaviors that makes it a much more flexible category than the more prescriptive and sometimes discriminatory term mental illness. While a study of the last thirty years of the twentieth century is instructive for thinking about the "credibility struggles" (to borrow a term from AIDS scholarship) of a range of mental health experiences, it is important to be attentive to who is speaking and what kind of health narrative is being constructed in order to test and explore the borders between biomedical, cultural, and political conceptions of voice.[1]

Mounting national interest in mental health at that time was reflected in an instructive report by the Centers for Disease Control and Prevention, *Mental Illness Surveillance among Adults in the United States*, which estimated that a quarter of the population was facing diagnosable forms of mental illness and another quarter was likely to experience prolonged psychological challenges during their lives.[2] This 2011 report assesses the costs of treatment and prevention (an estimated $300 billion per year), considers related chronic health issues, and uses state-by-state data to identify regional variances, finding that there are higher instances in poorer states in the Southeast than in other regions. It concludes that "increasing access to and use of mental health treatment services could substantially reduce the associated morbidity," but provides no easy answers during a phase when the "global burden" of noncommunicable diseases such as depression was on the sharp upswing.[3] At the same time, debates about mental health and gun control, following a wave of horrific shootings, have raised pressing questions about the relationship between equitable access to services, undiagnosed conditions, drug use, and the responsibility of families.

These questions were not new, of course, and they returned national attention to one of the major events that occurred late in President Clinton's term of office: the Columbine High School shooting of April 1999 in which twelve students and a teacher in Littleton, Colorado were killed in a carefully planned attack by two senior students (one was taking the anti-depressant Luvox and the other was experiencing depression and paranoia; they each committed suicide half an hour after the shootings). First Lady Hillary Clinton called the cold-blooded school massacre a wake-up call that "pierced the heart of America."[4] Little changed, though. And well over a decade later, President Obama was still pressing the nation to discover "the ability to act and to change" in his memorial speech for the victims of the 2013 Washington Navy Yard shooting. This crime again linked deadly violence to paranoid delusions, just two years after another shooting in Tucson, Arizona left Democratic congresswoman Gabrielle Giffords with a severe head injury and six others dead.[5] At that time, Obama warned against sharply polarizing debates in order to ensure "that we're talking with each other in a way that heals, not a way that wounds."[6] But media fascination with these and subsequent explosive events has tended to perpetuate stereotypes of mental illness and, as I aim to show here, needs to be set alongside more everyday stories that also pose serious questions about health—as Obama made clear in his opening remarks of the June 2013 National Conference on Mental Health, held fourteen years after the inaugural White House event on this topic.

To explore these factors, *Voices of Mental Health: Medicine, Politics, and American Culture, 1970–2000* extends the chronology of my 2013 book *Therapeutic Revolutions: Medicine, Psychiatry, and American Culture, 1945–1970* by discussing how key medical and social issues that intersected in the postwar years became part of the national conversation after 1970.[7] There are some shifts of emphasis between the two books, particularly the downplaying of Freudian language in *Voices of Mental Health* to reflect the fact that neurology and biology superseded a psychoanalytic framework late in the century. There is also a sharper focus on federal politics and national policies at a time when mental health was becoming more politicized than ever. This was most obvious in the late 1970s during the Carter presidency and the second term of the Clinton administration, which regained momentum on mental health advocacy and reform after some lean years under Presidents Reagan and Bush. I also discuss how the emergence of patients' and ex-patients' voices in the 1970s and 1980s—in survivor narratives, through advocacy and support groups, and within previously silenced or underrepresented communities—helped both to politicize and personalize health culture, linking individual experiences to narrative patterns and shared histories that sometimes enriched and at others challenged textbook case studies.

The concept of voice is central to this book, not merely because mental illness and disability became politicized in the 1970s but also because published accounts of suffering and care from the perspectives of patients and doctors proliferated, opening up often intensely private experiences to a broader readership. This is partly the legacy of the "literature and medicine" movement of the 1980s and the rise of cancer and AIDS memoirs—including moving testimonies by Audre Lorde and Paul Monette—and partly because an emphasis on voice reemerged around the millennium, after two decades when scholars in the humanities and social sciences downplayed it in favor of theories of embodiment.[8] Emblematic of this renewed focus on voice is the Faces and Voices of Recovery addiction support group, founded in St. Paul, Minnesota in 2001, and the "Voices of" anthology series from the independent publisher LaChance, which, since 2006, has offered first-person accounts of illnesses that range from alcoholism and autism to bipolar disorder and breast cancer.

This tendency can also be interpreted as a shift away from the "two cultures" model that captured the polarities of the Cold War years toward a pluralistic culture in which diversity and particularity replaced more universalizing terms, due, in part, to the emerging social movements and identity politics of the 1960s. While it is overly simplistic to think that the two cultures rhetoric simply vanished, the emergence of narrative medicine in the 1980s and the development of medical humanities research in the 1990s and 2000s have also helped transform the binaries of the mid-twentieth century into layered patterns of understanding. This transformation of knowledge structures finds a parallel in anthropologist Gregory Bateson's recommendation that integration and flexibility should be recognized as key markers of health. Although he was not writing explicitly about voice and narrative—and he did not discuss the risks to the self of becoming fragmented or unmoored—one can see how Bateson's model of health in the early 1970s as an "uncommitted potentiality for change" lays the groundwork for a narrative mode in which the individual is actively transported by open stories instead of being trapped within pathology.[9]

We can also, then, begin to see connections with the opening discussion of *Silver Linings Playbook*. The first scene portrays Patrick reading aloud the letter he has been composing to his wife, earlier drafts of which, as the novel makes more explicit, had been confiscated by his doctors.[10] Framed against an outside window but lacking a clear view, Pat reads the letter and insists (to his absent wife, to himself, and to the audience) that he "is better now" and ready to resume his normal life. He revises this draft letter to his wife throughout the film in an attempt to reconnect with his now-lost former existence and slowly comes to recognize that there is no normality as such to which to return. By the end, Pat sees that not only does he have a future—with all its messiness and contradictions—but also a voice that speaks to his new orientation, as dramatized when he reads a much shorter letter that he has written to Tiffany with its final line: "I just got stuck."[11]

One might dismiss this denouement for being as false as Pat's preferred ending of Ernest Hemingway's World War I story *A Farewell to Arms*, in which the heroine Catherine Barkley manages to survive death, but it is clear that he now has a better grasp of his place within a psychosocial matrix. Pat's voice here is a personal one, yet it also resonates through the lives of his family and friends, making authentic communication, however problematic, more enabling than institutional care or custodial enforcement, a message that actor Bradley Cooper and director David O. Russell took further in their efforts to raise public awareness of mental health challenges.[12] We will find as many stories of stasis and fragmentation as accounts of integration and healing in *Voices of Mental Health*, but the search for a voice that both anchors a therapeutic narrative and emerges from within that story is a motif that runs through this study of late-twentieth-century U.S. culture.

VOICES OF MENTAL HEALTH

Introduction

MENTAL HEALTH IN AN AGE OF FRACTURE

One of the central arguments of this book is that the 1970s are more important for understanding the horizon of mental health in the United States than is often recognized. As a decade, the 1970s has been more difficult to historicize than others in the twentieth century, largely because it lacks a compelling political and cultural arc. This is one reason why historian Daniel Rodgers sees it as the beginning of "an age of fracture," in which strong metaphors that undergirded postwar social values weakened and identities became "fluid and elective."[1] The vision of a world in fragments has a number of echoes, including cinema historian Robin Wood's reading of 1970s films as "incoherent texts" and Walker Percy's portrayal in his futuristic 1971 novel *Love in the Ruins* of a dysfunctional nation that is "broken, sundered, busted down the middle."[2] Rodgers's metaphor also chimes with the view that the social ideals of the 1960s floundered in the wake of the assassinations of 1968 and within the paranoia of the Nixon administration.[3] Whether or not we wish to identify faltering political leadership or broader socioeconomic transitions as the trigger for these fractures, the shift from high ideals to hard realities during what President Nixon called an "era of negotiation" was particularly evident in the arenas of medicine and healthcare.[4]

The primary focus of this book is mental health, but framed within a broader crisis in healthcare, which the liberal magazine *The New Republic* recognized in January 1970 through Nevada surgeon Fred Anderson's claims that Americans were "paying more" yet "getting less" for their health dollars and that the whole system was in bad shape.[5] We should, however, be careful when picturing the 1970s as a fall or fracture not to indulge in a nostalgic view of the 1960s as a high-water mark for medicine. The reputation of medical science was being threatened in the late 1950s and early 1960s by the Cold War suspicion that patients were being manipulated by the system in the name of national security, not long after the triumph of Jonas Salk's polio vaccine suggested that American medicine was still enjoying its golden age. Although the landmark health reforms of Presidents Kennedy and Johnson restored some public faith in the medical system, the respected Illinois pediatrician Julius B. Richmond claimed that the 1960s witnessed only a "fragmented approach" to health reform, at least until 1964–65 when new legislation stimulated broader social programs.[6] Richmond approved of the policy shift from inpatient care to community outpatient facilities during the Johnson administration, but he was concerned about inefficiency and worried that federal, state, and local initiatives lacked coordination and integrated planning.[7]

The financial and logistical realities of community healthcare often grated against its idealistic conception at the grassroots level, especially by the early 1970s when, as medical historian Gerald Grob has argued, "many chronically and severely mentally ill persons . . . were often cast adrift in communities without access to support services or the basic necessities of life."[8] This was a major reason why, in his 1969 book *Currents in American Medicine*, Richmond advised physicians and health administrators to search for new synergies between the institutions and practices of healthcare. Richmond promoted a collaborative model of medical research centers and community health services—a view that informed his health advocacy through the Office of Economic Opportunity in the mid-1960s and as surgeon general during the Carter administration.[9] Perhaps stimulated by activist Ralph Nader's critique of community mental health as a "Band Aid approach to a number of social sores that will continue to fester regardless of the amount of first aid," Jimmy Carter echoed Richmond's rhetoric in his 1976 presidential campaign, calling healthcare a "haphazard, unsound, undirected, inefficient non-system" that had been worsened by the partial dismantling of Johnson's reforms during two Republican administrations.[10]

This was a far cry from President Nixon's vision of where the nation would be at the bicentennial. In his first State of the Union address in January 1970, he envisioned a peaceful country that would have "abolished hunger," could offer a "minimum income" for all families, and would have "made enormous progress in providing better housing, faster transportation, improved health, and superior education."[11] The Nixon administration instituted a review of healthcare in summer 1970 and released a white paper setting out a comprehensive federal health policy, promising to increase medical aid for schools and for underserved and low-income families and to invest in research on disease prevention.[12] A spring 1972 federal advertisement stressed that the president was advancing effective healthcare "on many fronts," but the average American would have found it difficult to find evidence of Nixon's utopian predictions, especially as he was seeking to minimize "government-run arrangements" and to scale back Johnson's welfare and health reforms, which he viewed as "a monstrous, consuming outrage."[13] When Nixon presented an ambitious health insurance plan to Congress in February 1974, it was with the admission that reform was moving too slowly on his watch and that medical costs were too high for both individuals and the state.[14]

His successor, Gerald Ford, tried to shift the agenda, seeing the end of prolonged conflict in Vietnam as an opportunity "to bind up the Nation's wounds, and to restore its health and its optimistic self-confidence."[15] Ford inherited Nixon's cuts to health spending, including a curb on funding for the community health center program that was at the heart of Johnson's reforms. However, these reductions did little to dent already-committed federal health dollars, which Ford noted had increased from $5 billion in 1965 to $37 billion in 1975. By February 1976, when Ford delivered a message to Congress on healthcare legislation, he realized that the whole health system was under financial strain, but he nevertheless recommended better catastrophic care for the elderly and the disabled, funds for drug abuse prevention, and further improvements to medical services in disadvantaged areas.

Thus, if President Carter inherited a "non-system" when he took office in January 1977, it was due to the unfeasible combination of hard economic realities and the idealistic goals of the mid-1960s. In his inaugural address, Carter, like Nixon, called for national renewal and "a new spirit among us all."[16] Given his health work during his term as governor of Georgia, it is surprising that Carter did not mention medicine or healthcare explicitly. Instead, he avoided both the high ideals of the 1960s and direct mention of the Nixon and Ford years by diplomatically referring to "our recent mistakes," a view that tallied with the opinion of the 77 percent who thought that things were going badly in a spring 1975 poll.[17] With this in mind, Carter looked to renew confidence in the federal government and encouraged fellow Americans to look outward, where he was sure that they would see signs that the freedoms that were now being sought around the world and a commitment to basic human rights closely mirrored core national values. This modulated speech, modestly delivered three weeks after the end of the bicentennial year, was arguably the right tone for the era of negotiation that Nixon had set out at the end of the 1960s, a speech in which Carter attempted to refocus a nation that had weakened in spirit yet retained the ability to place "fresh faith in the old dream."[18] If this was an age of fracture, as Rodgers suggests, then Carter looked to heal the fissures by outlining a socially progressive but moderate vision of national healthcare that could be attentive to the actual experience of health and illness, not simply to the fiscal considerations that troubled Ford.

This vision was echoed by President Clinton's renewed emphasis on healthcare and his proposals for a Health Security Act in 1993–94 that harked back to a workshop he convened on health policy at the Democratic midterm convention in Memphis in December 1978. It is significant that Massachusetts senator Edward Kennedy and Carter's health secretary, Joseph Califano Jr., both participated in this Memphis workshop because, as my first chapter discusses, Kennedy and Califano offered different visions of health reform to Carter. However, at least during the first two years of his presidency, Carter's "efficiency and competence" won out over the more overt rhetoric of these two outspoken figures.[19] This did not mean that Carter was dispassionate about healthcare, despite the fact that he had detractors on both sides of the aisle. But perhaps Governor Clinton of Arkansas learned important lessons by participating in the 1978 workshop: that a passionate voice such as Ted Kennedy's needs tempering by Jimmy Carter's mode of pragmatic health reform.

Personal and Collective Voices

President Carter's inaugural address focused on two undergirding structures: a strong narrative and a supportive community that can together give shape to personal and collective stories. These structural elements are particularly important for those experiencing illnesses that go undetected or for those in which bodily symptoms mix with complex psychological and behavioral conditions. It is these illness experiences at "the borderland between the medical and the social," as described in a 1972 science advisory committee report, that became increasingly politicized in the late twentieth century.[20] Although mental health was often overshadowed by the perennial political headache of health insurance, its emergence on the national agenda in the mid-1970s and its prominence in the Carter administration marks the last quarter of the twentieth century as a distinctly politicized phase of health history.

This does not mean that mental health was always on the federal radar, especially during the Reagan years, but that specific health conditions resonated through medical reports and psychiatric manuals, policy commissions and political speeches, the mass media and popular culture. Historicizing the connections between different texts and media is vital for understanding the development of, and impediments to, a public health culture. It also helps to prevent psychiatric diagnostics or top-down health policies from having the final say on the where, what, why, and how of mental health—especially given that its etiology is often more obscure than is typically the case for physical conditions. This composite approach chimes with Johns Hopkins psychiatrist Paul McHugh's call for a layered public mental health culture that takes equal account of diseases (the presence or absence of pathology), dimensionality ("individuating characteristics of intelligence, temperament and maturation"), behavior (both private and public), and encounters (often expressed through stories).[21]

We can see the groundwork of such a public health culture (if not its full realization) most obviously during Jimmy Carter's four years in the White House, which this book sees as a pivotal phase in advancing mental health policy and advocacy. The Carters had prioritized healthcare as early as the 1950s and promoted mental health during their tenure in the governor's mansion in Atlanta, particularly Rosalynn Carter, who offered practical help on the psychiatric ward of Georgia Regional Hospital in the 1960s. The couple's personal investment in mental health is linked to the fact that two of Jimmy's relatives had been patients at the Central State Hospital in Milledgeville, Georgia, where they encountered unsanitary conditions and untrained staff, as journalist Jack Nelson highlighted in his 1959–60 investigative reports for the *Atlanta Constitution*.[22] In the period 1970–74, Governor Carter attempted to reduce the risks to isolated patients facing long-term incarceration in poorly equipped, badly designed, and understaffed state hospitals, both those who had been diagnosed with a mental illness and those who had been institutionalized on the basis of "mental retardation," a term commonly used at the time that has since been superseded by more specific descriptors of intellectual and developmental disabilities.[23]

The Carters were not the only ones to focus on mental health as a public discourse. This was just one element of a more complex history in which common feelings of isolation and loneliness were offset, yet not eradicated, by an increasing emphasis on support communities, sometimes focusing on family-based therapy and other times on alternative group structures. This trend had been institutionalized with President Johnson's community health program and emerged in the late 1960s through grassroots community centers. But twenty years later, when Gerald Grob looked at the turn of the 1970s and saw a version of the "non-system" that Carter bemoaned, the health crisis was due to the floundering of progressive initiatives in the face of economic realities, leading "many patients with serious mental illnesses to survive in homeless shelters, on the streets, and even in jails."[24]

Evidence for Grob's view can be found in a 1970 report *The Health of Americans*, which pictured a crisis that was attributable to inefficient and uncoordinated services. The report predicted that community health might not survive into the 1980s, given the "retrenchment and decentralization" that had started to take effect during the Nixon administration.[25] Nevertheless, the achievements of some community centers (albeit on a more modest level than Kennedy and Johnson planned) and the emergence of new health advocacy groups that were suspicious of medical specialization, helped widen the ambit of health culture, even though this risked drifting away from a biomedical understanding of illness in favor of popular forms of therapy that did not sit comfortably with organized medicine.[26]

Among the new groups that emerged at the turn of the 1970s was the San Francisco–based National Free Clinic Council, which, from 1970 to 1974, offered a community-based alternative to what its leaders called "our moribund, bureaucratized healthcare and delivery system" via a grassroots drop-in service.[27] Elements of the outpatient community model were absorbed into the medical mainstream during the 1970s, even though some neighborhood practices withered away for financial reasons or because of a weakening commitment to activist politics. Such integration can be seen in a positive light in that it pushed the medical system to be more responsive, augmented by free clinics that served previously neglected communities with both direct and indirect services.[28] Despite this trend, however, by the mid-1970s an impartial observer might conclude that the belief in alternative health services as an engine for social change was vanishing into a flatter consumer culture.[29]

Such dilution led novelist Tom Wolfe and sociologist Christopher Lasch to diagnose a culture of selfish individualism in their famous phrases "the 'me' decade" (Wolfe) and the "culture of narcissism" (Lasch).[30] It is also a reason why Daniel Rodgers detects a shift from contextual metaphors of "circumstance, institutions, and history" to individualized ones of "choice, agency, performance, and desire."[31] We may choose to valorize these individualistic beliefs, as did many of the interviewees in a 1976 national survey that sought to assess "help-seeking patterns" and "psychological adjustment" in contemporary American life.[32] But we must recognize, too, that these beliefs fueled what Peter Marin called in his widely read 1975 essay "The New Narcissism" a world view "centered solely in the self with individual survival as the sole good" rather than a commitment to "human reciprocity and community."[33] This concern was shared by the social critic Philip Rieff, who proposed in 1973 that "inwardness" had become "an aberrancy," leading to "the kind of naked life in which everything is exposed and nothing revealed."[34] Rieff worried that this meant a loss of authenticity and a blankness of tone from which it was hard to retreat.

Many of the critiques of popular therapy at mid-decade, such as Edwin Schur's *The Awareness Trap* (1976), shared the suspicion that a cult of "simple-minded" therapeutic enlightenment and "personal growth" was blinding followers to the communal and political implications of health and illness.[35] Schur was critical of "large-scale bureaucracy and technology" but was equally worried that "the current awareness movement often seems to be pushing us away" from values of community, "at least as much as towards them," with its emphasis on self-searching.[36] This kind of jeremiad chimed with the malaise that President Carter captured in his July 1979 speech "Energy and the Crisis of Confidence," which drew directly from sociologist Christopher Lasch's rhetoric of crisis and from Berkeley sociologist Robert Bellah's view of the need to reforge the social covenant.[37] For some critics, Carter's speech reinforced the sense of national malaise, but others applauded the president for speaking out about spiritual matters.[38] Bellah, in particular, was troubled by the fact that the nation relied increasingly on a technocratic contract model rather than on the covenant of a civil religion. It was the mix of insular individualism and the "excessive optimism" of new ageism that worried Lasch, Rieff, and Schur, a concern that Tom Wolfe captured in his description of "the third great awakening" as an intoxicating mix of religion and therapy.[39]

The retreat from civic engagement in favor of an individualistic journey of discovery was symptomatic of the early 1970s, when texts such as *A Separate Reality* (1971) by Peruvian anthropologist Carlos Castenada and *The One Quest* (1972) and *The Healing Journey* (1974) by Chilean psychiatrist Claudio Naranjo privileged personal questing over group experience. It is easy to identify social trends that explain this retreat: a lack of confidence in the political, legal, military, and medical establishments; a sense of betrayal over the Vietnam War; distrust of corporate life; and rising divorce rates. However, we might now question the legitimacy of the mystical teachings of Castenada's Mexican guru Don Juan or the flight of self-perfection of the outcast seagull in the 1970 novella and 1973 film *Jonathan Livingston Seagull*, which appear to illustrate Lasch's opinion that the "therapeutic jargon" of the 1970s "celebrates not so much individualism as solipsism, justifying self-absorption as 'authenticity' and 'awareness.'"[40] Lasch argued in *The Culture of Narcissism* that an environment of surfaces and pseudo-events was replacing depth models of understanding.

This kind of jeremiad was persuasive, but there were other, more searching voices to be heard too that challenged the view that personal questing was simply a passing fad. For example, in one of the decade's most widely read books, *Zen and the Art of Motorcycle Maintenance* (1974), the philosopher Robert Pirsig charts a trip of self-discovery on a road trip from Minnesota to California in the hope that he can rescue an authentic voice from within his troubled personal history. Pirsig's protagonist is accompanied on his motorcycle trip by his son and, for a time, by his neighbors, whose commonsense approach to life act as a counterpoint to the narrator's intellectualism. Early on in the text, he fears that "the stream of common consciousness seems to be obliterating its own banks, losing its central direction and purpose" in a culture of materialism, and he calls for "some channel deepening" to shift the silt and debris of tired thinking.[41] Pirsig's narrator spends little time describing natural scenery and more in meditating on ontological questions, which the reader later comes to realize links to the electroconvulsive treatment he had undergone five years earlier, when his introspection had tipped over into psychosis (this reflects Pirsig's own experiences and hospitalization in Illinois and Minnesota in 1962–63). Set against this hidden story, the protagonist begins the trip adhering to classical philosophy and practical reason, but he realizes en route that emotions and intuition cannot be denied without diminishing the self. Indeed, he believes that a rationalistic view of the self has led to an impasse in which personality has been "liquidated without a trace in a technologically faultless act"—a statement which echoes both his psychiatric treatment (described as "Annihilation ECS") and critiques of the threat the Cold War posed to personal agency.

At its heart, the book advocates a philosophy of balance based on a mix of romantic and classical elements. Pirsig sees this quest for "quality" as essential to the rebuilding of the distinctly "American resource" of "individual integrity, self-reliance and old-fashioned gumption."[42] Thus, the narrator comes to view the practical side of life as a necessary counterpart to the channel deepening he seeks. This example is very much a personal narrative, and yet the search for balance and value in an age of fracture implicates a shared moral realm in which questions of health—especially mental health—take center stage. *Zen and the Art of Motorcycle Maintenance* identifies psychic and moral resources that can be drawn upon to offset debilitating conditions. But it also hovers between a humanist faith in authenticity and the psychoanalytic view that the self contains deep-rooted schisms and fractures.

Health Advocacy and Social Transformation

These intellectual and cultural currents help explain the paradox of American medicine in the 1970s. It was both a time of deepening crisis for the medical establishment and a time of renewal that propelled the quest for health far beyond the biomedical sphere. This paradox draws us toward the central conceptual focus of this book: the importance of voice within the sphere of mental health. In addition to voices from within the medical profession (such as the civil-rights-focused Medical Committee for Human Rights, which launched a "National Health Crusade" in 1971), this can most obviously be seen in the 1970s in the form of the public profile of groups that directly opposed the medical establishment (in the case of the Insane Liberation Front in Oregon and the Radical Therapist Collective in North Dakota) and health advocacy groups for women and minority communities.[43] The Boston Women's Health Book Collective was one such early pioneering group for promoting women's health issues. The historic collaborative volume *Our Bodies, Ourselves*—first published in 1970 in a typed format with the title *Women and Their Bodies: A Course* and then in commercial form three years later—swiftly became a foundational text for the women's movement, bridging a concern for the female body (which was often neglected or overtreated by a patriarchal medical system) and a need to define individual experiences within the framework of group identity.[44] The rise of feminist health centers and the extension of health facilities within minority communities—prompted by recognition of inherent imbalances in health provision based on discrimination by race, class, and gender—offered a pluralistic model by which medical practitioners could, at least in theory, be more attentive to the needs of underserved social groups.[45]

The action and support groups that emerged in the early and mid-1970s point to a political dimension of voice that was less about self-expression and more about consciousness raising and the questioning of medical authority. Carol Gilligan emphasized the importance of breaking silence in her influential 1982 book *In a Different Voice*, while umbrella groups such as the National Women's Health Network gave rise to a potent collective voice—albeit, in this case, one that masked internal tensions about abortion rights (founded in Washington, DC, in 1975, it later adopted the slogan "A Voice for Women, A Network for Change").[46] Gilligan encouraged her female readers to reengage with and celebrate "nurturance," but the danger was that this attitude could easily elide differences of ethnicity, class, and region in favor of an essentialist notion of womanhood. The other extreme was just as problematic, though. Advocacy groups sometimes focused on special interests within a narrow ambit of experience, even though later editions of *Our Bodies, Ourselves* (1984, 1992, 1998) were much more representative than the original text in terms of race and age and more inclusive of both physical and psychological dimensions.

The increasing visibility of such groups as the National Alliance on Mental Health (which formed in Madison, Wisconsin, in 1979 as a family-focused body that sought to coordinate anti-stigma advocacy within states and communities) and the research on ethnic health issues under the umbrella of President Carter's Commission on Mental Health did not mean that all communities were represented or that medical services could flex sufficiently to deal with unforeseen rises in health needs. The influx of Cubans and Haitians from April to October 1980, for example, following a mass exodus from Fidel Castro's Cuba, brought 125,000 refugees to Florida, about a quarter of whom had obvious mental health problems or criminal records. When the administration detected that a high percentage of these refugees required treatment or custodial care, it quickly scaled back its open-door policy to prevent the country from being "used as a dumping ground" for criminals and those diagnosed as mentally ill.[47] The healthcare issues that arose from this influx suggested that only assimilated immigrant groups could hope for adequate medical facilities, and even then provision was uneven across regions. While the health crisis among Cuban and Haitian refugees can be viewed as a unique historical problem, the incident illustrates how inflexible the health system was, especially for Latino and Latina groups (the latter did not have representation until the National Latina Health Organization was founded in 1986), for whom language barriers and religious differences often impinged on diagnosis and treatment.

This point had been emphasized two years earlier by the task force of the President's Commission on Mental Health that focused on the health issues of Hispanic Americans, one of several focus groups that assessed the medical needs of minority groups. The report of the Hispanic American group acknowledged the nonsystem that President Carter had identified, calling it a "modern-day dinosaur . . . incapable of surviving on its own," and pushed for more attuned services for rapidly growing and heterogeneous Hispanic communities.[48] Not only did this task force—which was chaired by Raquel Cohen, a disaster victim specialist of Harvard Medical School—have "little valid and reliable information" about the mental health of Hispanic groups, but it marked this community as an "at risk" population beset by poverty, underemployment, poor housing and nutrition, urban crime, discrimination, and language barriers that together led to "undue stress."[49] The group also noted that appropriate healthcare services for Hispanic communities had been slower to develop than for African Americans (for whom medical training schools had been established by mid-century in Washington, DC, and Nashville). In addition, minority groups did not establish collective voices on issues related to the intersection of gender and race until the 1980s. The Latina Health Organization was preceded by the National Black Women's Health Project, established in 1983 in Atlanta, and the Native American Community Board, founded in 1985 in South Dakota.[50]

As I commented in the preface, the rise of these advocacy and support groups is a crucial part of the story of late-twentieth-century health culture, serving to highlight the stigma that clung to mental illness and the complex etiology of conditions for which it is hard to untangle biological, psychological, and environmental factors. Although there were many polarizing accounts of the self as a fortress against the micro-politics of power, there was also a broader recognition in the 1980s and 1990s that the self is a social and cultural (rather than just a biological) construct. While this view chimed with the model of "social medicine" promoted in Latin American countries, the weakening of the depth model of the self was both a problem and an opportunity for U.S. and European thinkers and practitioners to move beyond the tenets of Freudian psychoanalysis. For example, New York psychiatrist Robert Jay Lifton identified the emergence of a "protean self" in the face of fragmentation that possessed a more resilient and flexible structure than the "isolated self" that Marin described in "The New Narcissism," and was able to speak itself anew.[51] Conversely, though, French sociologist Jean Baudrillard was proposing in the mid-1980s that we should entirely abandon metaphors of the self because they had been coopted by a late-capitalist culture that sold health through advertising imagery.[52] This concern with surfaces led cultural historian Philip Cushman to argue that Ronald Reagan's public persona in the 1980s was the epitome of "the empty self," sold to the electorate as a supreme commodity within a narrative of national unity that promised to counter the fractures of the 1970s, whereas biographer Gail Sheehy speculates that Bill Clinton suffered from dissociative identity disorder based on the ways his personal life encroached on his presidency.[53] Despite the lack of clinical validity of these two opinions, the point is that the loosely conceptualized notions of "empty" and "dissociating" selves are just two more metaphors to line up with "isolated," "narcissistic," and "protean" selves at an unhelpful level of abstraction from lived reality.

This diffusion of medical and psychological categories formed one of the contexts for Princeton sociologist Paul Starr in his more traditional narrative account,

The Social Transformation of American Medicine, published during Reagan's second year as president.[54] In this book, Starr probes the structures that underpin the business of medicine, but he also accounts for its historical development and a range of external partners and providers that tend to be overlooked when the focus is squarely on the doctor and the patient. In response to the critical view that professional medicine was drifting away from human needs, Starr combines an account of diagnostic advancement, the authority of the physician, and the influence of the medical establishment over the health market with analysis of the disjointed nature of health reform.[55] Despite Starr's liberal politics (he was appointed as Clinton's senior health policy advisor in 1993), we can detect resonances between *The Social Transformation of Medicine* and Reagan's political narrative of reunification, especially because Starr largely ignores both personal accounts of illness and identity categories of race, class, gender, age, and sexuality that do not sit easily within a neat linear narrative.

Illness, Language, and Voice

Medical historian Jonathan Engel has argued that "the flowering of therapies" in the early to mid-1970s was "a grand conclusion to a passing era rather than an overture to a new one."[56] It is tempting to agree with Engel's view that alternative therapies such as "primal scream therapy, est, rebirthing therapy, and other bizarre approaches to mental health" were outgrowths of the "soul-searching of the previous decade."[57] However, we might instead interpret this period as a distinct historical phase that chimed with what political economist Robert Crawford called "new health consciousness." While Crawford was concerned that "the preoccupation with personal health"—or "healthism"—may lead to "elitist moralizing" about right and wrong life choices, it was the more expansive moral experience of illness that drew thinkers and practitioners from the humanities and medical sciences to explore common ground.[58] This was institutionalized in a new interdisciplinary journal, *Literature and Medicine*, launched in 1982 (the same year as Paul Starr's *The Social Transformation of American Medicine*), which set out to explore symbolic and ethical implications of the "strange marriage between literature and medicine."[59] It echoed the mission of the 1980 anthology *Medicine and Literature* that "insights of literature can help counter the thrust towards dehumanization in our health-care systems" while also recognizing that "experiences of medicine can help bring the often overly intellectualized humanist back to reality."[60]

Although the anthology and the early issues of the journal steered away from an institutionalized view of medicine, the contributors did not think that literature—or the arts in general—necessarily offered a more valuable frame of reference. Catholic physician Edmund Pellegrino valorized the power of literature to "evoke vicarious experiences," for example, but he claimed that both disciplines "need simultaneously to stand back from, and yet to share in, the struggle of human life." The volume set out an agenda that led to an increased focus on the intersections between medicine and the arts through the next two decades. This was often framed in terms of narrative and storytelling, such as Larry and Sandra Churchill's article in the first issue of *Literature and Medicine* that outlined the "dialectic of distance and intimacy" within storytelling that avoids both extremes of hard medical objectivity and empirically unverifiable forms of subjectivity.[61]

This intersection was not straightforward, though. This is best exemplified by Susan Sontag's *Illness as Metaphor*, originally published as three separate essays in the *New York Review of Books* in January and February 1978 and printed in book form later that year. Having been an active member of the New York Intellectuals in the 1960s, Sontag—like her former husband, Philip Rieff—was concerned about the dilution of therapeutic language and its shift away from the established vocabulary and practices of medicine. Sontag favored precise diagnostic terms for demystifying chronic illness instead of metaphors that sometimes distort what it means to be ill. She clarified this in a 1979 interview when she claimed that metaphors are a means "of stopping your thinking and freezing you into certain attitudes."[62] This is particularly relevant for the two "master illnesses" that she explores: cancer and tuberculosis.[63] Sontag was particularly suspicious of romanticized views of illness, which, as I discuss in *Therapeutic Revolutions*, led to a renaissance in the efforts of humanistic thinkers in the 1960s to counter the more technical language of medical science. Sontag was undergoing treatment for breast cancer when she wrote *Illness as Metaphor*, and her central point is that the metaphorical language of illness more often obfuscates than elucidates. She extended this critique further in her 1989 book, *AIDS and Its Metaphors*, in response to the negative metaphors of invasion and plague that were often evoked during the AIDS crisis of the 1980s—a book published the same year that the American Psychiatric Association began its commission to explore the intersections of AIDS and mental health challenges. Sontag gave voice to the frustration of a patient undergoing an aggressive illness and facing a schism between medical and social conceptions of it.

Sontag's essay raises a number of questions, but there are two with which she does not deal explicitly in *Illness as Metaphor*: the importance of the patient's voice and the need for a new language that is attentive to the patient's subjective experience of illness.[64] These were the kinds of questions that motivated the "literature and medicine" movement and led Roy Schafer, a neo-Freudian psychoanalyst, to call for a new language that attends to "the problems of perspective, subjective evidence and inference, and reliability and validity of interpretation."[65] In his book *Language and Insight*, published the same year as *Illness as Metaphor*, Schafer returns to the existential and humanist thinkers of the 1960s as a resource for constructing a "life history" that would furnish the patient and analyst with a language of action and a horizon for the emergence of a therapeutic voice. Instead of focusing on the Freudian emphasis on the past, Schafer consolidated his earlier volume *A New Language for Psychoanalysis* (1976) by outlining a future-oriented scenario that stressed choice and encouraged patients to develop a vocabulary by which they could become active interpreters of meaning. This did not mean that a cure could be enacted by simply redescribing an underlying condition, but that a new language of action and value could bridge scientific explanation and romanticized notions of authentic experience. This new language was no guarantee of health, but it increased the chances of becoming healthier. In so doing, Schafer shifted the debate, moving from a straight choice between rigid diagnosis and figurative language to an emphasis on verbs and adverbs: in other words, active doing and making rather than passive conceptions of "having" an illness or "being" treated.

One could argue that Schafer's focus on the psychoanalytic encounter does not easily translate to the medical sphere. However, if we return to our earlier discussion of the growing attentiveness to the patient's voice, we can identify some key characteristics. One of the problems with "voice" within the European philosophical tradition is that it is often seen as a metonym for metaphysical presence. This, at least, was the reason why French philosopher Jacques Derrida wished to replace the phenomenological view of voice as self-presence with the intrinsic ambiguity of the written word. Derrida's privileging of written texts over the spoken voice was widely adopted by humanities scholars in the late 1970s to the mid-1990s, but a countervailing trend in Anglo-American analytic philosophy emphasized everyday words and the human voice as a relatively straightforward means of communication that has the capacity to secure sense and meaning within specific contexts. Both positions are philosophically plausible, yet they suggest divergent paths between a European emphasis on *différance* and an Anglo-American focus on ordinary language.

However, there was a third way, which Derrida explored in a little-read essay on French surrealist writer Antonin Artaud, "To Unsense the Subjectile," first published in German in the mid-1980s. This essay provides the horizon for a mode of storytelling in which the self is both the voice of the narrative and an element within it by introducing the notion of a "subjectile" that paradoxically speaks to the subjectivity of the person and is exterior to the self, rather like a projectile.[66] Derrida warns us against thinking of a subjectile in terms of nonsense or madness (or "of someone mentally sick"), but he sees it as a key feature of a new language: the subjectile plays under the surface of words, revealing multiplicity rather than a single locus of meaning. The "I" of self-expression is never unitary, then, but contains within it traces of otherness and hints of its own destruction, while also offering the possibility of survival. In this way, Derrida, who at first banished voice as ontologically simplistic, allows it to return with all of the play and possibility that he assigns to the textual realm. This is particularly important for illness stories, not, as Sontag asserts, because metaphors obscure and confuse, but because words are often inadequate to describe health experiences for which such clinical terms as depression, borderline, mania, and dissociation fail to do justice.

In more straightforward terms, this is a theoretical echo of the emerging interest in literature and medicine in the 1980s as articulated in Jerome Bruner's *Actual Minds, Possible Worlds* (1985), Howard Brody's *Stories of Sickness* (1987), Arthur Kleinman's *The Illness Narratives* (1988), and the popular neurological case studies of Oliver Sacks. We might say that in the case of Sacks's most famous book, *The Man Who Mistook His Wife for a Hat* (1985), it is the dispassionate doctor who conducts the storytelling and there is none of the play of difference and surfaces that attracted Derrida. However, Sacks would argue that the engaged doctor should only speak for the patient when he or she has no voice or narrative pattern to connect fragmentary perceptions. Within this framework, *Voices of Mental Health* explores how medicalized literary accounts and "pathographies," such as Michael Ignatieff's 1994 lightly fictionalized Alzheimer's story *Scar Tissue*, offer rich source material for thinking about illness from the perspectives of both the experiencer and the caregiver. But these accounts do not represent a tightly bound genre and need also to be placed alongside the quest for a new vocabulary of mental health, such as Sacks's attempt to loosen the fixed subject positions of doctor and patient.[67]

Consciousness, Narrative, and Community

If, as psychiatrist Melvin Sabshin claimed, the turn to neurology and biological psychiatry in the late 1970s and 1980s was a key moment in the history of the medical sciences—foreshadowing President Bush's proclamation that the 1990s would be the "decade of the brain"—then it is interesting to note that many scientific thinkers (including cognitive scientist Daniel Dennett, philosophers John Searle and Thomas Nagel, and neurologist Oliver Sacks) started to reevaluate consciousness as both the most personal and most mysterious of concepts.[68] Searle, Nagel, and Sacks were all interested in regions of experience that behaviorism cannot easily reach, but Dennett is the most theoretically interesting of this group because his dislike of "final essences" chimed with the postfoundational trend in American philosophy during the 1980s.[69] In *Consciousness Explained* (1991), for example, Dennett argued that complex mental experiences cannot easily be reduced to a chemical or biological level, an insight that led him to develop an interest in storytelling and in cultivating an "intentional stance" toward others, as he called it in the title of his 1987 book. What this renewed interest in consciousness demonstrates is that there were theoretical alternatives to the critiques of social malaise and to the suspicion that narcissism and emptiness were symptomatic of debilitating cultural, economic, and ideological forces.

A growing interest in the narrative construction of health and illness in the 1980s was, in part, motivated by a desire to demonstrate that the sick self is never wholly isolated and is always embedded in a shared world of stories. This trend took on different forms, ranging from first-person testimony and survivor narratives to collaborative modes that connect the patient and physician to broader accounts in which family, friends, and caregivers fill in the gaps, especially in cases of dementia, depression, and trauma, when the patient's voice has been lost, obscured or fragmented, or for conditions in which the individual's view becomes radically distorted. This does not mean that narrative is a panacea that protects individuals from false, dangerous, or diminishing selves, but it can help dissolve the theoretical tension between inner authenticity and self-presentation that inflected Erving Goffman's sociological writings and, more recently, bioethicist Carl Elliott's 2003 book *Better than Well*.[70]

Whether or not this "narrative turn" represented the kind of "new language" that Roy Schafer, Carol Gilligan, and others were calling for is a central concern of this book. It can be understood as a facet of a sharper awareness of the social dimension of illness, but it can also be seen as a way of embedding patients within a network in which renewed agency emerges, if not always a new health horizon for severe conditions.[71] In more socially expansive terms, this is what the sociologist Robert Bellah and his team of researchers discovered in their extensive field study published as *Habits of the Heart* in 1985. This project followed Bellah's attempts to identify a civil religion during the "third time of trial" (the "military confrontation" of the Cold War and Vietnam that followed the first two trials of independence and slavery) that had intensified the need to renew the nation's core values.[72] Bellah concluded that many Americans were too wedded to the language of individualism and were ill equipped to see themselves as members of a community.[73] The overriding concern for his team was the erosion of the public sphere and a loss of "common dialogue."[74] This was an issue not merely for those who were labeled "sick" or in need of "care," but for a broad sweep of Americans, most of who function reasonably well yet lack a vocabulary by which they can bridge value systems and generate meaningful conversations. While a number of thinkers and public figures, including President Carter, were concerned about such a loss of faith, Bellah focused on the civic dimension of religion as the moral glue that can bind disparate individuals.

In a middle chapter of *Habits of the Heart*, titled "Reaching Out," Bellah's team considers the place of therapy in the late twentieth century. The discussion moves from the one-to-one therapeutic encounter to consider the everyday role of therapy, from business practices to home life. Suspicious of the "giving-getting" business model that seemed to be increasingly prevalent in the 1980s, Bellah's team point out that the ideal of the therapeutic encounter promotes mutual understanding within a community, even though Bellah reminds us that this may remain forever an aspiration.[75] On this level, *Habits of the Heart* offers a more positive account of cultivating therapeutic relationships than the suspicions of Philip Rieff in his influential 1966 book *The Triumph of the Therapeutic* or the proclamations of the social jeremiads of the mid-1970s.[76] Bellah does not talk explicitly about voice or narrative, but the ability of patients to articulate themselves is essential for a communication model that can negotiate divisive ideologies. Instead of empty, isolated, or narcissistic selves, then, a network of voices offers the possibility of purposeful lives, where individualism can coexist with community. As the preface discusses, voice is both the precondition of the narratives that bind together individuals and a quality that emerges from storytelling. We could argue that Bellah did not fully appraise the social and cultural pressures that inhibit or undermine the emergence of such a voice, but he was aware that formal therapy only goes so far in a "therapeutically inclined" community that requires a different lexicon from the technical language of medical science.[77] This, then, is both the return of everyday language by which to tell new stories and an action-oriented pragmatic language that helps individuals get things done.

In order to explore these contours in more detail, this book uses the organizing concept of "voice" as a means of assessing competing metaphors and narratives of mental health, focusing on conditions that came to public and media attention between the year of the moon landing and the millennium. This enables me to emphasize echoes and tensions between different voices: public and private voices, pained voices and healing voices, voices of strength and weakness, extravagant and diminished voices, split voices and multi-voices, raw and augmented voices, and voices of protest and "unspoken voices," the term therapist Peter Levine used to characterize trauma.[78] It is instructive to trace these voices through the final third of the twentieth century from the perspectives of health practitioners and patients. Sometimes these voices testify to accounts of suffering and survival and other times they raise public awareness of medical conditions in concert with others. We can locate some of these voices in clinical case studies, but we also need to look further to consider the broader role of culture in shaping awareness of mental health. This can be detected across a range of literary and cinematic accounts, which I draw upon to emphasize the importance of narrative as both the product of and the progenitor of voice.

In the eight chapters of this book, I move from medical case studies such as Oliver Sacks's account of post-encephalitic patients in *Awakenings* (1973) to the personal testimony in Barbara Gordon's *I'm Dancing as Fast as I Can* (1979) and Marya Hornbacher's *Wasted* (1998), biographical accounts of dementia such as Philip Roth's *Patrimony* (1992) and Michael Ignatieff's *Scar Tissue* (1993), and from novels like Philip Caputo's *Indian Country* (1987) and Deborah Hautzig's *Second Star to the Right* (1981) to consciousness-raising films such as *Rain Man* (1988), *Safe* (1995), and *Girl, Interrupted* (1999). These narrative sources—together with topical stories in the media that often centered on the health records of public figures or a succession of health crises—enable me to examine a range of historical experiences, inquiries, and voices that fall under the broad umbrella of mental health.

The discussion focuses more often on literature, memoir, and film than other forms of cultural expression as there is arguably a greater degree of self-reflexivity in these accounts than in, for example, television shows of the time. That does not make these cultural forms free from misconceptions about mental illness or immune from inherent biases: for example, published white patients' stories during this period are vastly disproportionate in number, given national demographics. But by looking at a spectrum of texts over a 30-year stretch—as well as the therapeutic role of music and art—I hope to go some way toward neutralizing biases in any single mode of representation. Moreover, the fact that the book spans three generations of writers means that I can encompass a diversity of responses instead of focusing on a single vanishing point. These writers include those born between the wars (such as William Styron, Philip Roth, Don DeLillo, and Donald Goines), writers born during or immediately after World War II (Philip Caputo, Tim O'Brien, Michael Ignatieff, Susanna Kaysen, and Amy Tan), and those born in the 1960s (David Foster Wallace, Chuck Palahniuk, Bret Easton Ellis, and Elizabeth Wurtzel). At times, my commentary addresses the public context of institutional care, policy priorities, new medical research, and emerging technologies, and, at other times, it focuses on the private stories of individuals and families struggling in the face of debilitating conditions or in environments that do not meet their health needs.

Trajectory and Method

Whereas the story of therapy in the post–World War II period covered in *Therapeutic Revolutions* maintains a strict historical spine, the period from 1970 to 2000—during which the U.S. population grew by 38 percent, topping 280 million by the millennium—requires a more panoramic perspective because awareness of certain conditions developed sporadically and research on physical and mental health revealed closer connections than has previously been acknowledged.[79] The interdisciplinary nature of this study is an attempt to do justice to the complex discourses, identities, and institutions of mental health and partly, to quote an important 2001 article by Catherine Prendergast, an attempt to find a "language with which to address the dilemmas and gaps in understanding that mental illness presents."[80] The central focus on voice enables me to draw together conversations about health, illness, and selfhood in which the struggle to find the right words with which to reorient the self goes hand in hand with the therapeutic need to give voice to health stories.

This book is also an historical account that draws upon archival sources and a range of late-twentieth-century print and visual media. To this end, I begin and end with two specific moments: the bicentennial year, when Jimmy Carter was running for president, and the pre-millennial year when President Clinton's second term of office was drawing to a close. The opening and closing chapters on 1976 and 1999 are more explicitly historical and political than the intervening chapters, each of which address a topical mental health condition that became part of the national conversation during these thirty years. In so doing, I trace a number of interrelating themes: the uneven development of healthcare provision at the federal level through four Republican and two Democratic administrations; the rise of professional and public awareness of Alzheimer's disease, autism, and anorexia during the Reagan and Bush years; tensions between the federal war on drugs and the addiction experience; and war-related conditions that emerged strongly in the voices of Vietnam-era veterans and were reprised in relation to soldiers' experiences during the Persian Gulf War. In addition, I chart how a succession of first ladies—from Betty Ford and Rosalynn Carter to Hillary Clinton and second lady Tipper Gore—played very visible public roles as health advocates. These roles often (although not always) dovetailed with the work of health activists and disability support groups whose mission was to show how inequalities based on gender, race, class, and sexuality often relate closely to inequities in healthcare provision. In pursuing these intersections, I draw implicitly from Kimberlé Crenshaw's work on the social dynamics of "intersectionality" (a term that Crenshaw developed in the late 1980s to link black feminism and legal thought), but I also seek to bridge the macro and the micro by juxtaposing political and medical conversations about mental health with personal expressions in spoken, written, and visual form.[81]

The first half of the book evaluates the health legacy of the 1970s from a national perspective. This was a period when debates about well-being and healing were taking center stage, and when war trauma, addiction, and dementia illuminated new cases of damaged and diminished selves. The questioning of what Jonathan Imber calls the "moral authority" of medicine to understand complex health experiences continues into the second half of the book.[82] But in these later chapters, the cultural politics of identity and community feature more prominently than federal politics and policy in order to reflect how selfhood and reality were becoming ever more slippery concepts for postfoundational and postmodern thinkers in the 1980s and 1990s. This discussion culminates in the final chapter, which turns to the national conversation about mental health during President Clinton's second term, a time when literary writers and filmmakers were exploring depression from both medical and cultural perspectives. With respect to national conversations on pressing health issues, HIV/AIDS figures less prominently in this book than might at first be expected. Although discussion of AIDS features in chapters 3 and 8, because the book's focus is primarily on mental (rather than physical) health, I discuss the virus through the thematic prism of voice and silence and in terms of broader mental health debates.[83]

The book also assesses the significance and impact of government policies, particularly the Mental Health Systems Act of 1980 (the culmination of the work of the 1977 President's Commission on Mental Health), which promised a new framework for mental health provision but which was dismantled only a year later at the beginning of President Reagan's first term. Within this 30-year narrative there are progressive phases during the Carter and Clinton administrations, but these need to be seen in light of publications and initiatives during the Nixon-Ford and Reagan-Bush years that are easily overlooked in a broad history and that serve to temper the charge of federal neglect at the hands of the four Republican administrations. In extending my discussion of the politics of mental health to the legal and medical spheres, I consider key pieces of legislation, such as the landmark 1975 court case *O'Connor v. Donaldson* and the Americans with Disabilities Act of July 1990, alongside the growing authority of the *Diagnostic and Statistical Manual of Mental Disorders*, particularly the third edition of 1980 (which included trauma in the wake of the Vietnam War and took a more scientific and organic approach to mental disorders) and the fourth edition of 1994 (in which personality disorders featured significantly).[84]

With closer attention to the specificity of mental health issues and the refinement of diagnostic terms, we may be tempted to tell a story of rising fortunes linked to the spread of advocacy networks for underserved groups. However, despite Bill Clinton's frustrated attempts to reform health insurance and his promise to forge "one America in the 21st century" by launching a presidential initiative against racial discrimination, not only was health insurance a more divisive topic in the 1990s than ever before, but the fact that worries about the status of psychiatric labels, the stigma of institutionalization, and "stereotypes of dangerousness" persisted through the decade is a reminder that the gap between mental and physical health did not close as much as advocates in the 1960s and 1970s had hoped.[85] Thus, at the millennium obstacles still remained in policy, treatment, and public awareness—a topic that the book's conclusion picks up by reflecting on the George W. Bush and Obama years.[86]

PART ONE

The Health Legacy of the 1970s

1 *Health Debates at the Bicentennial*

President Gerald Ford's Independence Day 1976 speech, delivered in front of a jubilant crowd at Independence Hall, Philadelphia, was a moving tribute to the founding fathers. The President's speech was both heroic and reflective. It took its momentum from the American Revolution Bicentennial Commission's traveling exhibition "USA '76: The First 200 Years" and the Freedom Train, which had begun its patriotic tour of the forty-eight contiguous states in April 1975 and was then traveling through Pennsylvania. The previous day, the *Washington Post* had noted that the country was "once again a nation in transition, sobered by new awareness of the limits of abundance, concerned about its future role in the world, uncertain of its social health and political vitality."[1] In contrast, Ford was keen to remain upbeat, especially after what amounted to defeat in Vietnam the month the Freedom Train began its trip from Wilmington, Delaware, and a constitutional crisis set in motion by the Watergate break-in still reverberating through the media. Ford's speech embraced three major themes of the Bicentennial Commission—heritage, festivity, and new horizons—but it had a sober undercurrent that tempered the gaiety of the celebrations.[2]

Halfway through the Independence Day speech, Ford asked rhetorically "are the institutions under which we live working the way they should? Are the foundations laid in 1776 and 1789 still strong enough and sound enough to resist the tremors of our times?"[3] In response, the final third of the speech focused on national goals under the rubric of what the *Washington Post* called social health: "a longer lifespan, a literate population, a leadership in world affairs." This potent mixture of idealism and pragmatism suggested that the president understood the pressing issues of the day and acknowledged that the nation's aspirations should be continually set higher. But, surprisingly, given his emphasis on national well-being, healthcare received only a single mention and the speech was less aspirational in terms of improved health than President Nixon's vision for the bicentennial year in his State of the Union address of 1970. While care for the elderly, immunization, and emergency medical services were all strands of the Bicentennial Commission's "horizons" theme, the question of whether federal institutions were fit for purpose hangs in the speech. This was not wholly masked by the rousing conclusion that returned to the founding ideals of the national "adventure" 200 years earlier.[4]

Ford's speech offers a snapshot of the bicentennial year that he was keen to maximize in order to promote himself as a safe leader who had the respect of America's allies. His rhetoric echoed that of intellectuals such as Robert Bellah, who saw the late twentieth century as a "third time of trial" that required both "responsible action in a revolutionary world" and a restoration of faith in the common good.[5] But while the Fourth of July speech promised national renewal, 1976 was a mixed year for President Ford. His attempt to affirm a strong narrative of accomplishment strained against alternative versions of the nation's past, as expressed in the ambivalent responses to the bicentennial celebrations from African American and Native American communities, for which "improving health" meant something quite different from the homilies of the Independence Day speech.[6]

Healthcare and National Politics

When countercultural icon Stephen Stills paid tribute to Gerald Ford at a Crosby, Stills, Nash & Young concert at Roosevelt Stadium in Jersey City on 8 August 1974 (on the eve of Nixon's resignation), it looked as if the mid-1970s were set fair for Nixon's second vice-president in a time of national healing.[7] We might be tempted to take "healing" as a keyword of the decade, particularly as Ford's 1979 memoir *A Time to Heal* revived a metaphor that he had first used during his controversial pardoning of Nixon for his part in the Watergate affair.[8] Ford claimed that he had decided to issue the pardon in order to heal "the wounds of the past," and he revisited the topic five years later, calling the pardon "necessary surgery—essential if we were to heal our wounded nation."[9] Healing did not necessarily mean party solidarity, though. When Ford sought the Republican presidential nomination in 1976, he could not have predicted what a tough contest he would face in the primaries from California's governor, Ronald Reagan. And when the narrowly victorious Ford was challenged by Democratic nominee Jimmy Carter in the race for the White House, the key issues were the economy and voter apathy, suggesting that public mistrust in the government was at an all-time high.[10]

It did not help the Republicans that Ron Kovic's Vietnam War memoir *Born on the Fourth of July* was published that summer, in which Kovic, a U.S. marine and, since 1970, an antiwar activist, wrote about the loss of his youthful ideals during his two tours of duty in Vietnam in the late 1960s, especially after a bullet left him paralyzed from the chest down on his second tour in 1968. Disgusted by Nixon's broken campaign promise to withdraw troops from Vietnam, Kovic became increasingly outspoken against inadequate medical treatment, leading him to disrupt Nixon's acceptance speech at the Republic National Convention in 1972 and to embark on a hunger strike in 1974. Two summers later, Kovic was invited to the Democratic Convention as one of the guest speakers. When he opened with the dramatic description of himself as "your Fourth of July firecracker exploding in the grave" and described the snake-pit conditions of Veterans Administration hospitals, he suggested that health and politics were closely bound in ways that Ford did not acknowledge in his Fourth of July address or in his acceptance speech as presidential candidate at the 1976 Republican Convention in Kansas City.[11]

Health was firmly on the radar of Democratic candidate Jimmy Carter during the election year, but it surfaced only occasionally in Ford's campaign. This apparent blind spot is ironic for two reasons: the first was that his wife Betty Ford had struggled with prescription drugs and alcohol for many years, and the second was that the Ford administration was embroiled in a health crisis throughout 1976. This crisis stemmed from fears of a pandemic of swine flu. The flu broke out in January when one soldier died and thirteen were hospitalized at a U.S. army base in Trenton, New Jersey. Fearing that this new outbreak would be similar to the influenza pandemic that swept through Europe and the United States in the late 1910s, the government's Center for Disease Control and the Department of Health, Education, and Welfare (HEW) were keen to develop a vaccine to prevent the outbreak from spreading. By the end of 1976, months after the Fort Dix crisis following a series of administrative delays, the vaccine had been given to 24 percent of the population at a cost of $135 million. Crucially, the vaccine led directly to twenty-five deaths, while over fifty more faced complications linked to the nervous disease Guillain-Barré syndrome.[12] What these circumstances showed was the need for much stronger coordination of federal healthcare programs, particularly as the distribution of Salk's polio vaccine in the mid-1950s suffered similar administrative failures.

Healthcare was not a prominent theme of the 1976 presidential debates, aside from Carter's criticism of Ford in their third and final debate, the candidate's differing stances on abortion, and Walter Mondale's assurance in his vice-presidential debate with Robert Dole that national health insurance was a distinct possibility.[13] However, Ford's files show his wariness about Carter's outspoken claims on health and early signs of Carter's desire to make healthcare "a centerpiece of his administration," as Joseph Califano, the secretary of health, education, and welfare from 1977 to 1979, later noted.[14] Carter's plans were initially galvanized by the criticism Democrats leveled at Nixon and Ford for eroding Medicare and Medicaid, abandoning support for the elderly, and overlooking the benefits of community healthcare in their efforts to cut costs, as evidenced by Nixon's failed Assisted Health Insurance bill of 1974.[15] Carter was particularly worried about the nation's underserved communities, which he sensed were becoming increasingly isolated and dislocated, a view that was reflected in the official publication of the 1976 Democratic National Convention.[16]

Carter found opportunities to tackle healthcare policy on the campaign trail.[17] This was most obviously the case in a talk to African American medical students in Washington, DC, where Carter claimed rhetorically that the most dangerous illness would not be discovered in any particular patient but in the "entire system" that spreads "from politics and society itself".[18] This is the speech in which he spoke about the "haphazard, unsound, undirected, inefficient non-system" of the Nixon-Ford years. His solution was to reorganize the over 300 federal health programs and to deliver services better by investing in more nurses and paraprofessionals and by improving medical technology and nutritional education.[19] Carter drew his talk toward a close by quoting the recently deceased theologian Reinhold Niebuhr on the need to tackle injustice. He said nothing obvious about mental health and made only passing reference to decreasing numbers of black students enrolled in medical schools, but he concluded in an ethical vein by stressing the need to open "many doors" across the health spectrum, while acknowledging the efficiencies required to slow down federal healthcare spending, particularly hospital costs, which were running at 39 percent of all health expenditures in 1976.[20]

This April 1976 speech can be read as a prelude to President Carter's four years in the White House, from 1977 to 1981, during which time he arguably did more than any other previous administration to promote health as a national priority. At the beginning of his term Carter was praised by the press for his energy and his legislative record as Governor and as an "embodiment of the new nation's hopes."[21] His disclosure in a *Playboy* interview that he had "committed adultery in my heart many times" did not help, but the interview also spanned the topics of abortion, homosexuality, preventive medicine, and the psychological pressures of the White House.[22] Aside from this interview, the press did not really interrogate the substance of Carter's views of healthcare and critics concurred with the opinion of the *Congressional Quarterly* that there had been not much change in federal health policy that year. However, this snapshot risks downplaying fiscal realities and it ignores the fact that when he entered office in January 1977, Carter built on the health initiatives of the previous three years that often go unnoticed in histories of the Ford administration.

It would be inaccurate to say that there was silence on the issue during Ford's thirty months in the White House. Following a 1973 conference sponsored by the President's Committee on Mental Retardation, First Lady Betty Ford hosted a reception in February 1975 at which she received a rug from Viola Hovel, an intellectually disabled Navajo girl from the Children's Rehabilitation Center in Brimhall, New Mexico. The president announced National Epilepsy Month in November, and two of his staff, William Baroody Jr. and Myron Kuropas, hosted a meeting on "Ethnicity and Mental Health" the following June. One of the keynote speeches at this meeting was given by Irving Levine, director of the Institute on Pluralism and Group Identity (a branch of the American Jewish Association), who reminded attendees from the education and health sectors why the mid-1970s were so pivotal to the reform of mental healthcare. Levine discussed factors of migration and urbanization, considered the impact of generational change on minority groups, and recommended a socially conservative approach that nevertheless respected "the pluralistic nature of our society."[23] Although Levine's model of pluralism was not especially progressive, the meeting took time to consider the needs of different minority groups, and the event was cited the following year as a source of the President's Commission on Mental Health.[24]

A more ambitious presidential committee report titled *Mental Retardation: A Century of Decision* was published in March 1976 as an attempt to "project the nation's needs in the prevention and treatment of mental retardation" over the next twenty-five years.[25] Secretary of Health, Education, and Welfare Forrest David Mathews commended the report to President Ford by focusing as much on the "human benefit" of mental health reform as on the need to keep healthcare dollars in check.[26] It argued that more effective medical interventions, training, and preventive care should link to better public information and improvements in legislation, building on the United Nations Declaration on the Rights of Mentally Retarded Persons of December 1971. The report is perceptive in identifying social, economic, and bureaucratic challenges and in encompassing a spectrum of experiences, from borderline conditions that might be managed by families and in outpatient facilities to severe impairment that requires extensive care.

In addition to considering the history and future of mental healthcare provision, the report offered personal stories to balance its formal analysis.[27] These vignettes were designed to combat stigmatizing stereotypes and to highlight "the competency of the retarded person to speak and act on his own behalf" or "to have a representative appropriately appointed" when he or she "is unable to exercise such choice."[28] Although preoccupied with health costs and the need to eliminate waste, the report profiled the individual's experience and upheld a developmental model of growth. It also covered human services, education, employment, mobility, and recreation and sought to combat the "loneliness and boredom" that accompany conditions in which the individual feels locked in or wholly dependent on caregivers.[29]

For these reasons, *Mental Retardation: A Century of Decision* is evidence that the Ford administration was taking health challenges seriously and that mental health and disability were critical topics, as symbolized by the first White House Conference on Handicapped Individuals in May 1977, which Ford and Mathews had originally planned for December 1976 as "a fitting climax to the Bicentennial year and the values that we seek to regenerate."[30] These examples offer a more variegated and responsible picture of the mid-decade than the more polemical sociological works of the time credit. As I discussed in the introduction, these accounts kept their distance from individual case studies in favor of the sweeping argument that many American citizens were indulgent and self-centered and lacked the social commitment of Americans of earlier decades.

Medicine and Psychiatry at the Bicentennial

This chapter will return to the contribution of the Carters to the field of mental health, but by way of context I want to consider the institutions of professional medicine and psychiatry in 1976, a time when both large state facilities and smaller community services faced fiscal and organizational challenges. The bicentennial year was not unique in this respect; budgetary concerns mark a line of continuity through the three presidencies of the 1970s. The rising price of healthcare had been Nixon's biggest concern, from an estimated $25.9 billion, or 5.2 percent of the gross national product, in 1960 to $118.4 billion, or 8.3 percent of the gross national product, in 1975. This meant that healthcare costs had risen 12 percent annually and that health had become the nation's third largest industry by mid-decade.[31] The cost of Medicare and Medicaid and increasing hospital overheads were two triggers, together with the mounting cost of medical technology, malpractice cases, and infrastructural bureaucracy.

Nixon claimed that Lyndon Johnson had been irresponsible to commit so much federal resource to healthcare and that the reforms of the mid-1960s were damaging the budget. He was justified to a degree and sought to lower growth from 12.2 to 10.4 percent toward the end of his first term—although one could mount the counterargument that the move toward localized community centers meant that the burden of healthcare was shared more broadly.[32] Inflation did not help matters and even California governor Ronald Reagan had to rethink his budget cuts of 1969 when it became apparent that a large group of frail patients had been released prematurely from state hospitals.[33] Johnson hoped that the Mental Retardation Facilities and Community Mental Health Centers Construction Act of 1963 (commonly known as the Community Mental Health Act) would establish a comprehensive system in over 2,000 catchment areas. But a decade later the National Institute of Mental Health (NIMH) believed that community centers were ill equipped to deal with severe mental health issues, particularly when psychiatrists found the environment in the centers to be deprofessionalizing and the number of qualified psychiatrists in these centers decreased.[34]

A lack of confidence in both the medical and political systems stemmed partly from the acknowledgement of a 1973 report by the Department of Health, Education, and Welfare (HEW) that it was difficult to measure the population's health and partly from a growing awareness of the multiple factors that shape physical and mental illness: "housing conditions, environmental defects, automobiles, conditions of employment . . . rapid urbanization and technological developments."[35] Nixon's Social Security Amendments of 1972, which extended Medicare to under-65s with severe disabilities, and the National Health Planning and Resources Development Act of 1974 were important pieces of legislation for addressing gaps in healthcare provision. The 1974 act sought to consolidate and regulate existing provision without adding another tier of administration. However, its lack of specificity rankled Thomas Watkins, president of the National Association for Mental Health, so much so that he wrote to the HEW department to argue that mental health itself is "not a narrow category," to emphasize that many physical illnesses have "a significant psychological basis or component," and to call for better coordination between mental and physical health services, particularly for underserved communities.[36]

Chiming with Watkins's opinions, the Government Accountability Office published a report in 1976 requesting more "coordination of effort" among federal agencies in "clearly defining objectives, roles, responsibilities, resource commitments [and] actions to be taken."[37] The report recommended a "presidential objective on deinstitutionalization" but offered no easy answers on how to improve a patchwork system while still making savings. This echoed Rosemary Stevens's view in her 1971 book *American Medicine and the Public Interest* that "ideas and proposals are whirling around in profusion, based on a variety of premises, and uncertain as to their ultimate importance and effect."[38] To counteract this, Stevens recommended that policy makers retain a historical perspective and avoid financial expediencies and short-term planning in order to rescue the true purpose of healthcare. This view was, in part at least, embodied by a set of amendments to the Community Mental Health Act in 1975. These amendments reaffirmed federal responsibility and emphasized aftercare and community living programs, but they did not allay concerns that the "dream of better care" for all Americans might drown in a "legal, political, and financial ocean."[39]

Within the more specific field of psychiatry, the mid-1970s were marked by two important trends. The first of these was the decline of invasive therapies in favor of pharmaceutical interventions. Humanistic therapists continued to promote drug-free treatments and stressed interpersonal trust at a time when public faith in national leaders was at a low. However, antidepressants such as imipramine (sold as Tofranil) were increasingly seen as a way of supplementing or replacing talk therapies and for tackling underlying chemical imbalances. This trend was given credence in 1964 by an experiment conducted at Camarillo State Hospital in Southern California by the British psychiatric researcher Philip May, whose conclusions were published in 1968 in *The Treatment of Schizophrenia*. May's clinical trials showed that psychotherapy on its own was less effective in dealing with schizophrenia than a combined course of psychotherapy and psychoactive drugs. While humanistic practitioners thought antipsychotic medication such as phenothiazine was no better than electroconvulsive therapy for treating mania and hallucinations, New York clinical psychiatrist Ronald Fieve was a key advocate of so-called safe drugs. His 1975 book *Moodswing* outlined psychopharmacological treatments such as the alkali metal lithium, which Fieve had been using to treat depression, mania, and alcoholism while working in the New York State Psychiatric Institute, a facility where Beat poet Allen Ginsberg had spent a number of months in 1949, the same year that Australian psychiatrist John Cade discovered that lithium carbonate was a potential psychoactive treatment for mania.[40]

The U.S. Food and Drug Administration (FDA) approved lithium treatment in 1970 (it had been previously banned in its earlier form in 1949). Lithium was a far cry from the effects of shock treatment and lobotomy that so worried Ginsberg and Ken Kesey. Graphic examples of their concerns were presented in the film adaptation of Kesey's novel *One Flew Over the Cuckoo's Nest* the same year that *Moodswing* was published.[41] Directed by Miloš Forman, the film polarized the forces of good (the patients) and evil ("the Combine" that rules the hospital), switching Kesey's focus away from the first-person perspective of an unspeaking Native American patient toward a wholesale critique of the medical system. Producer Michael Douglas defended the claim that the psychiatric conditions patients in the film faced in the Oregon State Hospital were too stark, saying that "the lines in the Sixties were drawn clearer, but now things just ain't that clear."[42] Nevertheless, the film melodramatically reveals how a combination of humiliation and hard-line medical intervention kept chronic and acute patients in a state of torpor and fear. Even the exuberant Randle McMurphy (played by Jack Nicholson), who tries to incite his fellow patients into an active state of well-being, is defeated by the fanatical regime of Nurse Ratched (Louise Fletcher) and ends up in a vegetative state following an enforced lobotomy.

A 1977 PBS documentary *Inside the Cuckoo's Nest* drew parallels between practices at the Oregon State Hospital in Salem (which Kesey used as a partial source

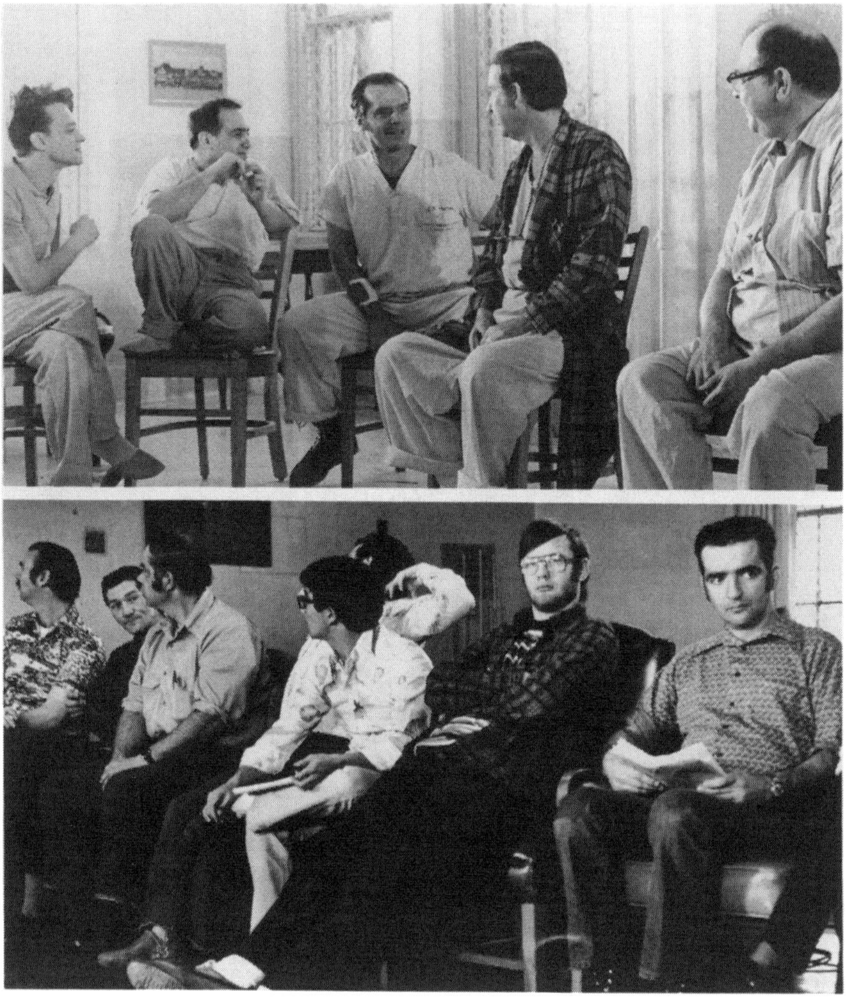

Figure 1.1 Publicity still for the PBS documentary *Inside the Cuckoo's Nest* (aired 8 September 1977). Wisconsin Center for Film and Theater Research.

for his novel) and scenes from the film. Despite this grounding in actual patient experience, these stereotypes of medical tyranny have been frequently recycled in the media since the mid-1970s and *One Flew Over the Cuckoo's Nest* is often cited as an example of the damaging effects of a psychiatric regime, even though the practice of lobotomy declined rapidly during the 1960s.[43] In contrast, Fieve was hopeful that psychoactive treatments could be both effective and humane in returning the patient's sense of selfhood: he upheld lithium as "the first truly prophylactic agent in psychiatry, one that can control, prevent, or stabilize the future lifetime course of a major mental illness."[44] Cases of lithium toxicity linked to impaired kidney function complicate this view, but despite a number of market alternatives in the 1980s, it is still seen as a relatively safe mood stabilizer (even though, as chapter 7 discusses, lithium is often prescribed in combination with other psychoactive drugs).[45]

Together with mounting concerns about prescription drug addiction, these positive accounts of drug treatment need to be set alongside the second trend: what Nathan Hale Jr. calls the "diminishing psychoanalytic realm."[46] In this account, the 1970s was a time of declining belief in psychoanalysis and psychotherapy as effective methods of treatment, partly based on methodological concerns and partly because experiments, such as those conducted in California and Massachusetts in the 1960s, revealed that psychotherapy had negligible effects in treating schizophrenic cases.[47] Close attention to biological and neurological factors led some psychiatrists away from psychoanalysis, particularly the Freudian emphasis on repression and childhood sexuality that often confused stressful circumstances with conditions rooted in early life. However, there was at least one associated benefit: although patients continued to seek swift relief from anxieties, the psychotherapeutic legacy encouraged doctors to treat more routine conditions with the sensitivity of an analyst. Yet, Hale detected that the debate between those who called for tighter diagnostics and those who were drawn to a broader psychodynamic understanding of health and illness was one of the major fault lines in psychiatry that helped shape the third edition of the *Diagnostic and Statistical Manual of Mental Disorders* (*DSM*).[48] Published in 1980, *DSM-III* was not alone in withdrawing from psychoanalytic categories; by the middle of the 1980s, straightforward psychoanalytic techniques had declined even at Chestnut Lodge in Bethesda and the Menninger Clinic in Topeka, two pioneering centers of noninvasive therapies.

As the next section discusses, there was still a great deal of anger on behalf of ex-patients, health advocacy groups, and radical thinkers, many of who thought that professional medicine was part of the problem rather than the solution. This view was encapsulated in Ivan Illich's description of "the medicalization of life" in his polemical 1975 treatise *Medical Nemesis*, in which he sets out his dystopian vision of a "medical-industrial complex."[49] Instead of simply critiquing invasive therapies or psychopharmaceuticals, Illich claimed that the whole medical system not only mistreated patients but was predicated on long-term dependency.[50] In Illich's bleak account of a "passive public that has come to rely on superficial medical housecleanings" there was little room for an individual to make choices when faced with a system that seemed more a menacing monopoly than an uncoordinated patchwork.[51]

Community health centers offered a partial answer to this jaundiced view of the medical establishment, both in terms of their responsiveness to the individual's needs and in their provision of greater choice for the underserved. Despite the problems of organization and finance many centers faced, as a socially progressive model of healthcare, they offered a counterpart to Illich's call for public scrutiny of the entire medical system.[52] This led to new designs for integrated hospitals that responded to the 1966 call of the National Commission on Community Health Services task force for improved communication, sanitation, transportation, and access, with doors that permitted patients to go out as well as in.[53] Such attempts to reconnect patients to their locality took the edge off critiques of medical authority and the dystopian vision of total institutions and pharmaceutical control, as epitomized by the film version of *One Flew Over the Cuckoo's Nest*.

Ex-Patients, Rights, and Stigma

Despite attempts to refine diagnostic language, it became increasingly clear during the 1970s that the boundaries between mental illness and mental health were becoming blurred, often in confusing ways. The growing legal interest in psychiatric cases promised some clarity, particularly in terms of who was responsible for making decisions to commit an individual to hospitalized psychiatric treatment. The most important piece of legislation stemmed from *O'Connor v. Donaldson*, a landmark federal case that ran through the first half of 1975. The focus was on Kenneth Donaldson, a 48-year-old ex-patient who had been interned in Florida State Hospital in a locked ward for nearly fifteen years on the grounds that he was experiencing paranoid delusions and auditory hallucinations. He petitioned eighteen times for release on the basis that he had been admitted without a full psychiatric examination and that his constitutional right to liberty was being denied. Even though he was suddenly released by the hospital in July 1971 (a fortnight before a pre-trial press conference), after five months of scrutiny and a four-day trial, the Supreme Court ruled that nonviolent patients such as Donaldson should no longer be held involuntarily if they were capable of living within the law.[54] This decision came after a wave of protests from groups calling for the abolition of involuntary hospitalization and state-level cases such as *Lessard v. Schmidt* (1972) that safeguarded patients' rights after over 4,200 individuals had been involuntary committed in the state of Wisconsin early in the decade.[55] The *O'Connor v. Donaldson* case, which was shaped by a significant amount of literature on the legality of involuntary hospitalization, informed *Kremens v. Bartley* (1977), which extended legal protection to children aged 14 to 18 to prevent their parents from institutionalizing them against their will.

In the spring of 1973, an article titled "Into the Abyss: Psychiatric Reliability and Emergency Commitment Statutes" called for an end to "emergency commitment, which authorizes detention on the authority of medical judgment alone, without judicial safeguards or a hearing of any kind."[56] Underpinning this view was a belief that psychiatry relied on vague concepts and often indulged in stereotypes based on class, gender, race, and sexuality. Writing the year the *Journal of Psychiatry and Law* and the *Bulletin of the American Academy of Psychiatry and the Law* (the first two journals dedicated to patient rights and advocacy) were launched, the authors drew on a number of legal cases from the early 1970s and sociologist Erving Goffman's comparison of the total institutions of asylum and prison. Their two central arguments were that the only cases of legitimate involuntary commitment are those when the law is violated and that due process needs to be established to properly assess such cases.

The relationship between psychiatry and the law was complicated by lurid headlines related to the dramatic Manson murders trial of 1970–72, and it was often tricky to decouple psychopathology and violent crime in media stories. These issues did not go away when Charles Manson was imprisoned for life in April 1971; four years later, a member of the Manson Family, Lynette "Squeaky" Fromme, was sentenced for attempting to assassinate President Ford in Sacramento, an incident that *Newsweek* described as "a helter-skelter touch of California evil . . . that summoned up all the worst vibrations of the murderous '60s."[57] Fromme thought that the president did not show enough concern for environmental causes, although she defended herself by maintaining that her gun was not loaded. A history of depression and drug use was known when Fromme was arrested in 1969 while attempting to stop witnesses from testifying at the Tate-LaBianca murder trial. Health issues were not fully explored, though, even when she was arrested again in 1972 on suspicion of being an accomplice in a multiple murder case. Despite her bizarre behavior, the *Newsweek* account does not mention mental illness (except for a passing mention of her "scrambled circuits"), and a psychiatrist was not brought in until some way into the trial of 1975, when an assessment that Fromme was "mentally competent" stripped her of her legal defense.[58]

The authors of "Into the Abyss" believed that it was essential to preserve an individual's civil liberties, arguing that plaintiffs should have the option of attending their own hearing and to "refuse medication prior to trial" or at least to have clear knowledge of its possible side effects.[59] However, the authors did not tackle the limits of dangerous behavior and the psychological triggers that might compel individuals to act in harmful ways or to absorb convictions that they might not otherwise hold, as was arguably the case for Lynette Fromme and Ford's second would-be assassin, the "estranged FBI informant" Sara Jane Moore, who narrowly missed shooting the president in San Francisco just seventeen days later.

These cases did not mean that situational influences were ignored. Psychology professor Philip Zimbardo's famous prison experiments at Stanford University in 1971 were designed to assess the effects of imprisonment on a group of volunteers who were asked to randomly play the roles of prisoners and guards. Planned as a longer experiment, the trial had to be halted after six days when the prisoners started to display extreme forms of anger and depression after being tormented, humiliated, and disciplined by the guards, many of whom were increasingly sadistic. The experiment pointed to both the psychological dangers of incarceration and how quickly individuals began to assume dominant or submissive traits. This led Zimbardo to conclude that it is easy "for ordinary people to begin to engage in evil deeds, or to be passively indifferent to the suffering of others" if the environmental conditions are right.[60] Zimbardo believed that situational conditions shape the likelihood of atrocity. Although his early reports noted variations in the behavior of volunteers who adopted the role of guards (some were tough yet fair, others were tyrannical, others were friendly to the prisoners), Erich Fromm suggested that the Stanford prison experiment did not compare well to the "spontaneous cruelty" SS guards practiced in Nazi concentration camps, where prisoners suffered long-term effects of incarceration.[61] Despite Fromm's criticism that Zimbardo's experiments lacked rigor, concerns about "depersonalization" preoccupied many thinkers, particularly in cases in which the individual is denied a voice or is faced with stigma for having undergone treatment.[62]

This trend was encapsulated by David Rosenhan's widely read and controversial article "On Being Sane in Insane Places," published in January 1973, which documented eight individuals (including Rosenhan himself) who pretended that they had schizophrenia as part of a covert experiment with the aim of recording the internal procedures of twelve psychiatric institutions. These pseudo-patients fabricated a story about hearing unfamiliar voices in order to gain entry but otherwise did not behave differently than they did before they were admitted. However, after the pseudo-patients were given an initial diagnosis of schizophrenia, it was virtually impossible for them to throw it off, leading Rosenhan to argue that "a psychiatric label has a life and an influence of its own."[63] Echoing Michel Foucault's *Birth of the Clinic*, his 1963 study of the disciplinary regimes of hospitals (which was first translated into English in 1973), the depersonalization that all the pseudo-patients experienced in the face of institutional pressures suggested that hierarchical hospital structures limited interpersonal contact and kept patients in a state of subjugation. Psychoactive drugs were shown to be a common mechanism in this process of depersonalization; Rosenhan argued that they convinced medical staff that treatment was being conducted effectively and that "further patient contact may not be necessary."[64] This led to three conclusions: psychiatric diagnoses are not always reliable, community health facilities might be more conducive to therapy than hospital wards, and mental health workers need to safeguard patients from "countertherapeutic" experiences.

Zimbardo's and Rosenhan's experiments suggested that the psychiatric infrastructure was largely unchanged despite the Community Mental Health Act and that the dehumanizing risks of the "total institution" that Goffman had identified in the early 1960s lingered into the 1970s. This is perhaps why the film *One Flew Over the Cuckoo's Nest* exaggerates the incarcerating forces that Ken Kesey had fictionalized a decade earlier. This popular (and, arguably, dated) critique of psychiatric regimes expanded on earlier accounts of malpractice, such as Jack Nelson's exposés of 1959–60 in the *Atlanta Constitution* that revealed the inhumane treatment of patients in Milledgeville Central State Hospital, Georgia.[65] This was the same hospital where Jimmy Carter's relatives had been treated for alcoholism, and it was still infested with rats and cockroaches when Rosalynn Carter visited in the early 1970s after her office received a call from a Milledgeville patient who claimed she had to leave to get well and that some patients were being mistreated in solitary confinement.[66]

Sandwiched between the glimpse of voiceless inpatients in large psychiatric facilities (it is notable that in *One Flew Over the Cuckoo's Nest*, the survivor patient, Chief Bromden, pretends he is mute) and the specter of drifting patients released prematurely from facilities in the face of health cuts was a wide-ranging sense that constitutional and citizens' rights should extend further, a process that would help transform the medical status of and the public attitude towards mental illness. Not all advocacy groups argued as forcibly as the American Association for the Abolition of Involuntary Mental Hospitalization, which Thomas Szasz, George Alexander, and Erving Goffman established in 1970 at Syracuse University. And not all activists shared Szasz's long-standing conviction that psychiatry was a dangerous profession that brutally coerced its patients into long courses of needless therapy. Nevertheless, in the first half of the 1970s, there was a marked rise in the activity of psychiatric reformers and protesters calling for more humane mental health treatments that did not simply look toward psychotropic drugs.

Among the ex-patient support groups were a number of organizations in Boston, New York City, San Francisco, and Vancouver that offered counseling and support for former patients and were linked to the consciousness-raising efforts of civil rights activists. One of the most significant challenges for these groups was communication between its members, which was aided by countercultural publications such as *Madness Network News* in San Francisco in 1972 and the first Conference on Human Rights and Psychiatric Oppression, which was held in Detroit in 1973 (both initiatives ran until the mid-1980s).[67] While the support network for ex-patients was seen as beneficial—and *Madness Network News* was interested in creative writing and art in addition to being strongly politicized—outspoken pieces on cases of malpractice, enforced drugging, and overtreatment offended conservatives and liberals alike because of their radical social agenda.[68] This was certainly the case for the short-lived Insane Liberation Front, which began in Portland, Oregon, in 1970 (and lasted for only six months) and the Radical Therapist Collective, which formed in Minot, North Dakota, that same year and argued strongly for a "total revolution" across the spectrum of American life.[69]

The main reason that these groups were short lived was because they strove to balance different agendas. For example, the Radical Therapist Collective split in half in 1972; the more outspoken faction moved to Cambridge, Massachusetts, where it amended its name to Rough Times (a name it gave to its journal that April) because its members believed that personal and political change were intricately linked. By 1972, articles on practical therapy had been superseded by angry pieces that made links between aggressive foreign policy and a denial of citizens' health rights, fueled by the belief that "mental hospitalization [derives] from the same established power that drops bombs over Hanoi."[70] A March 1972 article in this vein by psychiatrist Rick Kunnes, "Detherapizing Society," echoed Illich's 1971 book *Deschooling Society* in its call for an end to the "consumer-patient" mentality that pushes the "person-patient-consumer to hunger for a steady absorption of therapy."[71] Although *Rough Times* continued into the mid-1970s (before changing its name to *State and Mind*), it lost the potency of its early years, leaving a splinter group at the Berkeley Radical Psychiatry Center to publish more specific pieces on mental health in and beyond 1973 in their journal *Issues in Radical Therapy*.[72]

Away from these journals, there was a general feeling that ex-mental patients, especially those that had been hospitalized for lengthy periods, were liable to suffer in trying to reintegrate into everyday life. This was the case with the Velvet

Underground's lead singer Lou Reed, as voiced on his 1974 track "Kill Your Sons," a song he had written in the mid-1960s that reflects on the twenty-four electroshock treatments he underwent at Creedmore State Hospital in Long Island in 1959. He was only 17 at the time; Reed's parents had admitted him for violent mood swings but also because they were unable to accept his nascent homosexuality.[73] The song is full of bitter irony, targeted as much at Reed's self-righteous yet quietly disintegrating family as it was at the psychiatric profession and the pharmaceutical industry. The negative reaction to electroconvulsive treatment was encoded the following year by California neurologist John Friedberg in his cautionary book *Shock Treatment Is Not Good for Your Brain*. Friedberg, who had undergone a course of antipsychotic drugs and group therapy for "acute schizo-affective reaction" as a young man had become a devotee of Szasz's "myth of mental illness" philosophy, argued that shock treatment led to both memory loss and brain disease.[74] Even individuals who had not undergone invasive therapies but had an inpatient history often found that employment was tricky, as recounted in New York lawyer Bruce Ennis's *Prisoners of Psychiatry*, which conveys the voices of four individuals who had suffered after being labeled "criminally insane."[75]

Whatever the reason for psychosurgery and invasive treatments, the mid-1970s provided a moment when ex-patients started to speak out about their treatment and its aftermath. In a *New York Times* article in November 1977, Rosalynn Carter cited one such anonymized colleague who had been chosen for the President's Commission on Mental Health. Even though this individual was now committed to eradicating the stigma of mental illness, she claimed that she was "half in the closet and half out" and that "the people in the place where I live do not know, most of them, that I am a former patient. I didn't tell the manager this when I filled out the form [for a job]. When I told him later, he said he was glad he hadn't known because he would not have let me in."[76] Occupational health was being taken more seriously at that time, but there was still a knee-jerk reaction to disclosures of mental illness, especially when it was associated with particular forms of psychiatric treatment, as Mrs. Carter argued in a piece for *McCall's* the following June in which she quoted a former mental patient from Massachusetts: "You wonder after coming out if people can simply look into your face and see where you have been. Does it show?"[77]

The issue of stigma came to public attention with one of the most prominent ex-mental patient cases of the 1970s: that of a young Missouri senator, Thomas Eagleton, who was George McGovern's surprise choice for vice-president at the end of the long Democratic National Convention. Although Eagleton had been hailed as a rising star in late July 1972, when the news broke at the beginning of August that he had been hospitalized three times and given electroshock treatment in St. Louis and Minneapolis in the period 1960–66, McGovern did a volte-face. He initially stated that "Tom Eagleton is fully qualified in mind, body and spirit to be the Vice-President" and that the disclosure would not affect their professional partnership, but he dropped Eagleton a mere eighteen days after the nomination in the face of pressure from the media and some members of the Democratic Party and after he had had a conversation with Eagleton's psychiatrists. It is not clear how much detail Eagleton initially disclosed to McGovern, but he received scant support in the press, except for the 7 August issue of *Time* magazine that featured a poll in which over 75 percent of readers said the revelations had not swayed their views.[78] More generally, though, the media reversed their initially positive coverage of Eagleton; reports emphasized his intensity and speculated about excessive drinking, his tendency to perspire, and the instability of a potential vice-president who might need to have his finger on the nuclear button. The case was particularly poignant given the fact that McGovern's daughter Terry had been hospitalized for depression, alcohol abuse, and suicidal tendencies after an arrest in 1968 for smoking marijuana.[79]

More positively, later that year the American Medical Association saw the Eagleton case as an opportunity to organize a symposium to promote the reality of depressive conditions and the stigma associated with them. Ronald Fieve, one of the organizers, discussed the Eagleton case explicitly in *Moodswing*, speculating that the Missouri senator might actually be a "hypercompetent" manic-depressive who could function effectively for much of the time.[80] Fieve followed up on a question posed in the 1972 *Time* issue about the "strength and weakness" of public figures by considering other national leaders whose performance might have been enhanced by nonnormative conditions, ranging from President Lincoln's melancholy to the depression statesman James Forrestal suffered that led him to suicide in 1949, less than two months after he had resigned as President Truman's Secretary of Defense.[81] Echoing the arguments of radical mental health support groups, Fieve worried that ex-psychiatric patients were treated unfavorably compared to public figures with physical illnesses. He did not mask the erratic decisions that can be exacerbated by the pressures of high office, but Fieve argued that mood swings are often a feature of high-functioning leaders and that more attention should be paid to the spectrum of mental health instead of a specialist focus on pathology.

One could argue either way about how much the radical therapy groups helped the cause of raising consciousness about the consequences of institutionalization and invasive treatment, particularly at a time when gay rights activists were questioning the ethics of aversion therapy and demanding that homosexuality should be removed as a pathological category. (It was controversially retained in *DSM-II* in 1968 and then omitted in 1973 in the wake of events such as a "Psychiatry: Friend or Foe to Homosexuals" session at the American Psychiatric Association annual conference the previous year.)[82] Certainly, in the first half of the 1970s there were multiple circuits of communication at local and national level, ranging from countercultural publications such as *Madness Network News* and the revolutionary politics of the Radical Therapist Collective to coverage in the mass media, especially around the Eagleton affair. It is not clear how much the Carters would have been aware of these radical publications, but the stigma associated with bouts of mental illness that spill into the workplace was an agenda-setting issue for the 1976 presidential campaign and the initial years of the Carter administration.

The President's Commission on Mental Health

First Lady Rosalynn Carter played a central role in mental health advocacy in the late 1970s, and she set the bar high for her White House successors in raising awareness of the nation's health needs. She was extremely active in her husband's campaign for the Democratic presidential nomination in the spring of 1976, and even more so that autumn at a number of rallies. At one rally in Alexandria, Virginia, that October she spoke simply and plainly about her husband's rise to political office, in which he had moved from the hospital authority board and the Sumter County School board from the mid-1950s to the early 1960s (it was part of a segregated educational system during this time) to the Georgia planning commission, the state Senate, and then to governor in 1970. She stressed her husband's qualities as a simple working man who understood small businesses and would not tolerate "the waste and extravagance and unnecessary expense" of Washington and his commitment to health as epitomized by the Killers and Cripplers program of 1973–74 that committed $15 million to combat strokes and heart disease.[83] In addition to stressing her husband's credentials as a fiscal conservative, she mentioned her own role in raising awareness of Georgia's mental health needs after visiting nearly twenty state mental hospitals and clinics in 1971. Pointing out that from 1970 to 1974 the state had moved from the worst providers to one of the best providers of mental health services in the country, she highlighted the opening of eighty-four community centers stimulated by the Governor's Commission to Improve Services to the Mentally and Emotionally Handicapped (an initiative that Mrs. Carter herself had overseen).[84] Displaying a typically personal touch, she focused on the human cost of unemployment, shifting between statistics and personal stories, and claimed that her husband's greatest strength was to know "human beings," their needs, problems, and hopes.

When Jimmy Carter turned his attention to health on the campaign trail it was usually to criticize the nonsystem of the Nixon-Ford years or the need to improve preventive medicine. This did not mean that he avoided topics of mental illness or cognitive disability: Patrick Anderson, Carter's chief speechwriter in the election year, noted that he attended a Sunday school for cognitively disabled children near the University of Notre Dame, where Anderson observed Carter "amid the bedlam" of noise and movement, "smiling serenely, seeming to enjoy himself." Anderson surmised that the presidential candidate's serenity stemmed from his religious sensibility and a sense of ease that probably derived from encountering similar scenes during his tenure as governor.[85] This visit suggests that Carter often framed public issues in terms of personal experience, but it was Rosalynn Carter who directed her husband's thoughts to the treatment of mental health patients, perhaps because this was the arena in which she could make her mark by speaking for the underprivileged and the voiceless. Her experience, which stemmed from her volunteer work at Georgia Regional Hospital, led to her shift as first lady to a more business-minded approach toward health and gender equality, as was evident in her support of the Equal Rights Amendment that sought ratification at state level through much of the 1970s. Like Betty Ford, Mrs. Carter's role in the women's movement was not a straightforward one; however, her commitment to equality and her work on the ERA were key reasons why the president chose her to steer his Commission on Mental Health.

Given that Jimmy Carter did not actively campaign on this issue, it is perhaps surprising that as early as 17 February 1977, he announced the formation of his President's Commission on Mental Health. There is evidence to suggest that Mrs. Carter persuaded him that his success at the state level could be replicated nationally, although the conviction might have been instinctual or ideological rather than evidence-based.[86] This feeling of sympathy for the underserved was supported by comments the Carters made, for example in a March 1977 feature in the *New York Times* that quoted Mrs. Carter as saying: "I want to do everything humanly possible to help create a more caring society so that we can begin to counter the painful loneliness and sense of helplessness which has engulfed too many of our people."[87] Thus, while the commission was the first systematic overhaul of mental health provision since 1963, the motivations were at once both humanitarian and administrative. This overhaul was prompted by Georgia-based psychiatrist Peter Bourne's view that the nation needed "new and creative leadership for our health care system" and that the first lady should avoid "a quick, flashy operation that would get you and mental health a lot of instant attention" in favor of "a major venture looking at all aspects of mental health in depth" over the course of a year.[88] The plans for a commission evolved out of Rosalynn Carter's and Peter Bourne's community health work in the early 1970s, but it was slow to percolate into the presidents' speeches about health. For example, when he gave his Health Initiative Message to Congress on 25 April 1977, to introduce two new pieces of legislation (the Hospital Cost Containment Act to stabilize rising costs and the Child Health Assessment Program, which focused on children of low-income families), Jimmy Carter did not mention mental health explicitly, yet it was clear that it was an element of a broader plan that, when realized, would be founded on cooperation between private and public providers and would focus on outpatient care.[89]

By the time the president addressed Congress that April, the Commission on Mental Health was already two months old, following a ceremonial gathering at the White House on 17 February, at which Carter formally signed Executive Order 11973 and announced Mrs. Carter as honorary chair. The president opened the signing ceremony by commenting that "this is one of the most gratifying experiences that a human being could have—to deal with those who are at the mercy of governmental agencies . . . and then to see what apparently was an almost wasted life be enhanced and revived and a great spirit come forth."[90] This sentiment is in line with Patrick Anderson's assessment that Carter's religious sensibility drew him toward the disadvantaged and voiceless, perhaps stimulated by his mother's career as a nurse. Carter targeted his criticism at the failure of the medical infrastructure, and he reiterated this the following spring when he claimed that the American Medical Association was impeding progress by protecting the interests of doctors rather than those of patients.[91] He thought, too, that special interest groups were often as guilty as government agencies and national associations of building "tight walls" to prevent others from encroaching on their patch.

In her remarks at the signing ceremony, Rosalynn Carter spoke of her conversations with the electorate in Georgia in 1970 and across the nation in 1976 as the major stimulus behind the commission. Instead of seeing the moment as a starting point, she looked back to the Joint Commission on Mental Illness and Health of 1955, two years into the Eisenhower administration, as a key federal initiative that provided the groundwork for the community healthcare program. Despite progress on this front, she warned that only 40 percent of the population was currently served by health centers. Like her husband—and following the advice of Peter Bourne—she was keen to review the whole system to ensure that community services were effectively reaching the underserved.[92] Mrs. Carter emphasized fairness and what a few months later, in an address to the Washington Press Club, she called "a new philosophy" that would "bring mental health out of the closet" and a commitment that it would be "for all of us."[93] She stressed this "new attitude" in an article "Removing the Mental-Illness Stigma" for the *New York Times*, published in November, in which she moved from citing personal testimony and her experience as a volunteer in Georgia to outlining the strategic priorities of the president's commission.[94]

With this notion of recalibrating the whole system in mind, the 1977 Commission sought to address seven key areas: first, to what extent "the mentally ill, emotionally disturbed and mentally retarded . . . are being underserved, and who is affected by such underservice"; second, how emotional stress could be effectively addressed in the final quarter century of the twentieth century; third, the role of the federal government; fourth, how a coordinated approach could be achieved; fifth, what kind of research would be necessary; sixth, ascertaining the collaborative role of "educational systems, volunteer agencies and other people-helping institutions" in order to "minimize emotional disturbance"; and, seventh, to work out how such programs could be financed.[95] These goals were partly pragmatic, undergirded by a pluralistic philosophy that spanned many regions and individuals from different backgrounds. The health challenges of particular communities were not explicitly raised at the February meeting, but the Carters' comments about their experiences in Georgia imbued the commission with both a compassionate sensibility and a pragmatic plan for the formation of thirty task panels. The vast scope of the enterprise was a challenge to this pragmatic approach, but the commission's main objective was to develop enabling federal structures and a framework that would help silent voices speak for themselves in line with the president's comment about "the great spirit" issuing forth.[96]

Peter Bourne helped the Carters choose Thomas E. Bryant as the director of the commission. Bryant represented a line of continuity with the previous Democratic administration; he had managed President Johnson's Emergency Food and Medical Services Program, located in the Office of Economic Opportunity. After 1969, Bryant's work was largely in the sphere of alcohol and drug abuse; he was appointed president of the Drug Abuse Council in 1972, in which role he challenged the hard-line view of the Nixon administration that, to Bryant's mind, myopically linked marijuana use to criminal activity.[97] Bryant had advised the Carter campaign team in the fall of 1976, arguing that it was important to project a message that "'good health' is dependent upon both environmental/personal disease prevention factors *and* the provision of medical care" and urging Carter to take a "sensible" rather than a "radical" line on offering too many health panaceas.[98] He also informed the rhetoric of the nonsystem that closely echoed Bryant's 1975 volume *The Politics of Drugs*, in which he described drug control as "a patchwork" of confusing "policies, strategies and law."[99] A passionate champion of patients' rights, Bryant offered intellectual and ethical leadership to the Carter administration and in the mid-1980s to Rosalynn Carter as she was setting up the Mental Health Taskforce at the Carter Center in Atlanta (the center was established in 1982 to house President Carter's papers and as a hub for promoting human rights and mental health issues). He was also critical of psychopharmacological solutions to mental illness, which he believed had worsened in the 1980s when deinstitutionalization to reduce hospital costs (which were higher in the United States in 1982 than any other country) was not supported by "appropriate community facilities to care for those released."[100]

One of Bryant's concerns was the health of underserved communities and minority groups. Writing on this topic in June 1978—two months before the World Health Organization advocated "health for all" as a basic human right and pressed for government action—Mrs. Carter identified a number of problems within primary care, including inadequate access to mental health facilities for Hispanics, Asian Americans, and Native Americans and the lack of understanding of cultural heritage among health funders and providers (in the latter case this persisted despite the Indian Health Care Improvement Act that President Ford had signed in September 1976).[101] The fact that Mrs. Carter represented her husband on diplomatic visits to Central and South America in spring 1977 might have sharpened her awareness of international health issues, particularly among Hispanic groups, although there is no evidence to suggest that she discussed national health agendas on these visits.

Running alongside the first lady's international responsibilities was the commission's commitment to compile health reports on each minority group through its thirty task groups. These ambitions did not prevent criticism of the commission for not conducting a full sociological examination of the relationship between mental health, racial prejudice, unemployment, and lack of equal access to educational opportunities. Bryant defended the commission's approach at a National Coalition of Hispanic Mental Health and Human Services Organizations Conference in August 1977, following correspondence with Ford Kuramoto, the chair of the Asian Pacific subpanel, in which Bryant said that he was confident that "the Commission has sought the participation and heeded the advice of more ethnic and racial minority individuals and groups than any similar Commission."[102] He regretted that "no Asian or Pacific American" had been selected as a commissioner but pointed to the range of "highly qualified" representatives on health

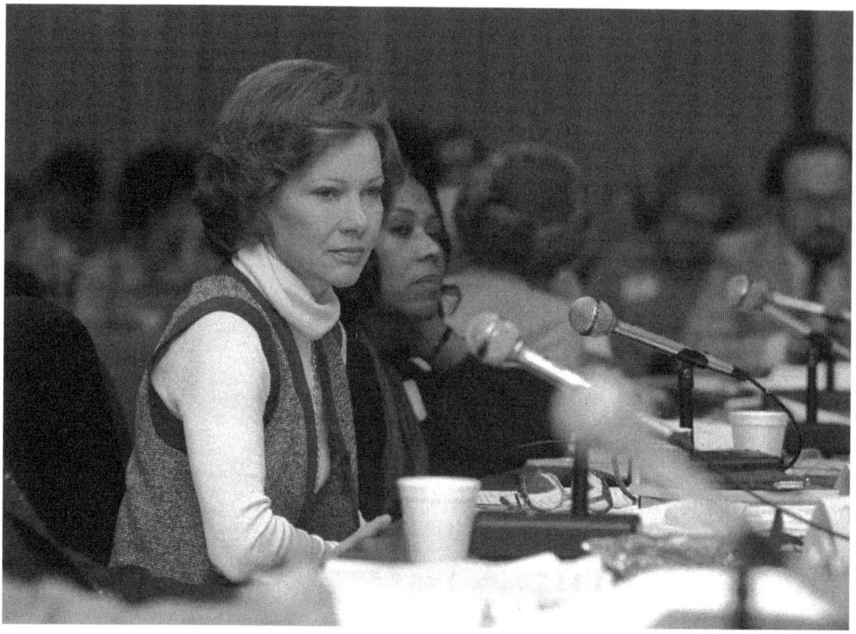

Figure 1.2 Rosalynn Carter chairs the final hearing of the President's Commission on Mental Health, Washington, DC, 17 January 1978. Courtesy of the Jimmy Carter Presidential Library.

task forces, including groups that focused on Asian Americans, African Americans, Euro-Ethnics, Native Americans, and Hispanics. The task groups delivered their findings at three hearings Mrs. Carter chaired from October 1977 to January 1978, and their reports helped shape the commission's final report.

Despite the lack of focus of some task panels, President Carter praised the commission's final report of April 1978 for assimilating information on mental health services for underserved communities and for making proposals for better coordination at the federal, state, and local levels. When Carter commended the report to Senate a year later, he stressed its flexibility and innovation, highlighted prevention and training, and pointed out that the nation's research capacity had been eroded during the Nixon-Ford years.[103] This legislation would be crucial, he argued, in protecting civil rights and clarifying the federal role in health advocacy. However, as the final section of this chapter will recount, all was not well in the Carter administration in 1978–79, particularly on the subject of healthcare.

The Health Legacy of the Bicentennial

The same month that former First Lady Betty Ford publicly announced her addiction to prescription medication and alcohol and admitted herself to Long Beach Naval Hospital, Congress was announcing "budgetary austerity" and a "new conservative spirit" in its April 1978 quarterly report on health, education, and welfare.[104] This view was fueled by the federal cost of healthcare, which had spiraled to $800 per U.S. citizen per year compared to the $600 per person that Carter had estimated in the third presidential debate of October 1976.[105] The congressional review also noted the rift between the president and Edward Kennedy, the chair of the Senate Subcommittee on Health, a rift that had begun in 1977, when Carter had told Kennedy that his health insurance bill was too expensive and would interfere with a balanced budget. Tensions between Kennedy and Carter mounted during 1978 on the subject of health insurance, which Kennedy had been championing since 1971 and which he was now calling the "missing promise" of the Carter administration.[106] Carter was keen to proceed in a "step-by-step" manner, particularly in the context of an unresponsive economy and high health costs, but the more liberal Kennedy wanted a sweeping mandatory health plan that would fix the "nonsystem" in one go, and he attacked the president at the Democratic midterm convention for jeopardizing the party's integrity.[107]

This disagreement had been exacerbated by George McGovern's public criticisms the previous May that Carter had broken his campaign promises on a number of domestic issues. The sense of disunity was inflamed in the White House by increasing tensions between the Carters and Secretary of Health, Education, and Welfare Joseph Califano, a longtime friend of Kennedy and Vice-President Walter Mondale.[108] Although Kennedy saw himself as the champion of the voiceless Americans that the democratic socialist Michael Harrington had identified in his 1962 book *The Other America* (particularly on employment-related healthcare), Mrs. Carter thought that Califano lacked the patience to listen carefully to the voices of the underserved and those who had close-up experience of mental illness as primary caretakers. President Carter asked Califano's office in late 1977 to find additional funds for the commission, but the truth was that the Carters trusted Thomas Bryant, a fellow southerner, much more than the outspoken HEW secretary.[109]

All in all, these disagreements did not provide a healthy backdrop to the president's announcement, following the submission of the commission's final report, that $500 million would be spent over three years on improving the mental health system for the estimated 10 to 15 percent of the nation's population with some form of mental illness—a total of 20 to 33 million people, in addition to an estimated 6 million with cognitive disabilities—particularly as budgetary constraints were high on the agenda.[110] Although this was a fairly modest federal commitment, Califano and Kennedy both thought that the president should rethink his priorities. Califano believed that it would be better to focus on disease prevention, immunization, and Medicare initiatives; Kennedy that national health insurance should be top of the president's agenda.[111] There were some points of agreement, such as Califano's support for the Green Door community program that began in Washington, DC, in 1976 to help foster independence for individuals with severe or persistent mental illness in predominantly African American neighborhoods.[112] However, relationships worsened to such a degree that Carter asked Califano to resign in July 1979 (purportedly for trying to undermine a bill that separated health and welfare from a new Department of Education), while Kennedy continued his vocal opposition

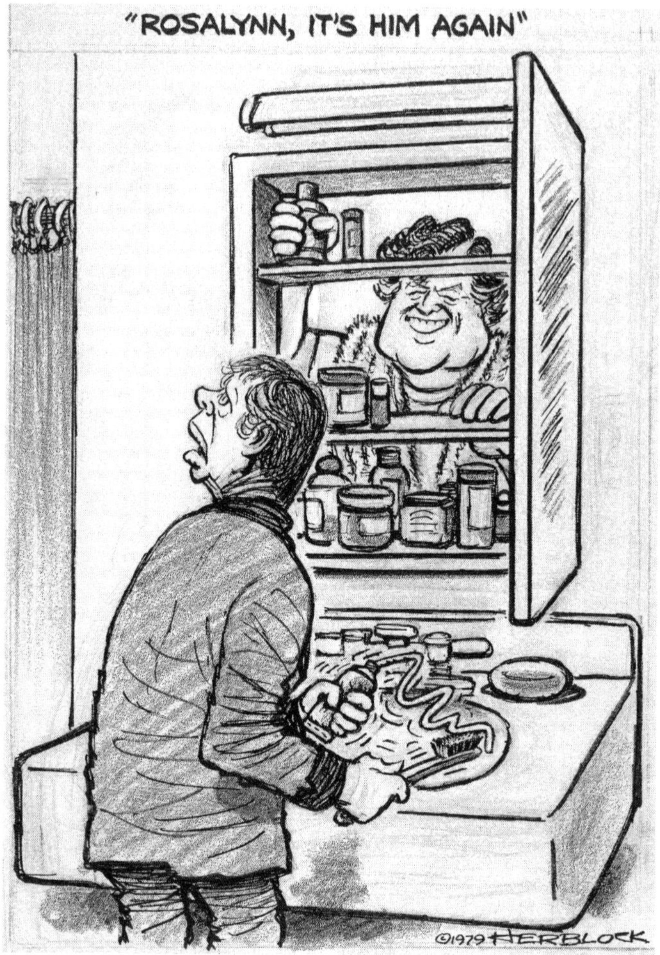

Figure 1.3 Herblock, "Rosalynn, It's Him Again," *Washington Post*, 12 September 1979. Courtesy of the Library of Congress Prints and Photographs Division, Herbert L. Block Collection.

to Carter's health insurance plans and chose to run against him for Democratic presidential nominee in 1980. *Washington Post* cartoonist Herb Block captured the rivalry in his September 1979 political cartoon "Rosalynn, It's Him Again," in which Kennedy's smiling face appears in Carter's medicine cabinet.

Added to these mounting tensions between Carter, Califano, and Kennedy was the resignation in July 1978 of the president's advisor on health issues, Peter Bourne, who had worked with the Carters through the decade and had informed the healthcare policies of the Carter-Mondale ticket in 1976. Bourne resigned when it became known that he had used a false patient's name in a prescription for fifteen tablets of the sedative Quaalude for White House employee Ellen Metsky, even though he claimed it had been to protect patient identity. (Quaaludes had been restricted since 1973 and were often used recreationally to stimulate euphoric states, in addition to being used as a sleeping aid.)[113] The case was just one in a series of public embarrassments for the president in 1978–79. Perhaps more important, Mrs. Carter believed that Bourne's role was vital for coordinating the commission, and she later pinpointed his resignation as a major reason why the transition from policy to legislation was so slow.[114]

Nevertheless, the president's announcement presaged what would eventually become the Mental Health Systems Act, which he presented to Congress on 15 May 1979. Hearings were held that summer, including Mrs. Carter's appearance before the Senate Subcommittee on Health, but disagreements and wrangles slowed down congressional approval. This was finally granted the following September, by which time Carter was deep in his reelection campaign. Nevertheless, the signing of the law at Woodburn Center for Community Mental Health in Annandale, Virginia, on 7 October 1980, was a joyful occasion for the Carters, and the president pointed out that this was the most important piece of relevant legislation since the Community Mental Health Act of 1963. After the tussle in the Democratic primaries between Carter and Edward Kennedy, the event marked another moment of healing when the president thanked the Kennedy family for their work on healthcare over two decades and, probably biting his lip, he introduced Senator Kennedy as a "man of compassion and sensitivity."[115] However, Carter's overwhelming defeat to Reagan in the presidential election four weeks later meant that the legislation that the Carters believed would have developed a more integrated system floundered almost immediately. Reagan thought that this was just another instance of state overregulation, and Congress replaced it with a block grant that reduced federal support for many social programs. Mrs. Carter commented that "the funding for our legislation was killed by the new President. It was a bitter loss," made worse because the deadline for passing the Equal Rights Amendment expired the following year, three states short of the thirty-eight approving states needed for ratification.[116]

If, as Califano and others were arguing, the Carter presidency was a passionless affair that mirrored the malaise of the late 1970s, this view overlooks the energy and commitment that went into the President's Commission on Mental Health and what promised to be a major moment in mental health reform.[117] One could argue, as did Ted Kennedy, that only comprehensive health insurance would repair the nonsystem that Carter inherited. However, at least in the sphere of mental health, the commission focused on integration and implementation while remaining sensitive to the voices and needs of underserved communities. Carter's plan was certainly not the radical dismantling of a medical system that ex-patient groups demanded, but their militant attacks were faltering by 1980, symbolized by the final issue of the journal *The Abolitionist* in the summer of 1979 (the journal spared Carter's mental health reforms the vitriol with which it attacked the "therapeutic state").[118]

For a short few months at the beginning of the 1980s, there was real hope that the president's commission would build on the previous commissions of 1955 and 1963 and achieve some concrete goals. Despite the delays, the Mental Health

Systems Act and the accompanying and more action-oriented National Plan for the Chronically Mentally Ill were examples of what Robert Bellah was calling "responsible action in a revolutionary world" in which the government makes a "commitment to the common good" and renews its moral and spiritual covenant with the American people.[119] This did not mean that a second-term Carter administration would have offered any panaceas. In the context of high inflation and unfavorable unemployment figures, rampant urban crime, and a controversial—if peaceable—foreign policy, it is important to keep mental health reform in perspective.

In assessing the healthcare legacy of the Carter years, it is hard to say more than the fact that the phenomenal amount of work that went into the commission report, the passage of the Mental Health Systems Act, and the December 1980 release of the National Plan for the Chronically Mentally Ill went to waste.[120] Reagan cut funding to the NIMH early in 1981 and Congress subsumed Carter's reform into the Omnibus Budget Reconciliation Act that August, reducing federal allocations to states in order to let them decide how to spend the limited funding. More than just another piece of legislation, the Mental Health Systems Act promised to foster citizen participation and community support measures as vital elements in the "new attitude" to a "caring society" that Mrs. Carter had advocated.[121] Reagan's pledge to trim the fat from government meant that such programs were seen as just more federal debt; he stuck to his belief as governor of California that measures to ease the reintegration of institutionalized patients were unnecessary to offset the closure of psychiatric facilities, even though an NIMH-funded study of ten cities showed that a third of homeless in Los Angeles and over half in St. Louis were suffering from clinical mental illness.[122] Although Reagan had spoken firmly about the need to provide care for Vietnam War veterans in August 1980, as the nation's fortieth president he closed some of the newly opened Vet Centers that supported outpatients experiencing war trauma, as the next chapter discusses.

Despite Reagan's belief in market forces it is, in fact, difficult to identify a coherent health plan during his first term: some commentators think that Reagan's twin commitments to privatization and price control were in tension with one another and that actually more federal control was required in order to prevent health costs from spiraling.[123] The formation of the Office of Minority Health in 1986, following a report on black and minority health spearheaded by Reagan's second health secretary, Margaret Heckler, was an important federal development that raised the profile of disparities and inequities in health services.[124] However, there is little in the Heckler Report that focuses specifically on mental health outside the topic of suicide, and it was clear that many progressive mental health initiatives struggled during the 1980s, leaving Joseph Califano to muse ten years after the bicentennial that "the human and economic issues are so vexing that many of us who have grappled with them have created problems in our quest for solutions."[125]

When President Carter and Governor Reagan met for their single debate in Cleveland, Ohio, on 28 October 1980, at least they gave healthcare some attention, although there is little detail in Carter's briefing notes. Carter stressed the importance of outpatient facilities and catastrophic care and again raised the possibility of national health insurance, while Reagan sidestepped any forthright statements about Medicare, occupational health, or health insurance. Perhaps Reagan knew that Carter would be stronger on health policy or that he could not blame the government for ignoring health. However, it is more likely a blind spot in his campaign and one that Carter might have better exploited. Evidence of this could be gauged when President Reagan gave his inauguration speech three months later. Once again, a new president promised renewal, less than five years after President Ford's bicentennial address, but the only time that Reagan mentioned the word "health" was in economic terms, promising a "healthy, vigorous, growing economy" for a new decade.[126] This did not mean that mental health issues went entirely underground. Indeed, the shooting of John Lennon by the periodically depressed and suicidal Mark David Chapman in December 1980 and the near-assassination of President Reagan by the ex-psychiatric patient John Hinckley Jr. in March 1981 returned violent psychopathology to public attention.[127]

More generally, it meant that the 1980s was a more troubled time for patients and ex-patients than the decade might otherwise have been. Stories of mental health remained fractured and much of the health activism of the 1970s, at both the grassroots and federal levels, waned or switched attention to AIDS, which loomed large after the initial cases of 1981, leading to an estimate of one million HIV-positive Americans by 1993 (nearly a third of whom had been diagnosed with HIV/AIDS) and the pronouncement by the National Research Council that AIDS was "the most profound challenge to the care of patients that has faced the health care provider community in modern times."[128]

One of my central arguments is that key issues arising from the 1977 President's Commission on Mental Health—particularly relating to stigma, parity of provision, and the health of underserved communities—returned to the political agenda in the late 1990s, following initial consultation during Clinton's first term as president. But first, in order to better assess the major health challenges that shaped the national conversation in the 1970s and 1980s, the next three chapters examine issues that informed federal policy—war trauma, addiction, and dementia—in which both individual and collective stories come to the fore.

2 *Wounds and Memories of War*

Ronald Reagan took every opportunity during his 1980 presidential campaign to portray the Carter administration as rudderless, particularly on foreign policy. Jimmy Carter was proud of his international relations record, especially his peaceful diplomacy over the Iran hostage crisis of 1980. The freeing of fifty-two American hostages during President Reagan's inauguration speech was, perhaps, an ironic capstone to the one-term Carter administration. Although it vindicated Carter's nonviolent strategy in the Middle East, it did not prevent a number of hostages from being psychologically scarred after enduring prolonged mental and physical abuse.[1] Carter's peaceful foreign policy faced a major challenge when the Soviet Union invaded Afghanistan in December 1979, but the primary international conflict of the 1970s, the Vietnam War, did not affect his presidency as much as it had the previous three administrations. When he gave his inaugural speech in January 1977, eighteen months after the fall of Saigon, Carter avoided the specter of conflict in the Asian subcontinent, even though he had promised to pardon draft dodgers a year earlier and to "get the Vietnamese war over with."[2]

In contrast, Reagan was keen to discuss the Vietnam War in positive terms, as he did in his presidential campaigns of 1976 and 1980. Most famously, in August 1980, Reagan called the war a "noble cause," arguing that the United States had been "sleepwalking through history" since the bicentennial.[3] His aim was to reunite the nation after a period of malaise and the erosion of presidential power by Congress, but instead of echoing the language of healing Ford and Carter had used, Reagan said "we have to snap out of it, and with your help, that's exactly what we're going to do." Foreshadowing the "Morning in America" slogan of his 1984 presidential campaign, Reagan's upbeat tone was part of his strategy to free the nation from a debilitating "Vietnam syndrome." The president spoke about the bravery of those who served from 1961 to 1973, he talked positively about hospital care for the over 500,000 wounded veterans (a group that represented a 300 percent increase in casualties involving loss or damage to lower extremities compared to either World War II or the Korean War), and he was sincere when he said that "they deserve our gratitude, our respect, and our continuing concern."[4]

Reagan's August 1980 speech was received variably by the press, but he was consistent on the subject and exemplified an emerging revisionist perspective on the war. This view was best represented by neoconservative Norman Podhoretz's argument in his 1980 *Commentary* article "The Present Danger" and his 1982 book *Why We Were in Vietnam* that the war was morally justified. Instead of "a third time of trial" in which national honor was at stake, as sociologist Robert Bellah described it, the Vietnam conflict was merely a stage in a prolonged Cold War for Podhoretz and Reagan.[5] This revisionist mood was echoed in the president's speech at a Pentagon military ceremony in February 1981. Here, Reagan claimed that the soldiers had come back home "without a victory not because they had been defeated but because they had been denied permission to win."[6] This was stimulated by his belief that the North Vietnamese had successfully spread anti-American propaganda abroad, a view he had first espoused during his failed campaign of 1976.

Reagan kept his word about honoring Vietnam veterans, such as awarding a Congressional Medal of Honor to Master Sergeant Roy Benavidez, who had been badly injured during a patrol in South Vietnam in 1965. Although Benavidez was initially unable to walk after his injury, his condition improved and he returned to active service early in 1968, during which time he saved the lives of eight soldiers despite suffering additional severe wounds and being believed dead. Although he had earlier received the Army's Distinguished Service Cross, the additional award of the Medal of Honor was delayed due to the lack of an eyewitness account. When a report finally came through in 1980, it gave Reagan an opportunity to reinforce his vision of a noble war and to bestow the highest military honor on Benavidez, the son of a Mexican farmer and an Indian mother. However, despite Reagan's belief in the therapeutic potential of the "power of conviction" (to use the title of Peter Wallison's study of Reagan's public philosophy), when it came to the second pledge of his August 1980 campaign speech he was less than constant.[7] And when he came to trimming the fat from federal spending, the president was reluctant to preserve some of the newly opened Vet Centers, claiming that general hospital services for veterans were adequate. This led to a volley of criticism of the government and the Veterans Administration (VA) and a wave of protests, sit-ins, and hunger strikes through 1981.[8]

One important topic that Reagan overlooked in his early speeches was the escalating view of veterans, journalists, writers, and filmmakers that prolonged combat and the unusual conditions troops faced had created a swathe of unresolved medical, psychological, and social problems.[9] Avoiding what was referred to at the time in pathological terms as "Vietnam syndrome" (or sometimes "post-Vietnam syndrome"), Reagan's rhetoric of honor was an antidote to harsh portrayals of the war. Such views were exemplified in novelist Tim O'Brien's feature "The Violent Vet" in the December 1979 issue of *Esquire*.[10] This piece tapped into growing concerns about the rise of violent crime and its cinematic depictions—from sex crime in *Forced Entry* (1973) to gun crime in *Dog Day Afternoon* (1975)—in which veterans were invariably portrayed as dangerous and at times psychotic.[11] This trend prompted O'Brien to parody the media version of the veteran:

> Haunted by his complicity in an evil war, the combat veteran is given to fits of violence, succeeded by periods of almost catatonic depression, succeeded by more violence. His own children fear him. Neighbors lock their windows. . . . His nation, which has failed to support him in time of war, has now deserted him in time of peace—no parades, no ticker tape, no honor. The typical

> Vietnam vet turns cynical and bitter and angry; he is surely suicidal, probably murderous. He is unemployed. He is unemployable. He is hooked on heroin or booze—perhaps both—and to support his habit, he must finally turn to a life of crime.[12]

Middle-class readers of *Esquire* might have mistaken O'Brien's parodic tone, especially as it tapped into fears about a disenfranchised working class. Such fears were voiced in a number of stories in the media that centered on the pathologies of working-class veterans.[13]

Social reality in the late 1970s and early 1980s lay somewhere between the new president's attempt to reestablish a strong national message and O'Brien's parody of the psychotic veteran who brought the jungle home. Two iconic films from 1976 illustrate this kind of pathology. At the end of Henry Jaglom's tragicomic film *Tracks*, Sergeant Jack Falen (Dennis Hopper) reverts to combat mode when he returns home with his dead friend's coffin to find nobody there to welcome them. In *Taxi Driver*, the transformation of isolated Vietnam veteran Travis Bickle (Robert De Niro) from quiet cab driver to gun-wielding vigilante suggested that the triggers for violent behavior were unpredictable.[14] Martin Scorsese's film is often remembered for De Niro's "you talkin' to me?" monologue, but Paul Schrader's screenplay emphasizes Travis Bickle's lack of voice, describing him as having "wandered in from a land where it is always cold, a country where the inhabitants seldom speak."[15]

Post-Vietnam disintegration films continued to be released into the 1980s. They were overshadowed, though, by a group of popular films that remasculinized the war, most obviously *Rambo: First Blood Part II* (1985), in which Vietnam veteran John Rambo (Sylvester Stallone) is rehabilitated from the melancholic figure we see at the opening of the first film of the Rambo series, *First Blood*, which had been released in October 1982, just a fortnight before National Disabled Veterans Week.[16] The image of the hypermasculine Stallone lingers in popular memory, but Rambo is more victim than victor in *First Blood*: he has flashbacks to torture at the hands of the Vietcong and the film's original ending sees Rambo persuading his U.S. army "father," Colonel Trautman (Richard Crenna), to help shoot him after he has wrought revenge on the brutal police officials of Hope, Washington (the end of the released version shows Rambo undergoing an emotional breakdown). Rambo's guerrilla violence is justified in *First Blood*, as his is resurrection as a warrior in Southeast Asia in *First Blood Part II*, but it also aligns with Keith Beattie's argument in *The Scar That Binds* (1998) that as the long-term effects of the war came to public attention, the rhetoric of national unity clashed with "unmanageable, dangerous, anarchic, even unpatriotic" forces.[17]

It is open to debate to what extent the Vietnam War was a singular military experience and to what extent it repeated the combat and post-combat conditions of World War II and the Korean War, particularly for those involved in hand-to-hand conflict. I will turn to field research on combat stress later in this chapter, but lawyer-turned-historian Eric Dean Jr. points out that the number of Vietnam veterans experiencing post-traumatic stress disorder, or PTSD (an estimated 500,000 to 800,000), was similar in percentage terms to the number of World War II veterans (just over 450,000) who were either discharged or required disability benefits for combat fatigue and related neuropsychiatric illnesses (as they were classified at the time). Dean finds in the descriptions of the psychological symptoms of Vietnam veterans echoes of previous war experiences (his main comparison is with the American Civil War), and he outlines four factors that made the Vietnam War unique. First, the Vietnam-era soldier was thought to be damaged by the war, particularly after the Tet Offensive and the My Lai massacre of 1968. Second, unemployment rose sharply between 1970 and 1972, especially among working-class veterans. Third, a perceived heroin epidemic tarnished the veteran's image and amplified Nixon's concern about recreational drug problems. Fourth, as *Tracks* portrays, there was no hero's welcome for many returning veterans.[18] We can find earlier instances of "silent heroes," to quote Ford's phrase from his October 1974 Veterans Day Address, when he promised better employment prospects and improved healthcare.[19] But despite statistics that suggest that psychiatric casualties had been higher in World War II, these four factors and unprecedented coverage in the media suggest that the Vietnam conflict had a unique historical arc, from escalation during the Johnson administration to the wave of war films at the start of President Reagan's second term.[20]

Reagan's compelling rhetoric aside, Carter's mode of responsible governance held the moral edge in its attitude to postwar adjustment. Given that employment prospects for veterans during the Ford years had not improved markedly, Carter appeared to be serious about helping veterans. On the campaign trail in October 1976, he criticized the "unconcern and neglect of the veteran" during the Nixon-Ford years, particularly the poor employment rate for Vietnam veterans. Eight months later, he held a White House Conference on Handicapped Individuals and promised meaningful action for the disabled.[21] The President's Commission on Mental Health sought to gather medical details about post-combat experiences and assess the level of services available to veterans, and Carter proclaimed that the fourth week of May 1979 would be Vietnam Veterans Week so that the nation could "remember" the war "honestly, realistically, with humility."[22]

However, this view of Carter's proactive response is complicated by the fact that Vietnam Veterans Week was prompted by a slew of angry responses from veterans about a lack of employment opportunities and weak leadership of the VA.[23] The Carter administration was also criticized by an increasingly vocal group for neglecting "health, employment, education and psychological needs" and for not appointing a Vietnam veteran to high office.[24] Although Congress was seeking to launch a dedicated counseling program for an estimated 1.7 million veterans suffering from alcoholism, sustained drug use, and depression, many felt that this was too slow in coming—and the Vietnam Veterans Against the War (VVAW) vehemently rejected the president's claim that the majority of veterans had "successfully joined the mainstream of American life."[25] This was confirmed by the themes of readjustment and stigma at the National Conference on Vietnam

Era Veterans, held that same week. This conference led the head of the Council of Vietnam Veterans, Robert Muller, to announce that "the day of the voiceless Vietnam veteran is coming to a close."[26]

So much has been written on combat trauma and the Vietnam War that this chapter is necessarily selective. However, in keeping with the book's three primary themes—that health voices became more politicized during the 1970s, that the mental health reforms of this decade had a consequential afterlife, and that narrative medicine grew in prominence and significance—it is vital to historicize the post-Vietnam experience to assess the complex relationship between medicine, politics, and cultural expression during this time. Chapter 3 turns to drug problems Vietnam combatants and veterans faced in the early 1970s, whereas here I discuss four distinct phases that bridge the mid-1970s and the early 1990s.

First, the chapter considers some of the early voices of wounded Vietnam-era veterans that grafted personal hardships to a newly politicized sensibility and helped change the stereotype of veterans as silent and inarticulate. I then examine the mixed efforts of the Carter administration to care for wounded veterans in the late 1970s. These efforts were linked to the aims of the President's Commission on Mental Health but at a time when the effects of the military use of the defoliation chemical Agent Orange were first coming to legal and public attention.[27] The discussion turns to the reaction of the Reagan administration to "Vietnam syndrome" in the context of changes in psychiatric nomenclature, the backdrop of U.S. participation in new conflicts in Grenada and Nicaragua (which Reagan was determined would not be repeat scenarios), and the powerful messages of Vietnam War films of the mid-1980s. In order to place the aftermath of the war in a broader historical frame, the chapter concludes with a comparative consideration of post-combat experiences in the Persian Gulf War of 1990–91 with a specific focus on mental health and the diagnostic language of trauma.

Concluding the chapter with a reflection on these two wars is pertinent because 1990 marked the publication of the results of the National Vietnam Veterans Readjustment Study, which identified PTSD among 30 percent of Vietnam veterans, even though only 15 percent had served in the combat zone.[28] President George H. W. Bush was adamant that the new war in the Middle East would not repeat the mistakes of Vietnam, but it helped bring post-combat experiences into sharper focus (although it was another ten years before serious literary accounts of the Gulf War started to appear in print). Linking these four sections is a discussion of the symbolism of the Vietnam War, which became a shifting signifier during this period for a historical condition that deeply affected the health of veterans and their families.[29]

Discovering a Post-Combat Voice

Ron Kovic had just turned thirty when he endorsed fugitive Vietnam resister Fritz Efaw as the symbolic vice-presidential nominee at the 1976 Democratic National Convention at Madison Square Garden. It had been eight years since marine Kovic had been shot on his second tour of duty that left him with a spinal injury that paralyzed him from the chest down.[30] In his autobiographical account, *Born on the Fourth of July*, Kovic emphasized how his physical wounds were exacerbated by an equally debilitating disillusionment over his part in a conflict that seemed to have little purpose, especially after he accidentally killed a fellow marine in a friendly-fire incident a few months before he was injured. This combination of factors pushed Kovic away from his youthful patriotism and hostility to the peace movement toward a militant anti-war stance. Kovic's activist phase emerged at a particularly contested moment that coincided with Nixon's decision to invade Cambodia and the shooting of four student protesters by the National Guard at Kent State University in Ohio. After the summer of 1970, Kovic became increasingly vocal as a member of a strident phase of anti-war activism that was symbolized by the VVAW's march on Washington, DC in late 1969. Kovic's primary target was President Nixon, who was campaigning for a second term in 1972 on the promise of withdrawing troops, but Kovic was also disgusted by the inadequate medical treatment that he had received at the Bronx VA Hospital. This, to him, typified the VA system at large. He argued that in VA hospitals, "paralyzed men cried to be treated like human beings," such as the stroke victim, Erwin Pawelski, who was stuck in an elevator of Hines Veterans Hospital near Los Angeles for twenty-seven hours, "strapped in his wheelchair, unable to talk or move."[31]

Kovic was an outspoken member of an increasingly loud chorus that condemned the shambolic state of the VA, and he borrowed the guerrilla tactics and militant performances of the VVAW to ensure that his voice would be heard.[32] He had first entered the public eye in late August 1972 when he interrupted Nixon's televised acceptance speech at the Republican National Convention in Miami Beach, the same day that the *New York Times* carried a feature with the title "Post-War Shock Besets Ex-GIs."[33] Although this event was not as dramatic as the clash between police and anti-war protesters at the Democratic Convention in Chicago four years earlier, Kovic was successful in disrupting the big Republican gathering by drawing attention to the neglect of disabled veterans. Four years later, he claimed that he was a living reminder of war when he began his nomination speech at the Democratic Convention with the lines "I am the living death/the memorial day on wheels" (he also quoted these lines in the frontispiece of *Born on the Fourth of July*). At the 1972 Republican Convention, Kovic deployed different tactics, though, ensuring that his war story was conveyed to the camera in powerful phrases and joining a pair of disabled veterans in a noisy chant.

Born on the Fourth of July focuses primarily on bodies that are active, wounded, and maimed. Hollywood also tried to address this topic in Hal Ashby's 1978 film *Coming Home*, which matches a paraplegic veteran Luke Martin (John Voight) with the wife of a marine captain, VA hospital volunteer Sally Hyde (Jane Fonda), who slowly comes to acknowledge the realities of war as her feelings for Luke intensify.[34] Although a press release claimed that *Coming Home* avoided sentimentalism in favor of exploring "the living debris of war," Sally's love is portrayed as a "potent regenerative force" that helps Luke overcome his depression and what Christopher Lasch calls "a paralysis of the moral will."[35] Kovic avoids such sentimentality by

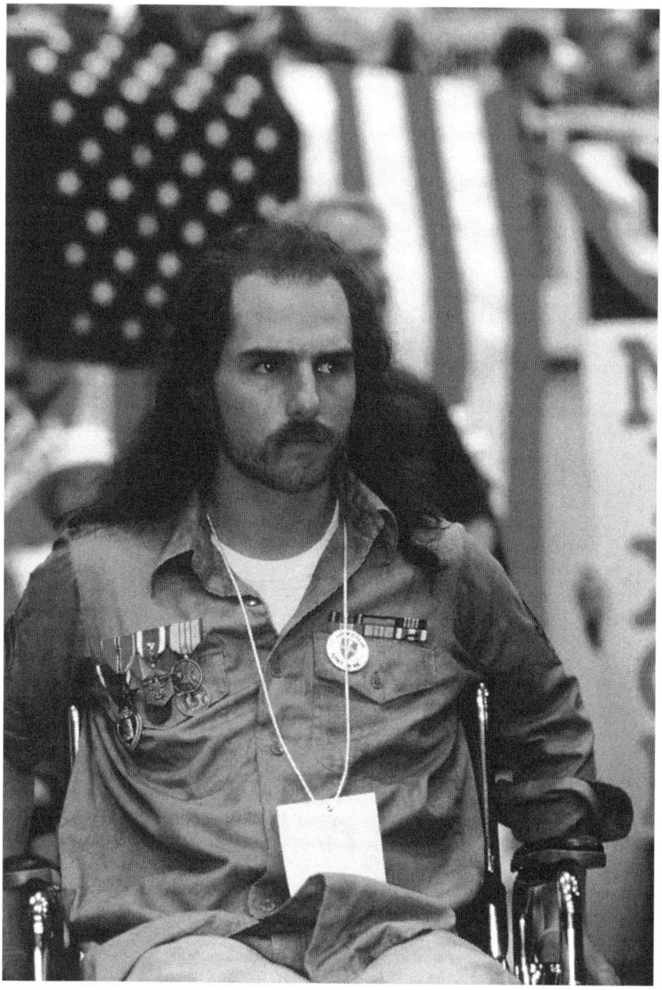

Figure 2.1 Tom Cruise portrays a protesting Ron Kovic at the 1972 Republican National Convention in *Born on the Fourth of July* (dir. Oliver Stone, 1989). Universal/The Kobal Collection/Roland Neveu.

emphasizing his personal journey from youthful enthusiasm to growing disillusionment with the war, making it a bleak coming-of-age narrative that pivots on a series of crises. This explains why Kovic does not begin *Born on the Fourth of July* with a depiction of his childhood in the working-class suburb of Massapequa, New York, but instead with the death of his comrade, the wounds he suffered on his second tour in 1968, and his dawning activism.[36] Reflections on his childhood years in the 1950s are an important inclusion later in the book, though, particularly as the text plays on memories that are both a source of pain and a means for him to gain some perspective.

Interestingly, Kovic's pronouns keep shifting: he uses the first-person voice in hospital, "we" for cultural memories, and "he" to describe combat experiences.

Not only does the third-person singular imply that he is an "instrument" in the war, it also allows him to distance himself from the most painful experiences—his inability to walk again and his bitter disillusionment with a war he once believed in.[37] This shuttling between pronouns is typical of illness narratives, but the danger of linguistic dissociation is that a strong ego can dissolve into fragmented memories that make it hard to recuperate a coherent self or a stable reality. A positive aspect of this same psychic mechanism, however, is that it prevents the self from hardening into a fixed perspective, allowing it to remain fluid, adaptable, and open to the future—a trajectory that Robert Jay Lifton later labeled "the protean self." This tendency also mirrors what Judith Herman describes as the double role of many trauma accounts—especially war narratives—that makes them both symptomatic and diagnostic.[38]

This pattern is typified by the coming-of-age story of the college-dropout recruit Chris Taylor (Charlie Sheen) in Oliver Stone's 1986 film *Platoon*, the first of a Vietnam War trilogy based loosely on Stone's own army experiences in 1967–68, which he had first attempted to make into a movie in the mid-1970s. Faced with his platoon's disintegrating morale, Taylor (like Rambo in the two *First Blood* films) is caught between good and bad "fathers," the redemptive comrade Elias and the corrupt sergeant Barnes, as he tries to make sense of the confusion of warfare. Although critics, such as veteran novelist Philip Caputo (who served in country in 1965–67), have been critical of this simplifying dualism, Taylor's role as an in-between figure highlights the moral ambiguity that some psychiatrists believe contributes to stress syndromes.[39] Early in the film Taylor's voice is indistinct and is only occasionally reflective in voice-overs and when he sends messages home to his grandmother, but a spate of violent episodes push him to suspect that Barnes is inciting the troop's disintegration. The "I" of the film is largely subsumed within the "we" of the group experience, yet the coherence of both pronouns suffers in the face of moral anarchy and debilitating terrain. Pivoting on Taylor's final words as he is airlifted from the jungle, "we didn't fight the enemy, we fought ourselves, and the enemy was within us," *Platoon* dwells on the ambiguous values of the coming-of-age story, in contrast to revisionist films such as *Missing in Action* and *Rambo: First Blood Part II* that tried to rescue the war as a noble cause.[40]

Platoon raises some profound questions about psychological preparedness and memory that resonate with other Vietnam War stories. Both Kovic and Michael Herr in his 1977 account *Dispatches* focus on distorted images of warfare that influenced young recruits and led some of them to think about the war in terms of acting, scenes, and special effects.[41] What Herr describes as images "locked in my head," Lifton sees as the "pseudomythology" that typically featured in the process of psychic stripping during training. This process of recreation was intended to enable recruits to face what would otherwise be unbearable encounters, but it also suggests a level of unreality that complicates the veracity of memories of wartime experiences. The act of remembering is crucial for engaging in shared war stories, but it is often complicated by the psychological screening that typically occurs in battle. This tallies with Marita Sturken's view that "the changeability of memory

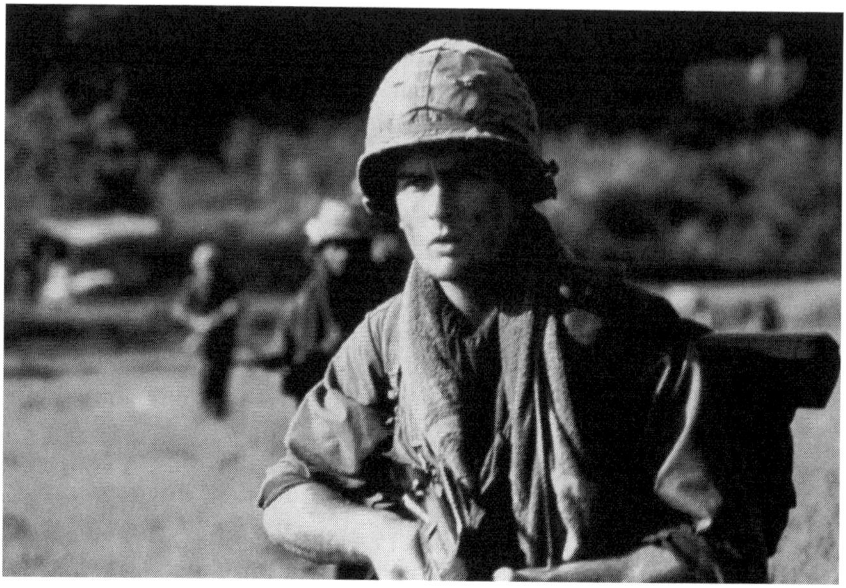

Figure 2.2 New recruit Chris Taylor (Charlie Sheen) faces his fears in an early scene from *Platoon* (dir. Oliver Stone, 1986). Orion/The Kobal Collection.

raises important concerns about how the past can be verified, understood, and given meaning," even as it expresses "collective desires, needs, and self-definitions" that are especially important during times of transition or crisis.[42] So while there might be a generational act of remembering for Vietnam veterans, we need to acknowledge that any expression of collective memory is replete with tensions where stories collide and sometimes break apart.

One of the recurring factors in war stories that focus on physical injury or psychological stress is the lack of narrative cohesion that can hold together combat and post-combat experiences. Some typical patterns of war stories—captivity narratives, a cyclical form, apocalyptic endings—are recognizable in accounts of the Vietnam War, yet there is also often a sense of incoherence and bewilderment, often shot through with despair or anger.[43] This was partly because the concept of "post-Vietnam syndrome" was fairly amorphous (at times linked to personal pathology, at others to foreign policy) and because its etiology was not fully articulated until *DSM-III* included PTSD as a clinical category in its own right. The complexity of this quasi-clinical category stemmed from the fact that the disorientation recruits experienced played out over a period of years, often in unpredictable ways.

The reason, according to Lifton in his 1973 book *Home from the War*, was that the stakes were much higher in Vietnam than in any previous war because "there was no genuine 'script' or 'scenario' of war that could provide meaning or even sequence or progression, a script within which armies clash, battles are fought, won, or lost, and individual suffering, courage, cowardice, or honor can be evaluated."[44] Such absurdist scenarios were not uncommon in World War II (Joseph Heller captured this phenomenon in his 1961 novel *Catch-22*), but Lifton identifies atrocities, such as the high body count of civilians in the My Lai massacre of March 1968 (an episode that did not come to public attention until November 1969), as part of a "malignant spiral of parallel illusion, deception, and self-deception" that played out during the ensuing two decades, even for those who had no part in that or other civilian massacres.[45] For Lifton, the fact that "killing and dying" could no longer "be placed within a meaningful system of symbols" is what made the postwar experience taxing for so many veterans.[46]

At a time when psychoanalyst Roy Schafer was seeking a language of action to return agency to his patients, many veterans felt that historical and psychological forces were hemming them in. This was not true of all veterans, but those who felt that they were victims—ideologically and militarily—often found it difficult to vocalize a coherent story. A retreat into private incoherence might be the result of distressing combat experiences and a unique war in which questions of purpose and conduct blurred ethical and personal boundaries. For example, the seemingly humanitarian Medical Civic Action Program that in 1965 provided aid to the South Vietnamese could also be seen as the therapeutic arm of U.S. propaganda rather than the embodiment of medical neutrality. Lifton describes this kind of ethical blurring as a "national descent" into "moral-psychological disintegration," as portrayed by the confrontation in *Platoon* between marine Chris Taylor and the corrupt father figure Sergeant Barnes.[47] Indeed, it was the "moral inversion" of the codes of war, together with the prolonged nature of the conflict, that made many Vietnam-era veterans feel more psychologically fragile than the veterans of previous wars.[48]

This issue of voice in *Born on the Fourth of July* and *Platoon* returns us to the primary focus of this book and is vital for understanding the trajectory of Vietnam War narratives. Keith Beattie argues that voice is more than just a synonym for the perspective of the narrator or character dialogue in these stories: voice is both a meaningful utterance and a metonym for an ideology that sometimes upholds a dominant perspective and other times contests a prevailing value system. This is particularly true of Vietnam War stories that meditate on silence and inarticulacy, as encoded in the colloquial expression "grunt"—a term that was often used to describe a foot soldier but also recruits who, as Tim O'Brien notes, were taught to carry "things inside, maintaining the mask of composure."[49] This inarticulacy might be associated with the youthfulness of the typical Vietnam GI, yet it also links to the combat stress that many soldiers carried with them beyond the war. Because the war lacked the obvious heroism of earlier conflicts and, for Philip Caputo, was characterized by monotony and tedium, "occasionally relieved by a large-scale search-and-destroy operation," it gave rise to a strange narrative pattern in which the struggle for meaning was punctuated with primal noises: "weeks of bottled-up tensions would be released in a few minutes of orgiastic violence, men screaming and shouting obscenities above the explosion of grenades and the rapid, rippling bursts of automatic rifles."[50] This pattern of silence followed by a burst of noise and then silence again meant that Vietnam-era veterans often found it difficult to pull together a story that could lend significance to individual and collective experience.[51]

Anxiety expert Mardi Horowitz catalogued in 1976 how veteran patients often swing between attempts to manage internal conflict and involuntary repetition, particularly following intense episodes of hand-to-hand combat, because the ego regression required for an effective soldier is unacceptable within the rules of civilian society.[52] Kovic's antidote to this was a concentrated phase of writing, which he describes as "an explosion, a dam bursting" in which "everything flowed beautifully, just kept pouring out, almost effortlessly, passionately, desperately."[53] The composition of *Born on the Fourth of July* proved cathartic for Kovic, though this did not mean that his anxiety instantly diminished: he suffered nightmares, heart palpitations, and clinging morbidity long after the writing process.

These symptoms and the struggle to articulate war and postwar experiences were common among male veterans, but were also true of women's war stories. An example is Patricia Walsh's 1982 novel *Forever Sad the Hearts*, which tackles the psychological effects of tending to the badly wounded and is based on Walsh's experiences as a civilian nurse in Danang in 1967–68.[54] Given that 37 percent of American women serving in Vietnam also experienced readjustment problems, Kathryn Marshall's 1987 collection *In the Combat Zone* argues that many such stories are "disturbed" by "fragments, images, severed piece of plot" that cannot easily be ordered into a coherent pattern.[55] Similarly, because post-Vietnam syndrome has no stable set of psychological markers, it was difficult to codify, even after the construction of the national Vietnam Veterans Memorial in 1982, which sought to symbolize reunification and mark the "moral legacy" of war.[56] The delay factor of PTSD meant that what Marshall calls the "nightmare geometry" of war persisted for some veterans, prompting the Vietnam Veterans of America to claim that a military visit to the memorial would be a therapeutic gathering point for many of the 2.7 million Vietnam combat veterans.[57] Indeed, one reason that Kovic turned his body into a memorial was that it was a reminder of the costs of war and a symbol of solidarity for wounded veterans who felt that their country had failed to protect or support them.[58]

The Nixon administration's inaction on the subject of veterans' health and welfare was echoed by President Ford's attempt to veto the Vietnam Era Veterans Readjustment Assistance bill, which sought to increase educational assistance for veterans by 23 percent and provide 18.2 percent more vocational aid for those with a disability. The president's veto stemmed from his worries about spiraling costs and the liberalization of veterans' educational opportunities, but the veto was overwhelmingly overturned in Congress. Despite the successful passage of this legislation in December 1974, when Jimmy Carter came into office just over two years later he was faced with Ford's fiscal cuts and a badly organized VA run by inept leaders who had been chosen during the Nixon and Ford years. Newspapers were regularly critical of the VA, noting that its "spiraling growth has come at the expense of efficiency," but Penny Coleman argues that silence rather than disorganization had the biggest impact on the health of veterans.[59] She points out that the relatively few official cases of war-related suicide cited in the 1990 National Vietnam Veterans Readjustment Study were at odds with President Carter's concerns about high veteran suicide rates in his October 1978 speech to Congress.[60] In her study *Flashback*, Coleman tries to reinstate the forgotten stories of veterans' families that were affected by suicide. In doing so, she pushes the historical and clinical narrative of PTSD to the foreground in order to offer "some healing, both in the telling and in the hearing, for all of us."[61]

The broader question regarding the therapeutic value of writing about war and postwar experiences is a vexed one. The pouring forth Kovic described suggests that the dam that had built up during his tour of Vietnam and the early years back home could be released. Caputo offers a different perspective, though. When *A Rumor of War* was published nine months after Kovic's account, Caputo was shocked to find that the manuscript, which had traveled with him many thousand miles, had suddenly transformed a private experience into "public property."[62] In a postscript he describes feeling "naked, invaded, and empty." During a book tour and a demanding interview schedule, he tried to escape these intense new feelings by drinking heavily and smoking marijuana, but this did not prevent a breakdown that led to a hospital stay, where he recuperated with the aid of Thorazine. After that experience, he boldly stated that writing *A Rumor of War* "was a trial" and "living with its publication an ordeal" rather than a healing process.[63] The act of writing may have had some therapeutic benefits for Caputo, but Kovic realized in 1970 that expression wasn't enough: political action was also needed to overcome deep war wounds, for which he believed the whole nation was responsible.

Vietnam, Mental Health, and the Carter Administration

Before returning to the issue of political responsibility and an assessment of how the Carter administration responded to veterans' physical and mental health needs, it is useful to consider the medical and psychiatric research of the time in order to better understand shifts in war-related clinical nosology. The key national figure who linked mental health research and treatment during the escalation phase of the Vietnam War in the late 1960s and the development of federal policy in the years following the bicentennial was Peter Bourne, Carter's special advisor on health. Bourne's work on war stress was formative in understanding the differences between Vietnam and previous conflicts.

In his groundbreaking book *Men, Stress, and Vietnam* (1970), Bourne explored the shocks recruits experienced as they adjusted to military life, particularly those who arrived straight from home. Bourne had a year's first-hand experience as a military psychiatrist in South Vietnam that began in October 1965, during which time he carried out scientific investigations when there were few mental health facilities for U.S. forces outside the Navy Station Hospital in Saigon.[64] Although his work was attuned to conditions of warfare (he had joined the anti-war campaign of the then-fledgling VVAW in 1967), Bourne was critical of narrow medical specializations and helped identify broader psychological processes. His analysis sometimes borrows sociological concepts, such as Erving Goffman's notion of total institutions, to conceptualize the requirement that recruits undergo an experience of mortification and subjugation during training.[65] Bourne focused particularly on the stripping and rebuilding of identity and the ways that soldiers in high-risk jobs protect themselves from unbearable processes. He noted that some war experiences are not unique (such as physical disaster situations), but he also noted how combat stress manifests itself psychologically and physically, especially when threats are prolonged or are linked to extreme conditions.[66]

In 1969, Bourne edited one of the earliest studies of mental health in the Vietnam War, *The Psychology and Physiology of Stress*, which brought together psychiatric specialists in the army such as Albert J. Glass, who had conducted extensive work on combat stress during World War II and the Korean War. Glass made the perhaps surprising claim that neuropsychiatric casualties among U.S. troops stationed in Vietnam were fewer than these two previous wars, even in the wake of the Tet Offensive of January 1968, which is commonly seen as a low point for morale. This did not mean that frustration and depression were uncommon or that combatants easily avoided anxiety and acculturation problems; just that these feelings rarely led to full-blown neuropsychiatric conditions, perhaps because there were fewer large-scale battles than in earlier wars.[67] Glass suggests that the relatively low casualty rate was due to better preventive measures (including tools for early detection and a twelve-month rotation policy for recruits) and what he calls "the brief, episodic nature of the fighting."[68]

Glass's policy in Korea had been to ensure that casualties were treated as near as possible to the combat zone in order to maximize the chances that a soldier would return for more treatment. Expectancy of recovery also informed practice in Vietnam, as did a belief that environmental factors (rather than personal weaknesses) were the primary cause of combat fatigue, together with "nonbattle factors" such as "isolation, boredom, inadequate diet, chronic physical discomfort, exhaustion, and physical illness."[69] Psychiatrists disagreed about the extent to which preexisting conditions were triggered by war. It was clear from research conducted in the 1950s at the Walter Reed Army Institute of Research that environmental factors were not the sole cause, particularly for those who did not return to combat after being moved to one of the numerous U.S. hospitals that were established in South Korea (and later in South Vietnam during the buildup period of 1965–67). Glass noted that underlying psychoneurotic conditions and personality disorders had been detected in the few soldiers who had been evacuated from battle in 1967–68, but his statistic of four casualties per month in each division was lower than statistics of those who had been removed from divisions that operated away from the combat zone.[70] Although the use of MASH facilities in the Korean War continued in Vietnam, the inhospitable terrain meant that it was not always easy to evacuate casualties who required more than thirty days of treatment.[71]

Despite the message of *The Psychology and Physiology of Stress* that useful lessons had been learned from the two previous wars, the contributors acknowledged that it was too soon to assess the long-term psychological impact of the war. Bourne's *Men, Stress, and Vietnam* noted that while high levels of anxiety often arose among soldiers who were hospitalized for physical injuries, some combatants learned how to behave like patients as a strategy for escaping active combat.[72] Given that displays of anxiety were even less acceptable among Vietnamese troops than among U.S. troops, *Men, Stress, and Vietnam* offered the concept of thinking about stress as a culturally specific condition. However, what both of these early volumes lacked was a consideration of the delayed shock that arises long after the journey home, an assessment of how the twelve-month tour of duty prevented soldiers in many troops from forming strong ties, and how soldiers who were dismissed on disciplinary grounds might have actually been suffering from neuropsychiatric conditions.

This, of course, proved to be the case, especially as some estimates suggested that 30 percent of veterans experienced delayed or periodic symptoms.[73] Research published in the period 1973 to 1975 revealed a delay of up to two years between withdrawal from combat and the emergence of nightmares and restlessness, leading Mardi Horowitz to conclude that the "relaxation of defensive and coping operations" often led to a "painful phase of intrusive recollection."[74] Canadian psychiatrist Chaim Shatan released an important report titled "The Grief of Soldiers" in 1973 that described varied symptoms that could be traced back to the war: guilt, "the feeling of being scapegoated," indiscriminate violence, "psychic numbing," alienation, and lack of trust, among other symptoms.[75] Shatan noted that it was tricky to carry out widespread statistical analysis on post-combat trauma, but he drew data from a series of rap groups for Vietnam veterans that he and Lifton held in autumn 1970 in New York City, while he was a professor at New York University.

There are examples to counter the view that these delayed symptoms were endemic, especially as a high percentage of the nearly 600 prisoners of war who returned in spring 1973 through Operation Homecoming did not show obvious symptoms of trauma. The Nixon administration focused on the stories of these unaffected POWs in order to divert attention from the anti-war protesters, though it was surprising that a significant number of long-term captives did not display high levels of psychological symptoms, despite the fact that many of them had endured imprisonment, torture, and loss of morale as the war dragged on. For example, prolonged captivity in Hỏa Lò Prison did not seem to debilitate navy pilot John McCain over the long term. When he returned home after over five years as a prisoner, McCain was judged to have "adjusted exceptionally well to repatriation," even though he continued to undergo psychological tests into the early 1990s.[76] Whereas social stigma was hard to avoid, both for veterans who turned against the war (such as Ron Kovic) and for those who continued to support or serve in an increasingly unpopular conflict, POWs such as McCain returned as heroes and were valorized for their patriotism and resilience.[77]

Nevertheless, from 1971 onward, a number of veterans found it difficult to adjust. These individuals often wound up involved in gun crimes, like the two veterans whose stories hit newspaper headlines: Dwight Johnson in Detroit and Johnny Gabron in Los Angeles. In early 1971, even though Johnson had been diagnosed by a Valley Forge Army Hospital psychiatrist as having "depression caused by post-Vietnam adjustment problems," he discharged himself. Several weeks later, he was killed when he pulled a gun on a liquor store manager in Detroit.[78] Three years later, Johnny Gabron, a trained sniper, escaped from the VA hospital in Brentwood, California, where he was being treated for suicidal tendencies. Believing that he was back in Vietnam, Gabron held two rangers and a hiker hostage for six hours in Griffith Park. Even though 100 policemen eventually surrounded Gabron, he would not release the hostages until his psychiatrist, Leonard Neff, agreed to come speak to him.[79] Neff was an influential figure in identifying the nosology of PTSD, but at the time these incidents and national newspaper headlines such as "Postwar Shock Is Found to Beset Veterans Returning from the War in Vietnam" suggested that the psychic numbing, insomnia, and potential psychosis that Vietnam veterans experienced outstripped the casualty experiences of veterans of previous wars.[80]

President Carter was not blind to these events and was aware of the complex domestic and occupational challenges Vietnam veterans faced. Bourne had worked with him from the 1970, and by the time Carter entered the White House he wanted to ensure that war wounds should not be left to "fester," as he announced to the American Legion in August 1976.[81] This informed his campaign pledge to pardon draft dodgers, although he held back on full amnesty, to the annoyance of veterans such as Fritz Efaw, who was skeptical about Carter's moderate language of forgiveness. While Carter was criticized for not doing enough for veterans, his job program of 1977 was part of the administration's commitment to deal fairly with those who "refused to serve out of conscience" and "those who honorably served in the armed forces but have had difficulty finding employment," based on the realization that World War II and Korean War soldiers had returned to a much more buoyant economy.[82] A January 1977 memo from Carter's domestic policy advisor Stuart Eizenstat reveals that the job program was devised to offset public criticism and to address unemployment rates that were much higher for young veterans than for civilians: the unemployment level for minority veterans was 50 percent higher than for their civilian counterparts, and a report of October 1978 suggested that 50 percent of severely disabled veterans were unemployed. Eizenstat recommended that the Department of Labor employ disabled veterans as paraprofessionals in outreach units. Around 2,000 veterans participated in this scheme, but the policy did not really tackle psychological issues of unemployment or the ongoing strain on families. While Carter proclaimed that the wounds of war must be bound up for the good of the nation, he also realized that many veterans were returning from Southeast Asia "with scarred minds or bodies" and that their ordeals continued through lack of job opportunities and the "indifference of fellow Americans."[83]

It was widely acknowledged that there was a gulf between Bourne's research on the stresses of combat and that facilities for veterans during the presidencies of Nixon and Ford. Even though Lifton's influential book *Home from the War* identified some of the psychological, moral, and social dilemmas veterans faced, these two administrations made no attempt to develop an overarching system of support for those with lingering psychological symptoms. Social lobbyist Stuart Feldman recognized this and wrote to Carter in December 1976 to remind the president-elect that it was the responsibility of "the people that managed the war" to speak up "on behalf of the veterans" and counter the "negative policies" of the early 1970s and the anonymity that the *Washington Post* article "The Invisible Vietnam Veteran" had bemoaned earlier that year.[84] However, it was not just severe cases of alcoholism and suicide that worried Carter's advisors. Counseling programs for those with milder readjustment problems were thought to be a necessary supplement to medical support.

The month of October 1978 was an important moment for the Carter administration in renewing its commitment to veterans, especially those with disabilities and others who experienced readjustment issues. Following his State of the Union announcement that there would be a comprehensive review of veteran support programs, the president spoke passionately to Congress about the need to "acknowledge our debt to those who sacrificed so much . . . and to repay the debt fully, gladly, and with a deep sense of respect." His emphasis was on physical disability ("there is no legislation that can . . . restore arms, legs, eyes to those who lost them in service"), but he also recommended the implementation of counseling programs on readjustment, collaborative research between the VA and the National Institute of Mental Health, and the establishment of halfway houses to better treat veterans with alcohol and drug problems.[85] Rather than putting the war to rest, then, Carter realized that there was work to be done to bridge the shortfall in the provision of healthcare and to address the unique circumstances of the war. This included a review of public portrayals of the Vietnam-era veteran, which underpinned the president's opinion that the "image of the Vietnam Veteran as unbalanced, unstable and drug-dependent is simply not borne out by available information."[86]

This endeavor did not satisfy many angry and disillusioned veterans, such as reporter Ward Sinclair, who wrote a scathing attack on the Carter administration for the *Washington Post* in April 1979. Sinclair claimed that Vietnam veterans saw themselves as scorned strangers and targets of lingering resentment over "a war that pleased no one," and he blamed Carter for not delivering the "special help" that veterans deserved.[87] The problem with this view is that it pushed veterans toward the role of helpless victims, waiting for a supportive hand to allow them to reenter the "mainstream of American life," to recall one of Carter's phrases. To counter the view of the victimized veteran, Lifton and Shatan aimed to stimulate a therapeutic culture through their New York rap groups, which chimed with Roy Schafer's attempt to encourage his patients to cultivate action language. Lifton says that his primary objective was to help veterans achieve "self-generation, the need on the part of those seeking help, change, or insight of any kind, to initiate their own process and conduct it largely on their own terms so that . . . they retain major responsibility for the shape and direction of their enterprise."[88] This version of "street-corner psychiatry" was an attempt to encourage openness within an enabling group structure.[89] Not all veterans needed a counselor or a group to facilitate the action language that Kovic's and Caputo's writing was geared to. But for those who did require facilitation, Lifton and Shatan's rap groups, which ran from late 1970 to 1974, were a prototype for other support mechanisms, even though these enabling structures were in short supply in the late 1970s, particularly for veterans from minority groups and those living in rural areas.

The War Goes On: Veterans, Ethics, and the Reagan Administration

Jacob Katzman usefully periodizes images of the Vietnam veteran into four overlapping phases. The first two phases run through the 1970s and pivot on the bicentennial year. During this period, the veteran as portrayed as an outcast who became increasingly disenfranchised and violent as the decade progressed. Fueled by such accounts as Tim O'Brien's "The Violent Vet," Katzman detects a third phase in the late 1970s and early 1980s when veterans began to be treated more sympathetically. This was followed by a fourth wave of realistic depictions that avoided caricatures of wayward and psychotic veterans.[90] To assess the ways that Vietnam veterans moved in and out of public focus, the discussion here concentrates on these later two phases, which coincide with Reagan's eight years in the White House and the rise of post-traumatic stress disorder as a more specific diagnostic term than post-Vietnam syndrome (a term that was frequently used to justify Reagan's foreign policy). While my analysis draws from Katzman's periodization, it also challenges the idea that straightforward realism became a dominant mode in the mid-1980s through commentary on Philip Caputo's 1987 post-Vietnam novel *Indian Country* and Adrian Lyne's 1990 film *Jacob's Ladder*.

It was apparent by 1978 that the end of the war did not mean closure. VA follow-up studies revealed that postwar readjustment was much trickier than had been predicted, even for those who had shorter tours of duty.[91] Studies of delayed and prolonged anxiety persuaded the authors of *DSM-III* to add PTSD as a diagnostic category, described as a "sudden acting or feeling as if the traumatic event were recurring (includes a sense of reliving the experience, illusions, hallucinations, and dissociative episodes)."[92] The previous section of this chapter discussed how Lifton, Shatan, and Horowitz detected dissociation among veterans in the early 1970s, predating what a 1980 study called the "painful dissonance of self-conception and personal identity."[93] *Legacies of Vietnam*, the results of a VA commission conducted by the Vietnam Era Research Project of the Center for Policy Research, which was published a year after *DSM-III*, supported both the lived reality and clinical nomenclature of PTSD. It claimed that around 50 percent of veterans were troubled by their war experiences.[94] However, the refinement of diagnostic language tells only half of the story. Ideological and medical agendas clashed through the 1980s, and politicians and doctors did not always concur on the best way to deal with readjustment problems.

In 1984, the editor of the American Psychiatric Association journal *Hospital and Community Psychiatry* noted that the Vietnam War had become a metaphor for the recognition of "political and economic decline" (a trend President Reagan was keen to reverse). However, "for psychiatry, it also represented the start of a re-examination of our views on stress, male bonding, drug predisposition, and situational ethics."[95] Even though the United States had entered new military conflicts in Grenada and Nicaragua, the president was adamant that post-Vietnam syndrome should not dominate the agenda or lead the nation into another war with no easy exit. In his 1990 book *An American Life*, Reagan claimed that the nation should not "remain spooked forever" by the Vietnam War "to the point where it refused to stand up and defend its legitimate national security interests" (intervention in Grenada, in this case), even if that meant deploying covert tactics.[96] Despite Reagan's commitment to improving relations in Central America and to avoiding the mantle of "the Great Colossus of the North," the role of the government and the CIA during the Nicaraguan conflict revived the specter of Cold War psychological operations that had blurred the lines between strategic and ethical activities in the late 1940s and 1950s.

In addition to offering military support to the rebel Contras, the CIA produced a controversial manual titled *Psychological Operations in Guerrilla Warfare*. Published in Spanish in 1983, the manual was based on studies from the late 1960s that analyzed the military tactics the Vietcong used. This study of guerrilla propaganda showed that while the Reagan administration clearly understood the psychological tools of modern warfare, it lacked a robust medical and ethical framework that might have led to better care for soldiers. This led a *Washington Post* editorial, published before the first presidential debate between Reagan and Democratic candidate Walter Mondale, to dub the 90-page pamphlet "The CIA's Murder Manual." The editorial argued that the manual represented "the darkest and least defensible tendencies of the Reagan administration's foreign policy" and that it incited "a whole style of terror and counter-civilian violence and deception" linked to the CIA's hand in planting land mines in Sandino harbor in Nicaragua.[97]

In spite of the furor around the CIA manual and the collateral damage it brought to the National Security Council, Reagan stormed into the White House for a second term pledging continued support for Vietnam veterans. At the beginning of his first term, Reagan had sought to achieve this by maintaining the integrity of the VA, providing better job training, and expanding the healthcare infrastructure, particularly for disabled veterans and those who were experiencing adjustment problems.[98] However, when Reagan sidestepped Carter's Mental Health Systems Act in 1981 and Congress replaced it, together with other federal health projects, with a block grant that left it to the states to decide how best to spend their reduced funding, it set the tone for a troubled decade of healthcare for veterans. It also threatened what Peter Marin in his high-profile 1980 essay "Coming to Terms with Vietnam" predicted would be an evasion of "our moral obligations" and a national inability "to confront and comprehend" the guilt about a war that should not have happened or at least went on far too long.[99] Marin's anger was shared by journalist Gloria Emerson, who covered the latter stages of the war and whose 1976 study of the effects of the war on a small Kentucky town, *Winners and Losers*, was republished in the mid-1980s. Emerson's reissued text highlighted the variety of problems that veterans—both men and women—faced a decade after the war and looked at "the reality" behind the statistics about suicides and drug and alcohol dependency in order to find a way forward that neither silenced the war nor indulged in stereotypes.[100]

By the time "Coming to Terms with Vietnam" was published, veterans who had been damaged by Agent Orange were slowly receiving reparation via the courts. But Marin worried that no one was asking searching moral questions about what the defoliation agent might have done to swathes of Vietnamese from both South and North. This perspective is not dissimilar to Lifton's view a decade earlier that the psychological scars of warfare were permanent and widespread. It also echoed Shatan's claim that "rehumanization" can emerge from postwar suffering; "by painfully 'breaking through the membrane' of military reality," veterans can "return to a new civilian reality [and] a new sense of life-purpose."[101] Marin did not go into detail about what was the most effective healthcare support (what Shatan called "emotional comradeship") or what model of postwar governance could lead the nation out of the psychological impasse that Lifton identified. Marin's point was that all Americans needed to accept culpability, regardless of their proximity to the conflict.

Published six months after a *Washington Post* feature "After Vietnam: Voices of a Wounded Generation," which explored the "scar tissue" beneath "the healed surface of American life" through the stories of seven veterans, Marin's article offered no easy solutions. An active voice is usually vital for moral awareness, but Vietnam War stories sometimes disappeared in a blizzard of flashbacks or were blocked by psychic defense mechanisms.[102] This tallies with the central message of Tim O'Brien's 1990 postmodern account of the conflict, *The Things They Carried*, that a "true war story is never moral. . . . There is no rectitude whatsoever. There is no virtue."[103] O'Brien did not mean that the effort to tell an authentic account of war has no value, only that the language of healing is always in danger of collapsing into sentimentalism or fantasy or self-justification instead of being oriented toward moral action.[104] This was not a totally accurate view. As we have seen, public testimony was an important means of bringing veterans' experiences to the attention of the media, such as Ron Kovic's political protests or the VVAW-organized Winter Soldier Investigation held in Detroit over three days in early 1971 that questioned the morality, brutality, and racism of the war through a series of personal testimonies and expert opinion from the likes of Lifton. (Although the mainstream media did not cover the event, it fed into a congressional hearing on foreign policy that spring.) Marin argued that such ethical activity was a vital antidote to the narcissism that he and others had identified in the 1970s, yet his article envisioned little radical change in the decade to come.

This ethical activity was complicated by the ideological agenda of the Reagan administration (which portrayed the Carter years in the worst possible light while scaling back welfare and medical support), but it can be more easily identified in personalized stories of the war that followed two epic films of the late 1970s, *The Deer Hunter* and *Apocalypse Now*. We have seen how in *Platoon* Chris Taylor struggled to find a voice amid the moral confusion of war, and Oliver Stone developed these twin interests in ethics and voice in the second and third instalments of his Vietnam trilogy: the 1989 adaptation of Kovic's *Born on the Fourth of July* and the reworking of Le Ly Hayslip's *When Heaven and Earth Changed Places*. Released in 1993, *Heaven & Earth* links the story of a Vietnamese woman to that of a retired

U.S. soldier whose voice is buried by his war experiences and becomes what Lifton called an "inner burden."[105] Stone's protagonists both wrestle with the "great ghostly fog" of war, as O'Brien described it, where "you can't tell where you are, or why you're there, and the only certainty is overwhelming ambiguity."[106]

While O'Brien treated "true" war stories with some skepticism and his fiction is haunted by memories of being in country, Stone's films situate the struggle to gain an authentic voice within medical and pathological frameworks: the profound physical injury sustained by Ron Kovic (played by Tom Cruise) and the flashbacks Steve Butler (Tommy Lee Jones) faces long after the war has ended. In *Heaven & Earth*, both Le Ly and Steve Butler have been victimized by the war. They find solace in each other during their time together in Vietnam, but after he returns home, Butler experiences uncontrollable rages and gloom that eventually propel him toward suicide. Whereas Le Ly draws resolve from her experiences of rape, brutality, poverty, and domestic violence in Vietnam (although she nearly loses her moral bearings in her experience of American consumerist culture), Butler is unable to make enough sense of his role in the war to construct a livable existence back home. Kovic finds two potent targets to rail against—unsanitary VA hospitals and corrupt politics—and he comes to appreciate the solidarity of other disabled veterans. In contrast, Butler remains isolated and dangerously unstable. Rather than the male veteran, then, it is the female Vietnamese refugee who discovers an authentic voice in *Heaven & Earth*, thereby marking a cultural shift in the early 1990s to a framing of the war in internationalist terms.

This sensitivity to other voices and the realization that the war was not simply a tussle between guilt and honor also comes through strongly in Caputo's novel *Indian Country*. Veering between melodrama, mysticism, and a realistic portrayal of PTSD, *Indian Country* explores the long arc of war, from the symbolically named Christian Starkmann's grief over the fact that his childhood Ojibwa Indian friend, Bonny George, has been killed in combat in 1969 (for which he blames himself) to the double life he leads back in Michigan in the early 1980s, where his inability to talk to his wife contrasts with a complex inner life full of painful memories, paranoia, and fear. Starkmann begins to experience nightmares in his early thirties that wage "a kind of guerrilla warfare on the life he had built for himself" and his family.[107] On his thirty-second birthday he wakens to find that his body is frozen; he feels like he is still lying in a foxhole and "his mind's eye held an image of the napalm—gobs of jellied gasoline spreading through the jungle like fiery marmalade."[108] Steve Butler experiences a similar visually intense flashback in *Heaven & Earth*, framed in terms of a violent confrontation with Le Ly, whereas Starkmann's nascent psychosis leads to a withdrawal from his wife and an internal psychodrama in which survival guilt and combat memories erode his ego boundaries. Although in this instance Starkmann regains self-control and manages to begin his working day for a local logging company, the grip of the war leads to the onset of distressing physical symptoms, including vomiting and loss of motor coordination.

Thomas Myers sees Starkmann as another postwar searcher who wrestles with his war wounds. But his malady seems untreatable, and he does not benefit from a visit to a clinical psychologist or participation in a veterans' support group.[109] He is particularly cynical about this rap session, calling it "linguistic camouflage, a use of casual contemporary slang to give the sessions the atmosphere of friendly get-togethers."[110] Although clinical research at the time suggested that a structured course of counseling could improve post-combat experiences, Starkmann thinks that confession only leads to shameful "exposure" and that repeatedly recounting stories is a dead end.[111] When an ex-special forces medic, Mike Flynn, manages to recall his story in "fragments, disconnected phrases interspersed with gasps," he ends up collapsing on the floor "choking and crying." He is taken to hospital and is never seen again, leading Starkmann to speculate that Flynn was probably incarcerated in a psychiatric ward. This compounds his belief that rap groups might be another therapeutic arm of the state that have the goal of tricking "the men into saying or doing something crazy so they could be put away . . . men indelibly stained by the muck and filth of where they'd been"—an expression that recalls the stigma debates of the 1960s and early 1970s.[112]

For Starkmann, then, clinical confession is deeply counter-therapeutic, whereas going to a Burger King after the sessions gives him a less formal atmosphere and a sense of safety that he only otherwise experiences "within his perimeter."[113] When Eckhardt, a psychologist, confronts Starkmann with the memory of an air strike in Vietnam that led to Bonny George's death, he responds violently, flinging Eckhardt across the room as a "half scream, half moan, shove[s] through his gritted teeth."[114] Although this primal noise could be viewed as the emergence of a deeply buried voice, the violent outburst leads to Starkmann being committed. Instead of finding release through formal psychiatric treatment, he does so by locating Bonny George's aged grandfather in the Michigan wilds. Starkmann realizes that Eckhardt had coaxed him toward a similar state "in somewhat different language," and his conversation with the tribal elder pushes him to discover a repressed inner voice and a more authentic form of expression than the "linguistic camouflage" of formal therapy.[115] By communing with nature and engaging with an ancient Ojibwa belief system, he realizes that he has unwittingly transformed "what had been, after all, a common misfortune of war into an apocalyptic vision of chaos, and himself into a murderer."[116] This insight is cathartic and enables him to achieve a psychological homecoming that he has denied himself for twenty years, renewing his hope for a world that he knows is "old and worn, full of death and pain."[117]

In combining a realistic portrayal of PTSD and mythical storytelling, *Indian Country* grapples with the "moral legacy" of the Vietnam War and challenges Jacob Katzman's view that realism became the dominant mode of the narratives of Vietnam veterans in the mid-1980s. This assertion is also problematized by Adrian Lyne's film *Jacob's Ladder* (1990), which explores the neuropsychiatric scars of the war and offers a scathing critique of the medical-military-industrial complex. The film, originally scripted by Bruce Joel Rubin in 1983, draws on the horror genre to amplify the disorientation that many veterans felt into the late 1980s and 1990s, filtered through a series of dreams and hallucinations in which the boundaries between reality and fantasy collapse. It is perhaps significant that Rubin wrote the

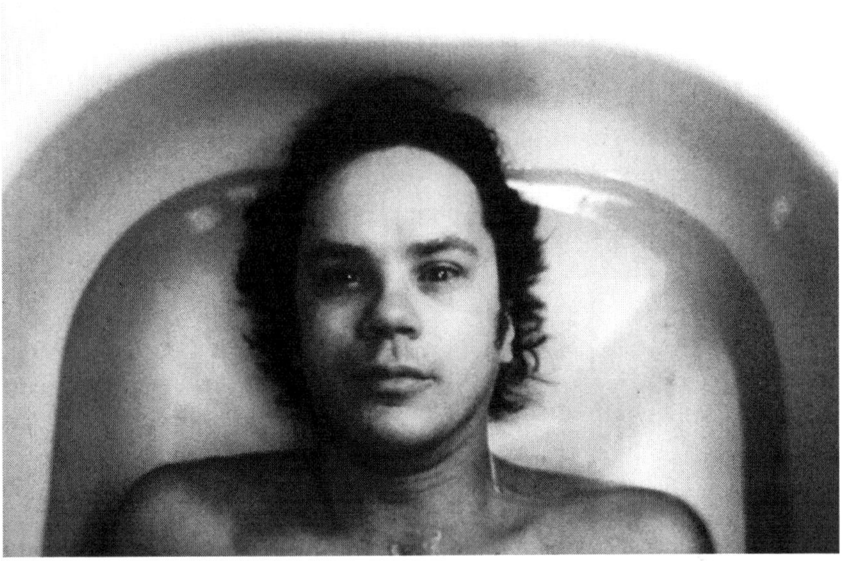

Figure 2.3 A hallucinating Jacob Singer (played by Tim Robbins) in *Jacob's Ladder* (dir. Adrian Lyne, 1991). StudioCanal Films / The Kobal Collection.

script after seeing *The Ninth Configuration* (1980), in which a disused psychiatric hospital is the setting for probing the politics of therapy in a nightmarish world of lost souls, at a time when research on the post-combat dreams of Vietnam-era veterans was coming to light.[118]

Jacob's Ladder recounts the story of veteran Jacob Singer, who has been badly wounded in combat in 1972. Four years later, he is experiencing dissociative states, a decreasing grasp on reality, and disturbing hallucinations and flashbacks filtered through the imagery of demons, decapitation, thalidomide deformation, and primitive Jungian imagery. Similarly to *Indian Country*, the descent into "ancient images" in *Jacob's Ladder* reveals the more primal psychology of warfare and acts as a counterpoint to Reagan's claim on Veterans Day 1988 that the nation could now hear with clarity the voices of Vietnam veterans after years during which they stood "in a chill wind, as if on a winter's night watch."[119] Reagan poetically claimed that the long cold night was now over for these "gentle heroes," but in *Jacob's Ladder*, released three years later, there is no healing narrative and no escape from Singer's paranoid nightmare in which even his wife metamorphoses into a threatening demon.[120] The erosion of the film's realistic frame mirrors the incoherence that Robin Wood identifies as a key trait of 1970s cinema and suggests that the rehabilitation of a stable self was a distant goal for many veterans fifteen years after the official end of the war.[121]

Vietnam Syndrome and the Gulf War

President Bush was determined that the Persian Gulf War would not be another Vietnam. He repeated this view through late 1990 and early 1991 in order to stress that a massive military strike on Saddam Hussein's regime would not only limit the imperialistic aims of the Iraqi leader after his invasion of Kuwait in August 1990 but would also banish the specter of the Vietnam War, which, as he admitted in January 1989, "cleaves us still."[122] Recognizing that war wounds were still lingering yet explicitly avoiding Ford's and Carter's language of healing, Bush said that "no great nation can long afford to be sundered by a memory." The reinvigorating image of a "fresh breeze blowing" in his inaugural address was a rhetorical attempt to overcome divisive partisan politics and to establish a New World Order that would reposition the nation after the Cold War, while the Iraqi invasion of Kuwait gave Bush the opportunity to reignite the country after the quagmire of Vietnam with a swift and precise military operation.[123] Casualties among U.S. troops were officially deemed to be "relatively slight," but statistics of soldiers "occupying military and VA hospital beds" after the war did not account for the veterans who were experiencing PTSD. It soon became apparent that there were marked continuities between Vietnam and Gulf War syndromes.[124]

The publication of the four-volume National Vietnam Veterans Readjustment Study in 1990—one year after the founding of the National Center for PTSD in White River Junction, Vermont—offered the most comprehensive view yet of the condition.[125] Based on over 3,000 interviews with Vietnam-era veterans conducted between 1986 and 1988, the findings in the Readjustment Study suggested that over twice as many veterans (30 percent) had suffered from a version of PTSD than those who had directly experienced combat, a statistic that was four times higher than the national civilian average of 7.8 percent. The National Comorbidity Study—a broad health survey conducted from 1990 to 1993 that was designed to test the nomenclature of the updated 1987 version of *DSM-III*—revealed that the overall national figure of PTSD was higher for women than men (perhaps because rape is a key trigger). In contrast, the Veterans Readjustment Study indicated that male veterans were twice as likely to be diagnosed as their female counterparts (15.2 compared to 8.1 percent), that 40 percent of male veterans had divorced, that nearly 40 percent had been identified with alcohol abuse, and that 34 percent had been arrested or had spent time in jail.[126] At the time the study was published, half of male veterans and a third of female veterans were facing PTSD between fifteen and twenty years after active service. The report also indicated that PTSD among Hispanic and African American soldiers was significantly higher than average, even though most cultural representations of postwar maladjustment focused on the experience of white veterans.

Cases of Gulf War veterans with symptoms of PTSD that emerged in the months following the publication of the Readjustment Study made the three clinical problems that Eric Dean Jr. identified in 1995 even more pressing: Was PTSD "a valid, free-standing disease construct"? Could the term account for varied symptoms of substance abuse, depression, panic attacks, anxiety, and personality disorders? And was there any evidence from clinical trials to indicate that PTSD could be cured?[127] The multi-symptom nature of PTSD was often the thorniest element because no simple therapeutic technique could unearth the root cause. Gulf War syndrome, as it emerged in the 1990s, had a complex symptomology that mirrored the experiences of Vietnam-era veterans but also had unique characteristics that included inflammation, rashes, diarrhea, migraines, and abdominal pain. While the use of the Agent Orange had led to a number of physical complications (cancer, digestive and respiratory problems, skin abrasions) that amplified the deep-seated anxiety many Vietnam veterans experienced, the psychological stresses the 532,000 U.S. troops serving in the Persian Gulf faced (7 percent of which were women, many of whom were closer to the combat zone than in any previous war) were compounded by their proximity to burning oil wells, pesticides, chemical weapons, and the effects of the bromide pills and anthrax vaccines administered to ground troops to protect them from nerve gas attacks.

Full case studies of Gulf War syndrome were only beginning to emerge in the final years of the Bush administration, whereas Bill Clinton was briefed during his election campaign of 1992 on the readjustment problems many Gulf War veterans were experiencing.[128] In a memo to Atul Gawande (Clinton's health advisor during the campaign), occupational and environment expert Jay Himmelstein (who had worked on veterans' mental health for Ted Kennedy) outlined the conditions many soldiers who had served in Kuwait and Saudi Arabia had faced that had led to a "mysterious environmental illness."[129] Himmelstein reflected on the significance of the Agent Orange Act of 1991, fourteen years after the first claims of exposure were filed by Vietnam-era veterans. Unlike the "anger, confusion and disaffection" that surrounded what he described as "the Agent Orange fiasco" (after unofficial hearings on the dioxin organized by the Vietnam Veterans of America), Himmelstein discussed the proactive response of the Department of Defense and the VA to the peculiar conditions of the Gulf War. He argued that "a large number of undiagnosed symptoms in gulf veterans" could not be traced to a single identifiable cause and advised Clinton not to buy into conspiracy theories about a cover-up of the scale of the psychological and environmental pressures of the war. In summary, Himmelstein outlined three points that he believed should underpin Clinton's campaign: a registry of veterans with symptoms relating to combat in the Persian Gulf, a robust framework for follow-up care, and an independent review to evaluate information on the health effects of active duty.

The framework of support for Gulf War veterans was arguably better than the support for veterans of previous wars, but this did not prevent them from feeling that the Bush administration had been sparing about the facts of combat. Although French sociologist Jean Baudrillard had audaciously claimed in 1991 that media spectacles had turned the Gulf War into a virtual war, for ground troops the conflict was as real as previous wars, just much shorter in duration. Ex-marine Anthony Swofford's *Jarhead*, published twelve years after the start of the conflict, serves as a counterpoint to Baudrillard's view, particularly as the reality of war zooms in and out of focus for him. The material reality of combat is symbolized by the sand that falls out of Swofford's map early in the book, which contrasts with his sense that at times this did not feel like a real war. Jenna Pitchford-Hyde points out that the contested nature of reality relates to unstable frontiers in the

Persian Gulf that were exacerbated by the use of new military and communication technologies.[130] The truth of the Gulf War became ever more slippery due to the disconnect between official rhetoric and the experiences of ground troops in the desert, especially as reports came out soon after the war that demonstrated a clear correlation between combat stress and deleterious postwar health issues.[131] The sense that troops were just as much victims as their counterparts in Vietnam and that the metaphors and realities of war often intertwine is powerfully rendered in the title story of Gabe Hudson's collection *Dear Mr. President* (2002), in which Lance Corporal James Laverne mixes mock deference to President Bush with the growth of a third ear on Laverne's torso (presumably the result of chemical exposure) and hallucinations that destroy his marriage when he returns home. This surrealist story is emblematic of the effects of Gulf War syndrome in which mysterious physical symptoms are linked to psychological maladjustment and distortions of reality; Laverne's extra ear suggests that warfare and its psychological effects are now heard differently.[132]

Jarhead, which was published in 2003, at a time when the United States was escalating a second conflict in the Middle East, explicitly links the Vietnam War to Swofford's experiences as a marine in the Persian Gulf. Early in the text, he recounts his military training in the spring of 1990 in the Mojave Desert, where the troops relax by watching a series of Vietnam War films. The antiwar messages of *Platoon* and *Full Metal Jacket* are largely lost amid the troops' enjoyment of what Swofford describes as the pornographic spectacle of combat, the effects of which are eerily reminiscent of the World War II films that Ron Kovic watched as a child. This initiation scene and the fact that Swofford was conceived during his father's R&R break from active service in Vietnam are emphasized early in the 2005 film of *Jarhead*, which is more explicit about the dangers of combat for mental stability. In the written text, Swofford notes that his father returned from the war only "partially disturbed," despite his emotional withdrawal, debilitating migraines, and the severe rigidity in his hands that he experienced in the early 1980s when he was faced by a "dead, cold" world "void of promise."[133] Although Swofford mentions that his father initially avoided psychiatric treatment, he portrays him as a figure for whom the wounds and memories of war never healed.

Swofford notes that the brief duration of the Persian Gulf War was the equivalent of a mere "long-range jungle patrol" in Vietnam, but at times he questions the official rhetoric of military command and the treatment of the enemy in ways that mirror the moral quagmire of the earlier war. In fact, rather than affirming the view this was a clean technowar with precise targets, Swofford's messy experience of hand-to-hand conflict differs little from the experiences of soldiers in previous conflicts, and he describes how he trained himself to close off his feelings just as he did to avoid exposure in the combat zone.[134] There is a sense of tacit acceptance of military authority through the text, punctuated by a questioning of defense policies and the intelligence that results in his troop being given pyridostigmine bromide (PB) pills to protect them against nerve gas attacks. However, all PB did was induce side effects that included cramps, vomiting, and diarrhea. The retrospective nature of the narrative is important because only after the war does Swofford realize that the troops should have been given the opportunity to provide informed consent before taking medication that had not been approved by the Food and Drug Administration.[135]

Although *Jarhead* is largely a realistic account, it is composed of short fragmentary sections and moves erratically between different states of mind and historical moments, as if Swofford cannot settle on a stable frame of reference. Swofford does not struggle for words as much as Chris Taylor in *Platoon*, nor does he turn to writing to contend with a profound injury as Ron Kovic does in *Born on the Fourth of July*. However, a more mundane sense of anxiety lingers under the surface of the text. And although *Jarhead* does not address Gulf War syndrome as explicitly as *Dear Mr. President*, it is important that he refers to Vietnam frequently, especially because the stories of father and son are entwined. The connection between the two wars is persistent, so much so that when the troop returns to California to a heroes' welcome, Swofford's comrade Crocket pulls a deadbeat Vietnam veteran onto their welcome bus, an incident that offers a moment of catharsis for a casualty of the previous conflict. When Swofford ends his penultimate chapter with the line "I hoped that even though the spectacle of the excited citizens was worth nothing to me, it might help the Vietnam vet heal his wounds," it is clear that the Gulf War—at least from this perspective—was a further phase of a military and psychological drama that had begun thirty years earlier.[136] *Jarhead*, then, can be either read as evidence of President Bush's claim that the Persian Gulf War put the Vietnam syndrome to rest or as a critique of a war that, despite military and technological advances, replayed the psychological stresses of Vietnam.

3 *Addiction and the War on Drugs*

While the health consequences of the Vietnam War have a long arc, the history of addiction in the late twentieth century has an even more tangled narrative, especially in relation to mental health. It is a story that links politicians and psychiatrists, school kids and middle-class housewives, street dealers and methadone clinic directors, law enforcement officers and combat veterans. Heroin use in the armed forces was the primary stimulus for President Nixon's war on drugs, yet this is just one strand of a longer story that reaches back to the federal response to narcotics smuggling in the 1930s and forward to attempts to improve treatment programs for an estimated 2.5 million hard drug users during the Clinton administration. The muscular speeches of Presidents Nixon and Reagan and three influential pieces of legislation—the Comprehensive Drug Abuse Prevention and Control Act of 1970 and the Anti-Drug Abuse Acts of 1986 and 1988—clearly outlined modern federal attempts to curb drug trafficking, but the medical implications of addiction are more complex, bringing together the stories of doctors, health workers, patients, families, support groups, and ex-addicts, especially in the 1970s when the social weight of addiction was strongly felt.

Public statements on the subject in the early 1970s tended to blur different types of recreational drugs. This led a Consumers Union report to speculate that the recent acceleration in rates of drug abuse could be attributed to anti-drug laws that linked marijuana use to heroin, based on the assumption that experimenting with soft drugs would inevitably lead to more addictive ones.[1] The media seemed to concur with this assumption. In the fall of 1973, for example, the *New Pittsburgh Courier* ran a five-month series titled "Drug Abuse and Society: The 'Chemical Cop-Out'" to raise awareness about the dramatic rise in drug and alcohol use in the area:

> Popular stereotype has it that the typical drug abuser belongs to a minority group and resides in the ghetto. This is not a correct picture. Generally speaking, drug abusers also include the middle-class businessman who finds it necessary to consume large quantities of alcohol to keep going, the over-weight dieter who misuses a prescription designed to curb his appetite, the otherwise healthy person who gets a refill of sleeping pills, the pre-teenager who sniffs glue, the pathetic old-ager, who, because of his loneliness, abuses his prescription for sedatives.[2]

While the authors emphasized multiple forms of drug use, the medical perspective was continually interrupted by a moralizing voice that reinforced the common view that abuse is a "manifestation of an inadequate personality unable to cope with the stresses of normal life," as a 1962 federal report described it.[3] Those who subscribed to this view often had only a hazy understanding of the psychopharmacological effects of recreational drugs and the complex networks in which they circulate. Inflammatory language was symptomatic of the time, especially when Nixon was calling drug abuse "public enemy number one."[4] Even the *Journal of the American Medical Association* asserted in 1971 that inhaling marijuana led to delusions, suicidal tendencies, and promiscuity.[5]

The first section of this chapter focuses on the war on drugs, which had broad implications not just for jobs, crime, social security, and the cost of healthcare but also for international relations as drug markets spread their networks across national boundaries. The early 1970s were a time of panic about heroin, fueled by public statements and newspaper columns that often transformed the regular drug user into a social deviant. Stricter control of prescriptions was one answer, yet the paradox was that drugs were sometimes the solution to addiction and sometimes the cause. Although the generally favorable attitude in these years toward the detoxification agent methadone plays an important role in this story, in his first term Nixon was focused on heroin abuse among returning GIs and the rise of multidrug use among teenagers.

The opening sections of the chapter discuss these topics and their implications for mental health and then considers the dramatic rise of prescription drug addiction. Even though the addictive properties of Valium were first openly discussed in the mid-1970s, prescription addiction often dipped under the political radar because it was rarely associated with violent crime. The final sections focus on the high-profile case of Betty Ford, a functioning pill and alcohol addict during her husband's presidency, and the revival of the drug wars during the Reagan and Bush administrations in which another first lady, Nancy Reagan, played a leading role. The chapter balances personal voices of addicts and former addicts and external voices of authority, as federal officials, medical professionals, journalists, and ex-addicts all spoke out with different stakes in this complex socio-medical issue. In addition to assessing federal drug policy of the time, this chapter discusses three narratives that explore the psychophysiology of dependency: the anonymously published *Go Ask Alice* (1971), filmmaker Barbara Gordon's *I'm Dancing as Fast as I Can* (1979), and Betty Ford's twin autobiographies *The Times of My Life* (1979) and *Betty: A Glad Awakening* (1988).

All these accounts could be said to respond to what sociologist Peter Conrad and political economist Robert Crawford (following Ivan Illich) have called the creeping "medicalization of everyday life."[6] However, medical treatment was sometimes at odds with federal drug programs, particularly during the Nixon administration, when special powers were awarded to the Office of Drug Abuse Law Enforcement to tackle narcotic smuggling and drug use as aspects of a criminal industry. Nixon was initially positive about the prospects of methadone for treating heroin addiction, a drug that had been in circulation since pharmaceutical company Eli Lilly began manufacturing it for commercial use in 1947 under the name Dolophine. But the approach of the Nixon administration to addiction, crime, and deviancy largely wrested control away from organized medicine and placed it in the hands of law enforcers. At a time when gay activists were challenging the nosology of pathology (especially the controversial framing of homosexuality as a deviant category in the 1968 edition of *DSM*), negative stereotypes of the addict turned self-medication into a disease that threatened to infect the nation and, from Nixon's perspective, needed to be stopped by punitive rather than by medical means.

The story is particularly complex because different narratives of drug use and abuse weave in and out of each other. Recreational drugs were the most politicized of addictive substances but were often taken in combination with prescription drugs, either legally prescribed or illicitly acquired. And as the case of Betty Ford illustrates, stories of prescription drug dependency were often linked to abuse of alcohol. My primary focus here is on drugs, but that is not to neglect research on alcohol, the "number one drug of abuse," according to a 1973 study.[7] In 1975, the Alcohol, Drug Abuse, and Mental Health Administration estimated that alcoholism affected 9 million Americans directly and 36 million more indirectly, causing 85,000 deaths per year and making cirrhosis the fifth most frequent cause of death, a figure that had doubled between 1950 and 1973.[8] Throughout the 1970s, alcohol abuse was on the federal agenda. President Nixon began the decade by announcing Alcoholism Information Month; the Department of Health, Education, and Welfare released a report titled *Alcohol and Health* in early 1972; and the Alcohol, Drug Abuse, and Mental Health Administration was formed in fall 1973 to help raise alcohol awareness during the Ford administration. Alcoholism was back on the agenda during the Carter years. It formed a significant strand of the President's Commission on Mental Health in 1977–78, at a time when research on controlled drinking was in tension with the abstinence philosophy of Alcoholics Anonymous.[9] Yet on the whole alcohol abuse was not as heavily politicized or as culturally resonant as drug stories in the 1970s and 1980s, even though it played a vital role in the development of a Cold War–style "alcohol and drug industrial complex" (as retired Iowan Senator Harold Hughes called it in 1974) and alcohol dependence was revealed to be nearly twice as prevalent as drug dependence in the first national mental health survey conducted at the beginning of the 1990s.[10]

The War on Drugs: Nixon and Ford

Drugs featured in both of Nixon's presidential campaigns of 1968 and 1972 as he pledged to bring law and order to an increasingly divided nation. In his August 1968 nomination speech, he was at his rhetorical best when he invited his audience to "look at America": "We hear sirens in the night. We see Americans dying on distant battlefields abroad. We see Americans hating each other; fighting each other; killing each other at home."[11] Within this context, he promised to "the real voice of America" that he would restore civil order and put an end to "the filth peddlers and the narcotic peddlers who are corrupting the lives of the children of this country." He did not mention heroin explicitly, but the growing number of addicts (estimated to number 250,000 at the beginning of the 1970s) worried him at a time when the influential founder of the Haight-Ashbury Free Clinic, David E. Smith, was warning his readers to avoid heroin, claiming "it's so good don't even try it once" in the title of his consciousness-raising book.[12]

Nixon's "public enemy number one" speech of June 1971 led to the establishment of a robust control and prevention program. In this speech, he outlined the massive investment the initiative would take, involving nine separate departments working on a broad front. The new efforts included the controversial Operation Intercept of September 1969, in which federal troops searched all traffic crossing the Mexican border.[13] The main impetus behind the topic in his 1972 reelection campaign was the outspoken anti-drug stance of New York governor Nelson Rockefeller, who set a tough example of drug control for other states.[14] Nixon only included a single line on drugs in his second nomination speech as presidential candidate ("We have launched an all-out offensive against crime, against narcotics, against permissiveness in our country"), but many of his public statements that year could be seen as intensifying a culture of fearmongering by eliding addiction, crime, and deviancy.[15] After he was reelected, Nixon capitalized on the passage of the 1970 Comprehensive Drug Abuse Prevention and Control Act (which raised the penalties for drug smuggling and offered detoxification treatment for new offenders) by founding the Drug Enforcement Administration and emphasizing an interventionist approach.[16]

The focus on Nixon's war on drugs was heroin, which films such as the Academy Award-winning *The French Connection* (1971) and *The Godfather* (1972) characterized as an international problem that involved mass smuggling, gang warfare, and gun crime. More neutral attempts to raise awareness of the narcotic properties of heroin included *Flowers of Darkness*, a 20-minute low-budget educational film in the NBC *Distant Drummer* mini-series made by George Washington University's Department of Medical and Public Affairs that aired in 1972 and was narrated by actor Paul Newman. More often, though, stories about heroin were linked to social unrest and criminal activities in urban ghettos and presented statistics that showed that arrests of male African Americans were on the increase.

In his 1996 book on the drug wars *Smoke and Mirrors*, Dan Baum notes that black crime in the late 1960s and early 1970s was nearly always linked to the stereotype of the heroin addict: "over thirty and male, usually but not always black."[17] Evidence for this could be found both in sociological studies of black ghettos (the 1964 field study *Youth in the Ghetto*, for example), articles in the black press (such as a 1970 feature in *Ebony*, "Blacks Declare War on Dope"), and African American cultural texts such as Donald Goines's 1971 novel *Dopefiend*.[18] Goines wrote this mass-market novel while serving time in Jackson State Prison in Michigan for drug-related crimes after becoming addicted to heroin while in the air force during the Korean War. Set in a Detroit ghetto, the story centers on heroin, the "drug of the damned" that leads to "slow death" for all its users.[19] *Dopefiend* offers no escape from this netherworld, not even for a middle-class couple who are drawn inexorably into a cycle of addiction and crime. Graphic descriptions of injection, lurid sexuality, and brutal exploitation revealed a new literary voice but were also symptomatic of the fears of Nixon administration officials about the affinity between crime and narcotics, an association that was hard to avoid when Goines was murdered in 1974. There were some anti-drug statements from the black community, such as the hard-hitting play *King Harlem*, which was revived in the spring of 1971 at a time when an estimated one-sixth of Harlem's residents were using heroin.[20] And it was not just an adult problem. In *The Littlest Junkie*, a 1973 WABC-TV documentary about growing fears of heroin addiction among unborn children, most of the addicts are black.

The dramatic case of Goines seemed to illustrate the links of returning Vietnam veterans to drugs and alcohol abuse, crime, and unemployment. Although Nixon warned the public that the drug threat "will not pass with the passing of the war in Vietnam which has brought to our attention the fact that a number of young Americans have become addicts as they serve abroad," the Vietnam War junkie became a stigmatizing stereotype that was almost as hard to shake as the black junkie.[21] Fueling the view that addicts were irrevocably scarred by the war were stories of drug pushing in VA hospitals and damaging headlines such as "Addict Runs Amuck with Rifle in Clinic," the story of a veteran with a heroin addiction who shot twenty-three bullets into the wall of a Bronx methadone center.[22] The media often blamed exposure to Southeast Asian culture for addiction among U.S. troops yet rarely examined the reasons why soldiers got hooked or why they switched from smoking to injecting heroin. This switch coincided with a new drug-testing regime in summer 1971 that made it more difficult for soldiers to obtain heroin in smokable form. However, Robert Jay Lifton thought that the government's search for a "technical solution" to the drug epidemic was a smoke screen to conceal the fact that the government was avoiding complex social and military problems.[23]

In his 2009 book *The Myth of the Addicted Army*, Jeremy Kuzmarov claimed that media coverage exaggerated the heroin epidemic, citing sensational headlines such as "The GI's Other Enemy: Heroin," "The Heroin Plague: What Can Be Done?," "The Smell of Death," "New Public Enemy No. 1." These headlines were influenced by the 1971 government report titled *The World Heroin Problem*, which estimated that between 10 and 15 percent of veterans were addicted to high-grade heroin.[24] Although a *Newsweek* column proclaimed that the Vietnam junkie was "condemned to a life of crime and early death," the numbers of veterans who were hooked on heroin and the numbers involved in drug-related crime were in fact very unclear.[25] Conservative estimates suggested that the former might be as low as 2 percent (including some service personnel who did not go overseas) and the latter 0.5 percent, although a more balanced estimate was a 10 percent addiction rate among U.S. armed services personnel in country.[26] Politicians and the media tended to clutch at convenient statistics that very often confused casual drug use, long-term addiction, the rise of urban crime, and unemployment among veterans.

Kuzmarov believes that Nixon responded positively to the wave of panic the media headlines of 1971 generated and that his drug abuse program gave equal attention to the medical treatment of addicts and the criminalization of drugs. Certainly the budget for drug and alcohol treatment rose rapidly in 1970.[27] Nixon appointed psychiatrist Jerome Jaffe of the University of Chicago as chief of the Special Action Office for Drug Abuse Prevention. The "abrasive" Jaffe convinced Nixon that methadone treatment could be used effectively to wean addicts off heroin.[28] This initiative contributed the most to the increased drug treatment budget and led to the establishment of 2,000 methadone centers by the mid-1970s. Some in the medical profession warned that methadone was equally addictive and should be used only when other treatments had failed, while others thought that the psychoactive plant extract ibogaine was a more effective anti-addiction agent (its reclassification as a Schedule I drug prevented fuller clinical trials.)[29] Based on positive accounts from Kentucky-based psychiatrist Marie Nyswander, Jaffe was confident that methadone was the best treatment model, partly because its effects lasted longer than heroin and it was a relatively cheap substitute. However, it could easily be abused, particularly by outpatients, and the dangers of overdosing were greater than heroin. By 1974, confidence in methadone treatment had dipped, leading Nixon to quickly discard Jaffe and cut funding for treatment programs. As rates of alcoholism and cross-tolerance increased among recovering patients, some even characterized methadone as a new killer drug, and by the time Ford took office it was no longer seen as the great heroin fix that it had seemed three years earlier.[30]

Realizing that Nixon's claim to be winning the war was premature, President Ford pressed for further sanctions, pointing to statistics that revealed 5,000 deaths a year from "the improper use of drugs" and that 50 percent of street crime was "committed by drug addicts."[31] Responding to a *White Paper on Drug Abuse* published the previous fall, Ford adopted a softer tone than Nixon had, describing in an April 1976 speech to Congress the "thousands who do not die but who are merely going through the motions of living," sitting in school "without learning" and growing "increasingly isolated from family and friends."[32] Although he used similar phrases to Nixon ("the drug menace," "a clear and present threat") and he pictured drug traffickers as "agents of death," Ford stressed that "national well-being is at stake" and made clear that his comments applied equally to housewives, teachers, and disadvantaged social groups.[33] Ford had recently enlisted cooperation on trafficking from the presidents of Mexico and Turkey—the latter was partly motivated by the serialization of the Pulitzer Prize-winning report "The Heroin Trail" of 1973, a piece of investigative journalism that linked the opium fields of Turkey to addiction in the United States.[34] Ford's speech to Congress focused not only on the need to curb the use of narcotics but also on the need to control barbiturates, amphetamines, and tranquilizers. He saw the trend of abusing these substances as "now almost as serious as the abuse of heroin." The president suggested that the federal initiatives of the early 1970s had not decreased recreational drug use and demanded a redoubling of efforts.

The 1975 *White Paper on Drug Abuse* confirmed that attacking the supply of drugs in order to control demand was the best strategy for making drugs "difficult to obtain, expensive, and risky to possess, sell or consume."[35] However, it also outlined a balanced program of which the federal role was only one arm. The main target was not the occasional drug user but the illicit commerce in drugs that have "the highest social cost."[36] Prompted by his health advisor Peter Bourne, President Carter took this need for improved coordination seriously. In August 1977, when he addressed Congress on the theme of drug abuse, he distinguished between grades of drugs and different types of recreational drug experiences, as he had while working with Bourne on a narcotics treatment program in Georgia in the early 1970s.

Ford was serious both about coordinating activity across existing offices and broadening the responsibility to include states and communities; he emphasized reform at the community level, envisioning programs where young people and adults would work together. This concern for the vulnerability of the young was nothing new. It echoed fears about teenage delinquency in the mid-1950s, but the stakes were higher at a time of economic decline and civil unrest when the underground market for illicit drugs was stronger than ever. The fact that drug dependency is largely invisible in its early stages fueled fears of a creeping epidemic that could blight generations to come, and in the early 1970s the stereotype of the young addict became almost as potent as caricatures of the addicted Vietnam veteran and the black drug pusher.[37]

Teenagers and Multidrug Use

The 16 March 1970 cover of *Time* magazine depicted a dreamy-eyed boy with a large green hypodermic needle superimposed over the left side of his face, with the headline "Heroin Hits the Young." The piece was triggered by reports that heroin had become the primary cause of death among New York City teenagers.[38] Titled "Kids and Heroin: The Adolescent Epidemic," the *Time* feature introduced a twelve-year-old Bronx boy, Ralph de Jesus, a heroin addict and a pusher. The six-page article, which included quotes from interviews with healthcare officials and reformed addicts, confirmed that heroin was widespread in inner-city areas. The piece strove for balance but edged toward a moralistic stance ("heroin, long considered the affliction of the criminal, the derelict, the debauched is increasingly attacking America's children") and inflammatory language ("something frightening is sweeping into the corridors of U.S. schools and onto the pavements of America's playgrounds"), describing heroin as "the notorious nepenthe of the most hopeless narcotic addicts."[39]

The feature began by outlining Ralph's group therapy with other teenage addicts at the Odyssey House in the Upper East Side of Manhattan, a social service facility for substance abuse and mental health issues that had opened its first branch in Harlem in 1967. Ralph had come to Odyssey House after contracting hepatitis from a dirty needle, yet he was a largely silent presence in the therapy sessions and was itching to return to the Bronx. The article did not examine the urban or economic conditions that led Ralph to taking heroin as a preteen; instead, its focus shifted to the rise of heroin use among middle-class teenagers (due to peer pressure, it assumed) and it conveyed the usual warning that soft drugs would lead to harder ones. The article lacked sociological depth and said nothing about Ralph's neighborhood or his parents, although perhaps that was because he barely spoke and did not seem to realize that "death or imprisonment" were the only alternatives to therapy.

A piece in *Newsweek* the following summer brought some heroin stories to life, but the lack of a voice among the estimated 250,000 American heroin addicts was nothing new, particularly given the sedative effects of the drug.[40] William Burroughs's famous exploration of his own habit in his 1953 novel *Junky*, for example, introduced a young painter, Nick, whose canvases became "concentrated, compressed, misshapen by a tremendous pressure" as his heroin sickness intensified.[41] Even though he realized that narcotics have damaging effects on creativity and he periodically struggled with heroin addiction, Burroughs was a great advocate of finding the next fix, wherever that might take him.[42] He did not change his view about the positive effects of drugs even when his son, who shared his name, became an amphetamine addict at age 15. As documented in *Speed* (1970) and *Kentucky Ham* (1973), William Burroughs Jr. took speed with other drugs and soon began drinking too much, to such a degree that he had to have a liver transplant in 1976 and died of cirrhosis in 1981 at age 33.[43] Other examples of drug experimentation suggest that poor parental relationships are not always the trigger. For example, *The Eden Express: A Memoir of Insanity* (1975) by Mark Vonnegut, son of Kurt Vonnegut, shifts from post-college experimentation with a hippie lifestyle in the Pacific Northwest to psychotic episodes that led to his committal in 1971 to a psychiatric hospital in British Columbia. When Vonnegut later discovered that his psychosis was caused by a combination of mescaline intake and bipolar disorder, he speculated that his case might not be atypical: "I guess there are probably as many disabled and deeply scarred ex-hippies as there are Vietnam Vets."[44] However, there is also an unexplored family history, which included his paternal grandmother's suicide (an overdose of sleeping pills) and the suicidal depression that later plagued his father.

Although heroin was frequently seen as the deadliest of drugs, worries were mounting over multidrug use. As one doctor in the *Time* article noted, the drug scene was changing rapidly every year. However, few longitudinal studies examined drug use in schools, and even when they began appearing in the early 1970s, conclusions tended to be muddied.[45] One aspect was clear, though: multidrug use meant that detoxification was trickier and the chances of recuperation slimmer, especially when addicts began using substances such as alcohol phencyclidine (PCP), an animal tranquilizer that stimulates hallucinations in humans. PCP use increased at a time when the quality of street heroin was declining and marijuana was scarce following police crackdowns in cities such as Baltimore.[46] PCP users required extensive detoxification programs and relapses were frequent.

It was evident from political, medical, and educational perspectives that it was important to dissuade children and teenagers from experimenting blindly with drugs. Nixon's drug abuse prevention program attempted to do this by issuing a range of print and media material.[47] Beyond government publications there were some balanced attempts to inform teenagers about the dangers of drug use. These included Mark Lieberman's *The Dope Book* (1971), which avoided "preaching" and "despair" in favor of providing drug awareness information for young readers in clear language. Lieberman's chapter on heroin was particularly modulated, even though it ended with the frightening image of "a path to a grim destination."[48] Advice books on drugs for teenagers had been around since the 1950s, but one publication had more effect than any other on shaping negative opinions about drugs in the early 1970s: the anonymously authored *Go Ask Alice*.

First published in 1971, *Go Ask Alice* is presented in diary form over a two-year period, from 1968 to 1970, and documents a middle-class teenage girl's descent into a world of multidrug use. It takes its title from the San Francisco band Jefferson Airplane's 1967 psychedelic song "White Rabbit," which explores the psychological and physiological effects of hallucinogens—the kind of pro-drug lyric that Nancy Reagan would criticize in public speeches during the 1980s.[49] *Go Ask Alice* is certainly not a countercultural text, even though Alice describes her first LSD trip in hackneyed psychedelic language. She shows great emotional range in the early diary entries and displays typical anxieties about boys, parents, schoolwork, and her weight, but the loss of childhood innocence and new drug experiences change her perspective. She expresses caution following her first LSD experience yet is still eager to explore: she injects speed ten days after her first trip, steals sleeping pills from her ailing grandfather, and begins a cycle of tranquilizers and Dexedrine.[50] Although Alice retains some of her initial exuberance, her diary entries swing between highs and lows and she becomes increasingly involved in drug pushing. After finding out that her boyfriend-pusher is gay, she runs away to San Francisco with her drug friend Chris. There she finds herself at a party where she takes heroin. On waking from her fix, she discovers that she has been treated "brutally" and writes that she has been raped, although she gives no details.[51]

Following her harrowing heroin experience, Alice manages to get clean and start attending school again, but she soon relapses. In desperation, her parents pressure her to see a psychiatrist and later to visit a health center, where she is diagnosed as being malnourished. As her drug use worsens, her diary entries become ragged. She loses track of time and starts to feel "shriveled and deteriorated" on the inside.[52] Although she never descends into complete incoherence, her language becomes more colloquial and visceral and her moods swings more extreme as she becomes desperate, particularly when she finds that she cannot distinguish between reality and fantasy due to increasingly vivid flashbacks.

Alice's problems worsen when she is hounded at school due to her reputation for being a druggie and her grandparents both die, leading to a breakdown. She thinks she is being consumed by worms, she barely recognizes herself when she wakes up in the state mental hospital, and her ability to find the right words is succeeded by "verbal rantings, useless, groping, unimportant."[53] Alice is eventually permitted to go to school on day release. She shows signs of improvement after group therapy and seems more like the teenager of the opening pages. She says goodbye to her second diary on the penultimate page, suggesting that she has learned that sharing her problems is more productive than recording them in diary form. But on the final page, written by the editor, we are told that Alice died of an overdose (either accidentally or premeditated) three weeks after deciding not to begin a third diary.

The editor rounds out the story with the hard fact that Alice "was only one of thousands of drug deaths that year."[54] Her death comes as a surprise, though, particularly at the end of the clunky 1973 film adaptation of *Go Ask Alice*, where we see a smiling Alice returning to school with her youthfulness intact before the image freezes and a caption marks her obituary. However, when the editor, Beatrice Sparks, emerged as the author (and copyright holder) of the text in 1979, doubts were raised about the diary's veracity.[55] It is now accepted that Sparks, a psychologist and Mormon youth counselor, ventriloquized Alice's voice, particularly because she failed to provide evidence to justify her claim that the diary belonged to one of her patients. The fact that Alice plummets toward a breakdown despite the support of her parents suggests that this is a cautionary account and the diary a covert means of instruction. Nevertheless, the widespread ban of the book in high schools from the mid-1970s through to the 1990s was due more to the use of profanity and the harrowing account of Alice's decline than it was to Sparks's act of textual deception.

What *Go Ask Alice* reveals is that certain myths and propaganda about drug culture were hard to resist, especially because there were few objective case histories of addiction among girls and women to draw upon. The book also suggested that soft drugs lead to hard drugs, that the casual drug user quickly becomes involved in a spectrum of stimulants and sedatives, that heroin is the worst of all and inevitably leads to the "slow death" that Donald Goines describes in *Dopefiend*, that drug use was infiltrating suburbia, and that the loving support of families was often not enough to save young addicts from a grisly fate.[56] The view that drug addiction was all consuming and needs to be stamped out at the source echoes the strident federal statements of the Nixon-Ford years and returned to prominence in the 1980s with a new political and moral agenda. Before looking closely at rehabilitation narratives and the revival of the war on drugs, it is important to consider the rise of prescription drug addiction that complicates the multidrug story and blurs the lines between licit and illicit drugs.

Prescription Drug Addiction

The visibility of heroin in the early 1970s overshadowed a creeping reliance on prescription drugs, a topic the melodramatic 1967 Hollywood film of Jaqueline Susann's novel *Valley of the Dolls* brought to the public eye. The film's three central female characters all turn to barbiturates to help them through difficult times. The most unstable of the trio, Neely O'Hara (played by Patty Duke), finds that she cannot function easily as a performer without a combination of uppers and downers (Dexedrine and Seconal), often washed down with alcohol. Only a few medical professionals, such as Stanford psychologist J. Maurice Rogers, were speaking out about the rise of psychoactive drugs at the time, even though reports suggested that up to 20 percent of amphetamines were ending up on the black market.[57] Media stories of prescription addiction were sporadic during the early years of the decade. But in 1976 the *Washington Post* revealed deep-rooted tensions between the pharmaceutical business and the medical profession, and the *New York Times* reported that in the period 1974 to 1977, twenty-seven New Jersey doctors had lost their licenses or had them suspended for diverting prescription drugs for street use.[58] The stories kept coming (such as an exposé in *People* magazine on the multiple drug habit and rehabilitation of television personality Carol Burnett's daughter Carrie), and by the end of the decade there were "hundreds of tranquilizer narratives" in the media and a number of malpractice cases in the courts.[59]

The question of who was responsible for prescription drug addiction was a tricky one, given that there were so many variables, but by mid-decade the blame had squarely shifted toward both the medical profession and pharmaceutical companies before an equally sharp swing back to the individual user during the Reagan years. Instead of the public excitement that greeted the appearance of Miltown, Librium, Valium, and other wonder drugs in the mid-1950s and early 1960s, there was a growing suspicion that pharmaceutical companies were putting profit over health, as was evident in the title of the 1974 book *Pills, Profits, and Politics*. Medical historian Andrea Tone points out that it was not just new studies of the addictive nature of psychopharmacological and anxiolytic drugs that roused suspicion but also a loss of confidence in "pharmaceutical panaceas."[60] The Controlled Substances Act of 1970 recategorized mood-stabilizing drugs and regulated prescriptions more tightly. However, personal narratives emerged that revealed a widespread everyday reliance on tranquilizers that was often linked to feelings of blame and abandonment.

Long-term use of Valium, the most prescribed drug of the 1970s, could be as damaging psychologically and physically as heroin addiction, but because it was a seen as a middle-class drug it posed little threat to law and order.[61] Although many women taking Valium thought the drug helped them maintain "the traditional female role of wife and homemaker," the rise of patients' rights groups and the growing popularity of exercise, aerobics, and yoga meant that by the end of the decade Valium was seen as part of the problem rather than the solution.[62] The deleterious side effects of Valium were more fully recognized by 1975, when a widely read article in *Vogue* highlighted its addictive properties and the Drug Enforcement Administration reclassified it as a Schedule IV controlled substance, but it remained a heavily prescribed drug.[63] Four years later, Ted Kennedy launched an inquiry into its use and misuse, the same year the mass-market book *The Tranquilizing of America: Pill Popping and the American Way of Life* compared the "chemical tranquility" of individuals like Carol, a 30-year-old airline stewardess who had become addicted to Librium and Valium, to the "real tranquility" that seemed to be in short supply in the 1970s.[64] Authors Richard Hughes and Robert Brewin argued that the widespread use of benzodiazepines was a feature of a growing sedativist culture for which suppliers, regulators, doctors, and patients (some of whom feigned symptoms) must all share responsibility.

The most significant narrative for raising the voice of the addict was television writer and director Barbara Gordon's memoir *I'm Dancing as Fast as I Can*, a personal story about the damaging effects of long-term use of Valium. Gordon started taking diazepam pills as a muscle relaxant for back problems, but by 1976 she had realized that she was an addict when her anxiety began to mount despite the medication. She experiences "feverish intensity" and feels that she cannot function without Valium. Her agitated state of mind contrasts with the cool and distant attitude of her physician, Dr. Allen.[65] He insists that the pills are not addictive, and when he recommends the antipsychotic drug Thorazine as an alternative she loses faith in his judgment, possibly because she associates it with a bewildered group of Long Beach mental health patients (the focus of a PBS documentary she had recently made) who are forced to fend for themselves after being released prematurely from their institution. A few days later, when she suddenly stops taking the pills, we hear two voices: the Barbara of the story senses the psychological effects of Valium, yet it is only Barbara Gordon the writer who can anticipate the dreadful pains of going cold. Barbara the character thinks that "in a few days I'd be fine, rested, refreshed, ready to face a new day"; Barbara the writer notes that "instead I blew my head open. But I was lucky: I could have died."[66]

Her withdrawal symptoms are dire: a burning scalp, spasms and tremors, dizziness, hot flushes, insatiable thirst, constant anxiety and terror, insomnia, and loss of self-esteem as she loses the will to get dressed, let alone leave the house. It is not clear to what extent Barbara is losing her grasp on reality, but her symptoms are exacerbated by the control she feels her partner Eric starts to exert in the home. Thinking that he is conspiring against her, she throws tantrums, leading Eric to take the role of the cruel patriarch. He hits her to calm her down, accuses her of insanity, and restrains her. After a series of violent struggles, Eric commits her to hospital, where she is diagnosed with depression and cyclothymia and is given the anti-depressant Sinequan. In the hospital, Barbara is keen to rediscover her former sense of self, but initially her memories are "jumbled" and her words are "incoherent" and the hospital doctor agrees to release her only if Eric moves out of the apartment.[67]

Barbara's search for an alternative psychiatrist leads her to another diagnosis—schizophrenia—and similar drug choices: lithium and Thorazine, which she eventually takes despite despairingly referring to it as "end-of-the-road medication."[68] A third psychiatrist tells her that she is not schizophrenic and that she is still experiencing Valium withdrawal, exacerbated by her decision to go cold turkey instead of trying gradual withdrawal. Eventually Barbara agrees to check herself into a specialist clinic. However, instead of discovering her inner voice she can only hear "sounds of wretchedness interrupted by anonymous mirth," "screaming women, shrieking like hyenas in the night," and the incessant sound of the hospital phonograph inside her head. She is nevertheless pleased to be able to talk with a female doctor, whose style of engaged psychotherapy contrasts with the austerity of her male doctors. Therapy is painful, especially as the doctor prompts her to keep talking about the same psychological issues, but she eventually comes to realize

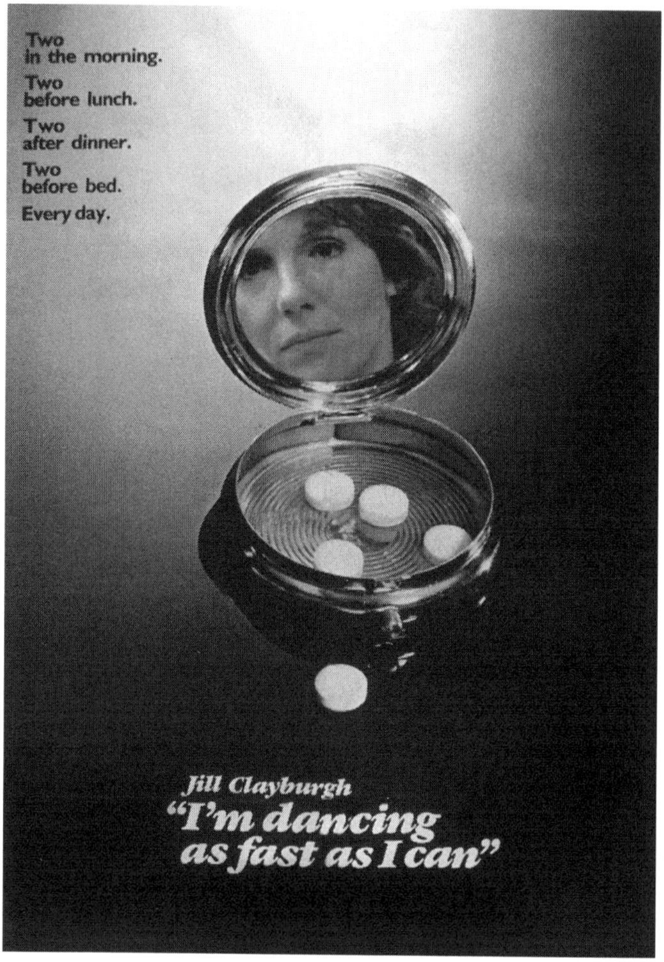

Figure 3.1 Film poster of *I'm Dancing as Fast as I Can* (dir. Jack Hofsiss, 1982). Paramount/Everett Collection/Rex Shutterstock.

that the pills had turned "small problems into giant conflicts, little demons into monsters."[69] Barbara is encouraged to take partial responsibility for her Valium addiction instead of simply blaming Dr. Allen's "treat-the-symptom" therapy or her domestic tribulations with Eric, although she finds it difficult to keep things in proportion. Art therapy helps check her emotional regression, yet she experiences separation anxiety when she is permitted to take outings and feels empty and helpless when she finally leaves. Struggling with reintegration into daily life, what "seemed like the nine thousandth doctor" advises Barbara that she is still "experiencing a schizophrenic reaction to drug withdrawal" over a year since she took her last Valium pill.[70] Further experiments with therapists, megavitamins, new friends, reorientation toward her parents, and a tricky return to work are all needed before she begins to feel whole again.[71]

Despite her long journey, in the afterword Gordon criticizes the "fragile science" of psychiatry and the "brutality" of what she sees as an uncaring medical system.[72] Writing *I'm Dancing as Fast as I Can* was both a form of self-therapy (she began drafting the book in February 1977 to ease her transition to life outside) and a way of exposing the sedativist culture that stimulated her breakdown and painful recovery. Her narrative is instructive because it connects gender roles, career issues, medical mismanagement, and a drug that anesthetizes emotions through the testimony of a patient who is unable to calibrate a safe dose. Gordon dedicates her story to women who were struggling with identity issues during the Valium panic, especially given the fact that doctors were much more likely to prescribe diazepam for women.

Perhaps because Eric was demonized in *I'm Dancing as Fast as I Can*, the real-life Eric, Anton Holden, wrote a riposte to Gordon's story that questions certain aspects of her account. Published as *Prince Valium* in 1982, the same year a simplified film adaptation of *I'm Dancing as Fast as I Can* was released, Holden places himself in a heroic role as he tries valiantly to contend with Barbara's breakdown. The book describes Barbara's memory loss and mounting anxiety, her propensity to wash down her pills with beer (a detail that is absent from Gordon's story and the film), Barbara's mental health issues earlier in life, and his feelings of helplessness. He too is critical of her doctor (a "Valium-dispensing machine"), but he focuses on Barbara's deception when she relapses into drinking and taking pills during cold turkey.[73] He does not avoid nasty scenes, calling her a "hard-core junkie" and reacting violently to her relapse and her childish tantrums. He casts Barbara as the violent one, describing her attacks on him with her fists and a pair of sharp pliers.[74] In the face of this onslaught, he portrays his decision to commit her as a last resort and he seems genuinely hurt when Barbara ends their plans to marry. He quickly moves on, though: she is not mentioned in the final two pages of *Prince Valium* and Holden leaves the story about a third of the way into Gordon's narrative.

Although this counternarrative seems reactive and self-justifying, it points to the danger of relying on first-person stories alone to understand the addict's experience. Addiction stories are more unreliable than other autobiographies because of their contradictions, deceptions, omissions, repetitions, and lapses. Holden was especially suspicious of the linearity of Barbara's story of her withdrawal, claiming that she was oblivious for much of the time. We might also be wary of her one-sided account of the relationship with Eric, but her story does not evade uglier emotions. The 1982 film version skirts over these narrative tensions, even though it depicts the disturbing scenes of Barbara convulsing on the beach and domestic violence with Eric. It also elides the two voices we hear in Gordon's written account: the Valium victim who cannot easily see outside herself and the resilient woman intent on showing that the stigma of mental illness persists into the mid-1970s. *I'm Dancing as Fast as I Can* is important because it shares a hidden story with other women of her generation, a point editor Burton Beals emphasizes (in the early 1960s, Beals had edited the founding text of second-wave feminism, Betty Friedan's *The Feminine Mystique*). Gordon's narrative sought to raise consciousness about the deleterious effects of a drug that she believed was possible to kick, even if doing so led to the collapse of her career and relationships along the way.

Betty Ford and Rehabilitation Narratives

Looking back at the history of addiction from near the millennium, historian William White detected that alcohol and drugs were "two worlds" until the second half of the 1970s, when treatment centers began to see a marked increase in cross-addiction.[75] The most important public story of the mid-1970s that served to raise the profile of cross-addiction was that of Betty Ford. As first lady, Mrs. Ford largely managed to avoid scrutiny into this aspect of her life. However, a personal story that began quietly several years earlier came to the media's attention in 1978, over a year after the end of Gerald Ford's presidency, but with the couple still in the public eye.

Betty Ford was well liked by the public, so much so that *Newsweek* named her woman of the year in 1975.[76] However, one occasion that aroused suspicions that all was not well behind the scenes was a *60 Minutes* interview with Morley Safer that screened in August 1975, in which the first lady admitted that she had seen a psychiatrist. The interview is remembered less for this passing mention and more for her candor on premarital sex, marijuana, abortion, and her active support of the Equal Rights Amendment, all of which made the interview much more political than anyone had anticipated. Worried that the interview might have cost him 20 million votes, the president issued a letter that smoothed out his wife's more forthright comments to the 20,000 respondents who criticized what they saw as Mrs. Ford's immoral and ungodly stance, particularly her pro-choice opinion on abortion.[77] Realizing that she could damage her husband's prospects, she was less outspoken during the election year despite her Equal Rights Amendment advocacy.[78]

The negative responses to her *60 Minutes* interview contrasted sharply with the warmth expressed by the 45,000 letters and cards she received following her mastectomy after being diagnosed with breast cancer in September 1974. This extended the generally favorable view of the first lady based on her reputation as a compassionate person, such as her charitable work for the Hospital for Sick Children in Washington, DC (a facility that opened in 1882 and had been specializing since 1968 in the rehabilitation of disabled children and teenagers) and her volunteer work with disabled children at the Mary Free Bed Rehabilitation Hospital in Grand Rapids, Michigan, in the early 1930s.[79] After Mrs. Ford spoke out on women's healthcare rights following her mastectomy, many women sought breast examinations in 1975, and the White House sponsored a conference on breast cancer the next year.[80]

But 1974 was not the first year that Betty Ford faced health issues. As the wife of a member of Congress, she was prescribed painkillers for inoperable pinched nerve in her neck and osteoarthritis. Her psychological condition deteriorated as she used alcohol to self-medicate, progressing from drinking every evening to adding vodka to her morning tea. She consulted a psychiatrist in 1965 during an emotional low linked to her physical ailments that was exacerbated by her husband's long absences. In her 1979 autobiography *The Times of My Life*, Mrs. Ford wrote that her visits to the psychiatrist increased her feelings of self-worth, helped her realize that she didn't have to be "the Bionic Woman," and encouraged her to take better care of herself. However, although she recovered her composure, she continued to take painkillers and drink heavily over the next thirteen years.[81] The media noticed her fragile health. An August 1975 issue of *Newsweek* focused on the strains of office and the course of chemotherapy after her cancer operation, but the piece hints at something else: "her movements often seem stiffer and more deliberate than before, her pauses longer, and there are new signs of strain under her eye make-up. . . . She appears to be thinner, and brittle as well."[82] Even a celebratory column in *McCall's* speculated that "the open and natural Mrs. Ford" was often "frozen stiffly into a pose that leads some observers to wonder if she isn't dazed on tranquilizers."[83] This comment and the *Newsweek* picture of a "limp and ashy pale" first lady took on a different hue when the news of her addictions broke three years later.

Ford's two autobiographies are instructive for assessing the arc of her addiction and recovery. She laid out her health problems in *The Times of My Life*, published a year after her children had convinced her to check into the U.S. Navy's Alcohol and Drug Rehabilitation Service in Long Beach, which had opened in the mid-1960s to deal with drug and alcohol use in the armed forces. She was 60 when she started her rehabilitation, but not until her second book, *Betty: A Glad Awakening*, published in 1988, did she look back on her long-term substance abuse with clear eyes. This second autobiography promoted the cause of the Betty Ford Center, an 80-bed inpatient rehabilitation facility that had opened in 1982 on the landscaped campus of the Eisenhower Medical Center in Palm Springs, California, for those suffering from heavy alcohol and drug use, at a time when there were few dedicated inpatient facilities for recovering alcoholics besides the 30-year-old Hazelden Center in eastern Minnesota.[84] Mrs. Ford's second book is evangelical in places, written from the perspective of an ex-patient who has plumbed the depths but now sees the light. This story of her "glad awakening" is absent from the commonplace prose of *The Times of My Life*, which deals more quietly with the fifteen years since her physical and psychological condition had begun to overwhelm her.

It is not until the final chapter of *The Times of My Life*, titled "Long Beach," that she broaches the subject explicitly. She did not want to deal with the episode at all, but her husband convinced her that writing an extra chapter would be a "proper conclusion. . . . There is no other responsible way to end the book."[85] With this in mind, she begins her final installment with the line "I had thought my book was finished. I had not expected to write this chapter." She is adamant in her claim that she could always carry herself with decorum in public life, counter to some stories that described her as a zombie, especially during one episode in fall 1977 when she delivered a drunken commentary on the *Nutcracker* ballet during a visit to Russia. She was partially receptive to her family's intervention, yet at first admitted only to her history of overmedicating, largely, she said, because her alcohol addiction "wasn't dramatic" and did not prevent her from fulfilling her role as first lady.[86]

Mrs. Ford claimed that she benefited from the military regime of the Long Beach rehabilitation facility, which had been designed for naval personnel. Initially she finds it hard to accept the twice-a-day group sessions, until one day when another patient's confession triggers her own, which she gave trembling and in a cracked voice. Despite her discomfort, the group gradually bonded and she felt grounded by the community of inpatients. She includes a short excerpt from her hospital diary before concluding that her recovery was successful and she could now enjoy ginger beer while her husband drank a cocktail, claiming with equanimity that "I've learned a lot about myself. Most of it is all right. When I add up the pluses and subtract the minuses, I still come out pretty well."[87]

This everyday description and analysis is colored by her compassion for others, particularly women who she realized while undergoing her mastectomy often suffered silently and with inadequate support facilities. Her conclusion that "I'm not out to rescue anybody who doesn't want to be rescued, I just think it's important to say how easy it is to slip into a dependency on pills and alcohol. And how hard it is to admit that dependency" is heartfelt and does not resort to the clichés of self-help or group therapy.[88] This tone contrasts with that of *Betty: A Glad Awakening*, which focuses more on the intervention and recovery. She describes withdrawal and detoxification in greater detail (although not as graphically as Barbara Gordon), the clash of cultures in group sessions (especially among patients from different class backgrounds), and the strength she draws from the Serenity Prayer, which was written by theologian Reinhold Niebuhr and adopted by Alcoholics Anonymous in the 1940s.[89] She values her family's love and the hospital staff and comes to appreciate her support group, but it is to prayer that she returns for the deepest source of strength.

The second half of her book focuses on the Betty Ford Center and is interspersed with reflections on the psychology of dependency and the necessity of ongoing treatment for alcoholics. She writes about the need for the clinic, particularly for women who do not fit into the macho culture of heavy drinking and who have "toughed it out" or "tried to straighten up on their own."[90] The tone moves from autobiographical candor to commonsense responses to addiction but occasionally turns to symbolism, such as her own take on William Blake's poem "The Sick Rose": "Like the invisible worm that eats at the heart of the rose, drugs and alcohol are dark secret lovers that destroy."[91] She reflects on the seductive qualities of pills and drink and her belief that psychiatrists often make dependency worse by prescribing drugs in combinations.[92] Ford can be criticized for not dealing with addiction in psychological terms and, like Gordon, for pointing the finger at a generation of male doctors, yet her experiences also lead her to the conclusion that "there was enough blame for all of us, the doctors and me."[93] She always returns to her religious faith for giving her the resolve to kick her habit and reminding her of the Christian mission to help others. While the text is never sanctimonious, it ends by seeing recovery as form of blessed rebirth in line with the AA twelve-step recovery program, which was extended from the treatment of alcoholism to the treatment of narcotic dependency in the early 1950s.[94] She does not offer a radical departure from this program, and although she focuses on gender, lifestyle, and class, other factors of race, region, and alternative belief systems are absent from both texts.

Betty Ford's $9.6 million privately funded drug rehabilitation facility rapidly became a major institution in the 1980s. She was not the only high-profile public figure with multiple addictions to catch the attention of the media. The tension between public demands and private life that Mrs. Ford experienced was arguably even more pronounced for celebrity musicians, leading to a number of well-publicized cases of drug and alcohol addiction. Two casualties of the excesses of the 1970s rock lifestyle are worth pausing on. Both Stevie Nicks, the lead singer of Fleetwood Mac, and David Crosby of the supergroup Crosby, Stills & Nash developed serious cocaine habits during the 1980s. They sang together on Nicks's 1994 song "Street Angel"—the year Nicks was undergoing rehabilitation for prescription drugs and Crosby had a liver transplant after years of drug abuse—but their stories and treatment arcs are quite different. Nicks first checked into the Betty Ford Center in 1986 to recover from cocaine addiction and by all accounts came out clean. However, a psychiatrist she saw soon after her release prescribed Klonopin (which was usually given to control epilepsy or anxiety disorders) and Nicks developed a much worse addiction to this benzodiazepine than her cocaine habit. She took Klonopin, Valium, and Xanax over the next eight years, finally seeking treatment in December 1993. In interviews since 2001 she has described her wasted years as a time when she lost her creative voice and felt that the drug was consuming her body. Her drug use led to weight gain and a reclusive lifestyle. With the help of her assistant, she put herself through what she describes as a "hellish" six-week detoxification program at the Exodus Recovery Center at the Daniel Freeman Marina Hospital, Los Angeles, and has since been outspoken about the perils of a reckless repeat prescription that she claimed wiped out her forties.[95]

David Crosby also sang about a lost decade in his 1988 song "Compass," which begins unsteadily with the lyrics "I have wasted ten years / In a blindfold." Crosby could not blame anyone else for an addiction that his peers were surprised he recovered from. Whereas the other members of Crosby, Stills & Nash used cocaine and marijuana, Crosby moved on to freebase, a pure and highly addictive form of cocaine. Heating cocaine in a spoon or pipe means that inhalation of freebase is purer, but it also stimulates a forceful yet short-lived high. (David Foster Wallace describes this high in both angelic and orgasmic terms in his 1996 novel *Infinite Jest*.)[96] Freebase often leads to binging due to the sharp down that typically follows an intense high, as comedian Richard Pryor burlesqued in his stand-up shows after sustaining third-degree burns while freebasing in June 1980. In contrast to the hardcore use of freebase, cocaine was seen as a lifestyle drug among urban yuppies in the mid-1980s, even though the belief that it was non-addictive was being challenged by Jay McInerney and Bret Easton Ellis in their debut novels *Bright Lights, Big City* and *Less Than Zero* and by Washington insider Richard Smart's 1985 account of his rampant cocaine addiction in *The Snow Papers*.[97] The kind of drug habit that Crosby had experienced for years did not come under media scrutiny until 1986, when the Reagan administration focused on crack as a highly addictive version of freebase that often led to drug-related violence, according to the National Institute on Drug Abuse. In October that year CBS aired a documentary *48 Hours on Crack Street* and the president called the "new epidemic" of crack use "an uncontrolled fire" that needed to be tackled with aggressive measures. Eighteen months later, in a new election year, an ABC news special called crack "a plague eating away at the fabric of America."[98]

By the late 1970s and early 1980s, Crosby was freebasing nearly all the time: in the recording studio, at the wheel of his car, and with his girlfriend, who also had a severe habit. When he was arrested for possessing drugs and weapons, Crosby tried to outrun the law and dodge rehabilitation. Only a prison sentence in 1985 after he caused a car crash while freebasing at the wheel broke his habit. The 1982 song "Delta" captures Crosby's hazy world of freebase, even though this was in sharp contrast to the irritable, self-absorbed, and selfish figure that he had become during his drug years. It was not until "Compass" in 1988 that we see a gap opening between his former life and the present: the lyrics identify a "still, sure, spirit" that he thinks has been hidden throughout his lost years.

Nicks and Crosby can be seen as self-indulgent victims of a music industry in which drugs were widely available, yet they have distinct stories: Nicks claims that her prescription drug habit (for which she did not accept responsibility) was more debilitating that her cocaine habit (for which she was responsible), while Crosby rehabilitated only when he was compelled to. This was unlike the response of fellow West Coast musician Jerry Garcia, lead singer of the Grateful Dead, who checked himself into the Betty Ford Center for heroin addiction in 1986 after slipping into a diabetic coma. Garcia did not last long as an inpatient, and although he survived into the mid-1990s, his last fifteen years were a struggle against drugs and failing health. These cases contrast with the more evangelical narratives of Ford and Georgia medical student Martha Morrison, whose 1989 book of recovery from heroin addiction, *White Rabbit*, concludes with an admission "that only God could help me" and a recitation of the Serenity Prayer.[99] In contrast to the honest ending of Barbara Gordon's account—she has "no epiphany, no single moment of synthesis and complete understanding"—Ford and Morrison presented strong voices of rehabilitation that played into the moral agenda that President Reagan advanced in the mid-1980s as he stepped up the war against drugs.[100]

The Reagans' War on Drugs

The Reagan and Bush administrations pursued similar tactics as Nixon and Ford had in pushing for a tough response to narcotics. In fact, President Reagan stepped up the criminalization of drug use and the federal crackdown on drug trafficking by tripling the budget for such efforts in the period 1981 to 1986. These measures were flanked by the portrayal of the war on drugs as a surgical strike against crippling illness and a widespread anti-drug-use education program, accompanied by a tendency to manipulate statistics relating to drug-related deaths and the number of "drug babies" affected by their mother's habits. Reagan's papers are full of briefings, policy reports, and communication strategies relating to the war on drugs. Along with high-profile initiatives such as the 1984 National Strategy for Prevention of Drug Abuse and Drug Trafficking and the February 1988 White House Conference for a Drug Free America, the administration emphasized the effectiveness of Reagan's leadership and tried hard to convince the public that the war was being won on multiple fronts: reducing the perceived threat to national security, strengthening law enforcement, and decreasing health risks.[101]

Even though a 1977 Gallup poll revealed that 60 percent of Americans thought that smoking marijuana would lead to harder drugs, President Carter distinguished between occasional marijuana use and the health damage caused by the sustained use of narcotics.[102] But the tendency to blur hard and soft drugs returned during the Reagan administration, influenced by marijuana expert Carlton E. Turner, his deputy assistant for drug abuse policy, who did not believe in this distinction. Turner published widely during his five years in the Reagan administration and made good use of the media to publicize the correlation between recreational drug use and health risks. For example, he appeared on *The Larry King Show* in October 1982 and a month later he participated in a televised panel discussion following an airing of the powerful documentary *Epidemic: Why Your Kid Is on Drugs*. When Reagan addressed the nation from the West Wing on 14 September 1986, midway through his second term, he capitalized on the language of crisis to justify an increase in criminal measures, claiming that during his first term marijuana use had gone down markedly and drugs in the military had declined by 67 percent.

Reagan's September 1986 speech is very important, not only because it linked closely to the first Anti-Drug Abuse Act, which focused on punitive measures for using drugs when it was passed the following month, but also because the president was not alone when he announced that "drugs are menacing our society. They're threatening our values and undercutting our institutions. They're killing our children."[103] With him in the West Wing was First Lady Nancy Reagan, who had hosted a White House Conference on Drug Abuse the previous year. She had adopted this as her special project early in her husband's first term, despite concerns among her advisors that it might backfire due to public negativity surrounding the issue.[104] Drug prevention did not stem from Mrs. Reagan's personal experience as naturally as women's rights and mental health did for Betty Ford and Rosalynn Carter, even though she had visited rehabilitation centers during her husband's 1980 campaign and it resonated both with her stepfather's medical background as professor of surgery and her work as a nurse's aide at college.[105] Harrowing accounts of drug use among teenagers and links to crime and prostitution in fictional depictions of the late 1970s, such as Jim Carroll's *The Basketball Diaries* and Hubert Selby Jr.'s *Requiem for a Dream*, made Mrs. Reagan's advisors nervous. Nevertheless, a survey suggested that campaigning against drug abuse in schools was a relatively risk-free project for Nancy Reagan. After four months of preparation and the encouragement of Carlton Turner, Mrs. Reagan's office launched the Just Say No campaign, which began with trips to Florida and Texas

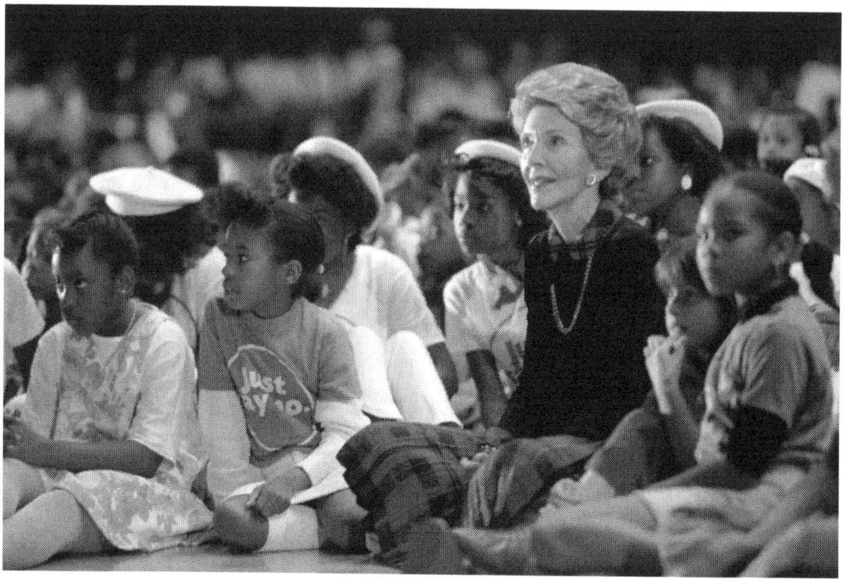

Figure 3.2 Nancy Reagan with California children at a Just Say No rally at the Kaiser Arena in Oakland, 26 November 1985. Courtesy of the Ronald Reagan Presidential Library.

in February 1982 and led to the proliferation of anti-drug-use school clubs by the summer of 1984.[106]

Over the next seven years, Mrs. Reagan played a prominent role in ensuring that drug use was treated as a moral issue, in contrast to Mrs. Carter's more obvious stress on caregiving. When she did mention health issues it tended to be in broad terms: "drugs can make you sick—so sick that you don't want to live anymore," she announced to 4,000 Oakland school children in November 1985, encouraging them all to chant "just say no."[107] The emphasis on communication and publicity was the biggest shift from the Nixon-Ford years. Mrs. Reagan gave primetime interviews early in the campaign, made a guest appearance on the NBC/ABC comedy show *Diff'rent Strokes* in March 1983, co-hosted an episode of *Good Morning America* in October 1983, and hosted *The Chemical People*, a PBS documentary that focused on addiction and rehabilitation, in December 1983.[108] These high-profile appearances and the Reagans' September 1986 speech brought together two powerful voices that defined drug abuse in ideological terms, reflecting Carlton Turner's claim the previous year that "when you buy drugs, you buy terror; when you buy a high, you buy a nightmare. Drugs are a threat to our national security, our health, our future."[109]

In her section of the speech, Mrs. Reagan echoed the president's rhetoric of crisis and epidemic. She began by portraying herself as a mother in the 1940s and 50s sending her children off to school, secure in the belief that they would be cared for in a warm environment "in which they could fulfil the promise and hope of those restless minds."[110] She contrasted this scene with her present-day fears that schools were no longer safe institutions that nurture "the brightness and life of the sons and daughters of the United States." As new research into children born to addicts began appearing in the mid-1980s, Mrs. Reagan portrayed drugs as the antithesis of life and pressed parents and teachers to "be unyielding and inflexible in your opposition to drugs."[111] Perhaps reminded of the *Go Ask Alice* narrative of terminal decline or news of eleven-year-old boys arrested for selling hard drugs in the nation's capital, she closed her address by appealing to children and teenagers to resist temptation. Instead of focusing on health issues, she played into the president's second-term campaign slogan, "Morning in America," by portraying drug use as transforming the bright colorful worlds of the young into shades of black and gray.

President Reagan concluded the joint address by characterizing Mrs. Reagan's work as part of a national "moral crusade" that included advice literature for schools and instructional fiction for children.[112] He stressed the need for a coordinated front ("a combination of government and private efforts") in order to achieve six goals: drug-free workplaces and schools; the development of tough rehabilitation programs (such as the Toughlove support network Mrs. Reagan favored); an expansion of international cooperation on curbing drug trafficking; stronger law enforcement; and heightened public awareness in order to bring about "a massive change in national attitudes . . . to take the user away from the supply." There was nothing here that explicitly addressed the mental health complications of sustained drug use. Instead, the emphasis on public awareness might have been triggered by scare stories about crack cocaine and, more subtly, linked to growing fears that AIDS would spread through inner cities via contaminated heroin needles.[113] The finale was the Great Communicator at his best. The president reflected on the importance of the home front during World War II and the need to "pull together again" through "clubs, service groups, and community organizations"; he encouraged citizens to report their neighbors if they thought they were taking drugs; and he likened reformed drug users to "combat veterans" who can "help others by telling [their stories] and providing a willing hand to those in need."

In addition to this emphasis on volunteerism and responsible citizenship, the president and Mrs. Reagan realized the need for positive stories of rehabilitation, such as the kinds of recovery stories former female addicts presented in the 1985 collection *A Woman Like You*, actress Ally Sheedy's testimony in 1986 about her drug experiences and rehabilitation at the Hazelden Foundation, Nancy Whittier Dudley's 1987 article "A Million Dollar Habit" in *The Washingtonian*, actress Carrie Fisher's semi-autobiographical novel *Postcards from the Edge*, and Martha Morrison's *White Rabbit*, which was published at the end of the Reagan administration.[114] Dudley's article, which candidly discusses her addiction to freebase cocaine and her three attempts at rehabilitation, led Mrs. Reagan to invite her to the White House. It was a hard-hitting piece that does not read like a conversion narrative. Nevertheless, certain phrases chimed with the rhetoric of the Reagans, such as the "wasteland of lies out of the rich soil in which my values had been rooted," "it is far less painful to accept and deal with one's feelings without drugs than to try to escape those feelings through drugs," and her concluding line: "Thankfully, I am beginning to gain a spiritual understanding of myself, to live with dedication to reality."[115] Such recovery stories could be used as warnings that might prevent what the president called a war that is "killing America and terrorizing it with slow but sure chemical destruction."[116] Reinforcing the point that there is no moral middle ground, Reagan challenged all citizens to participate actively in his anti-drug crusade and to uphold core national values of hope and freedom.

The Reagans' speech set in motion a shaping period in the war on drugs that continued to the end of George H. W. Bush's term in early 1993. Nancy Reagan had a prominent role to play in this. Her popularity was soaring by the mid-1980s, and during her husband's second term she was keen to preserve her legacy by developing the Nancy Reagan Drug Abuse Center. She envisaged this as rivaling the Betty Ford Center in raising consciousness about drug abuse and implementing more robust forms of rehabilitation. However, the final two years of the Reagan administration, when she was seeking a West Coast location for the new facility and establishing a foundation in her name, were not so kind to her image. Her falling out with the nonprofit drug treatment organization Phoenix House and an ill-advised publicity shoot in a South Central LA crack house in April 1989 raised suspicions that she was engaging a national health issue for the wrong reasons.[117] Despite the ideological battle lines of the 1980s, distorted statistics, and further exposés of drug use (such as revelations that child movie star Drew Barrymore was drinking at age 10 and taking cocaine age 12 before being admitted in the summer of 1988 to Malibu's ASAP Family Treatment Center), the figures suggest that drug use declined during the Reagan years, particularly among children and teenagers.[118] It was a matter of debate, though, whether this trend can be attributed to the Just Say No campaign; to propaganda such as the White House-sponsored anti-drugs issue of the DC comic *The New Teen Titans*, which was distributed to 35,000 elementary schools in spring 1983; or to increased measures to control crime.

The Bush line on drugs was similar to Reagan's Cold War zeal. During the Bush administration, most of the additional $2.2 billion in federal funding bolstered law enforcement and the prevention of drug trafficking, whereas much less was spent on drug research, education, and treatment. This attitude was on display in President Bush's inauguration speech of January 1989, in which he adopted a high moral tone about addiction, using rhetoric that was similar to Reagan's; he called cocaine a "deadly bacteria" that has "hurt the body, the soul of our country" and promised to focus efforts on stopping "the scourge."[119] It was not just teenagers, veterans, and black communities that concerned Bush; the general public needed education through such publications as the white paper *Understanding Drug Treatment* (which was deliberately written in plain language). He recognized that television could influence an estimated 20 million children between the ages of 5 and 11, an age group that he claimed was the target audience for schoolyard drug pushers.[120] Bush did not use illness metaphors as frequently as Reagan and he was not as bold as Nixon (he admitted that the war could not be won in his generation). He was willing to invest more in treatment, but was keen to remain vigilant in the face of 11 million regular drug users.[121] The second Anti-Drug Abuse Act, which was passed in November 1988, at the end of the Reagan administration, led to the comprehensive National Drug Control Strategy of September 1989, which embodied Bush's remarks that "drugs are sapping our strength as a nation," even though the strategy cited a 37 percent overall decrease in recreational drug use since 1985.[122]

In the second presidential debate of 1992, Bush claimed that his drug strategy was making good progress, particularly on interdiction (buoyed by the recent 40-year sentence of Panamanian general Manuel Noriega for drug trafficking), but he said that more effort was needed to deter "habitual drug users." Journalist Joseph Treaster was skeptical about the effectiveness of the administration in drying up supplies, though. Treaster argued in 1991 that the "grim saga of drug addiction is far from over," particularly as a highly potent blend of crack and heroin had appeared in cities two years earlier, as had a wave of new addictions that were difficult and costly to treat.[123] Instead of wiping out international cartels, the Bush crackdown was more successful in targeting street dealers, leading to a suspicion that the war on drugs was racialized and that federal initiatives were disproportionately targeting black neighborhoods. Drug-related arrests of African Americans doubled in the period 1976 to 1990, prisons were crowded with convicts from minority groups, and drug hygiene was a concern as AIDS spread in black communities through dirty needles at a rate that was triple the national average.[124]

When protest was heard, it was rarely from mental health advocates and more often pointed out that legalization of recreational drugs or harm reduction might prove more effective than the combative policies of Nixon and Reagan, given that estimates suggested that the war on drugs was costing the nation $35 billion in the early 1990s.[125] That is not to say that prevention and treatment had not improved over twenty years, and the fact that Clinton chose not to mention drugs in his inaugural address did not mean the war had been abandoned. Clinton's critics thought an invisible drug policy was worse than the urgency of Reagan and Bush, but the Clinton administration was certainly aware of new intelligence about drugs and urban crime. It continued to tackle drug trafficking from Mexico and Colombia. The Clinton administration's policy on marijuana was similar those of its Republican predecessors (despite Clinton's admission that he had smoked a joint without inhaling as an Oxford University student), and the government invested in highly visible anti-drug and anti-meth campaigns in 1998.

Despite the drama of the "This is Your Brain on Drugs" advertisement of 1997 (in which a smashed egg represents the neural effects of heroin), and the suspicion that policies and rhetoric on drugs and violence were racially coded (such as the mass incarceration implications of the 1994 Violent Crime Control and Law Enforcement Act and Hillary Clinton's ill-advised "super-predator" comment of January 1996), there was an important shift of tone.[126] The rise of right-wing media channels, the heroin-related death of Nirvana singer Kurt Cobain in 1994, and knee-jerk reactions to the vogue for the euphoria-inducing drug Ecstasy among students did not entirely help public health efforts, but on the whole, public information on the toll drugs took on health was more balanced in the mid-1990s and the voices of advocacy groups and former addicts were easier to hear.[127] However, when surrealist filmmaker Darren Aronofsky released his bleak film adaptation of *Requiem of a Dream* in 2000, its graphic portrayal of the deleterious effects of prescription pills, heroin, and cocaine on the mental health of four interconnected lives suggested that the realities of drug regulation and addiction had changed little since Hubert Selby wrote his novel in 1978.

4 *Dementia and the Language of Aging*

In his Thanksgiving proclamation of 1975, as the nation approached its bicentennial, President Ford urged all Americans to actively remember the elderly.[1] The president had expressed a similar sentiment the previous year, but in 1975 he was probably reflecting on the recent publication of Robert Butler's *Why Survive? Being Old in America*. As the founding director of the National Institute on Aging, Butler argued that although modern medicine was helping elderly Americans survive longer, it could not guarantee that their lives would be fulfilling ones.[2] Butler was particularly critical of the second White House Conference on Aging of November 1971 for failing to stimulate the same level of federal action as the inaugural conference had done a decade earlier in preparing the ground for Medicare and the Older Americans Act. What made it worse for Butler was the fact that although Senior Citizens Month was observed each May and President Nixon mentioned the elderly as "special participants" in his Thanksgiving speeches, Nixon's focus on Cold War détente, reducing unemployment, and controlling narcotics meant that the elderly often disappeared off the political radar.[3]

Sponsored by the nonprofit, nonpartisan volunteer organization No Greater Love, the 1975 Thanksgiving campaign pressed families to include the elderly in their celebrations and encouraged the young to visit nursing homes. On November 20th, as part of the campaign, honorary patron Betty Ford held a Thanksgiving dinner at The White House for fourteen guests aged 64 to 88 to focus attention on the isolation many seniors felt.[4] The campaign's promotional brochure, the tagline of which was "to age is human," estimated that the demographic of 20 million elderly Americans (10 percent of the population) was increasing twice as fast as the total population.[5] The ratio of 3.5 women to every man in this group pointed to both high mortality rates among middle-aged men and inadequate care initiatives for older women, particularly those susceptible to loneliness and understimulation.

Betty Ford sensed this lack of dedicated care for women in the 60-plus age range during her period of rehabilitation in the late 1970s, yet there had been earlier alarm bells. The Senate Special Committee on Aging released a report in 1971 calling for urgent action and recommending that events be organized every two years to prevent a lull between the White House conferences. The report warned that welfare and healthcare problems had grown in some regions despite the aim of the Older Americans Act to ensure coordination at the state level.[6] The committee was particularly worried that cost containment at the state level would restrict access to doctors. For example, although Californian seniors had previously been allowed to see a doctor as often as they needed, in 1970 Governor Reagan had

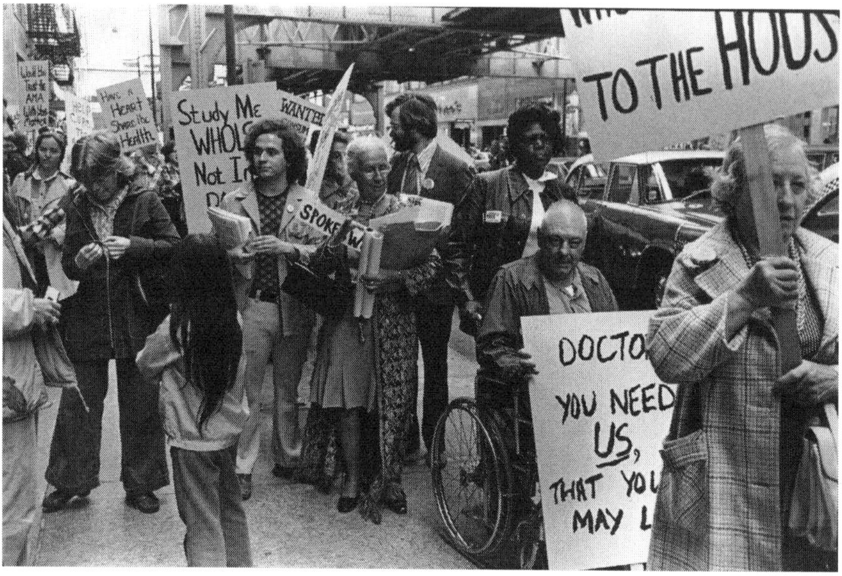

Figure 4.1 Gray Panther demonstration on Wabash Avenue in Chicago to protest the American Medical Association's lack of investment in gerontology, 25 June 1974. Image courtesy of the Gray Panthers Records, Urban Archives, Temple University, Philadelphia.

scaled back Medicare consultations to a maximum of twice a month. The National Health Planning and Resources Development Act of 1974 was an attempt to tackle inequality of access, but the lack of an integrated national policy prompted the militant activist group the Gray Panthers to stage a provocative piece of theater outside the American Medical Association convention in Chicago that year. On the day Vice-President Ford addressed the conference delegates, the Gray Panthers demanded that "the sick AMA" declare a country-wide healthcare crisis and immediately invest in new gerontology programs.[7] The founder of the group, Maggie Kuhn, thought that extreme tactics (such as protesting the lack of an African American presence at the 1971 White House Conference on Aging and pressuring the media to address ageist stereotypes) were needed to speed up a coordinated federal policy and threats to Medicare. The lack of such policies prompted Robert Butler to write despairingly that "nothing dramatic, compelling, innovative or surprising" emerged from the 1971 conference, particularly on mental health.[8]

These concerns did not go unnoticed. Butler was appointed to be the first director of the National Institute on Aging in 1975, funding for geriatric research increased in the mid-1970s, and aging became a key theme of Ford's reelection campaign. This focus was prompted by two factors: estimates that suggested that 26 percent of voters in the 1976 presidential election would be over 60 and Ford's concern that Medicaid and Medicare were inadequate to support catastrophic illnesses. Perhaps as a response to Butler's criticisms of the 1971 conference, one of Ford's campaign spots, "Aged Health Care," reinforced the message that the president had "sensitivity, concern, [and] a willingness to listen and to act."[9] The advertisement portrayed a series of fulfilling lives that contrasted with the typically negative portrayal of the elderly in commercials for prescription drugs. However, it sidestepped issues of nutrition, housing, and transportation and failed to address why so little of the National Institute of Mental Health budget had been allocated to the task of improving mental health or research on aging.[10]

Ford's campaign spot offers evidence that the administration was concerned about the effects of inflation on the finances of many seniors. At the heart of this reform was a proposal for catastrophic health insurance whereby anyone over 65 covered by Medicare would pay no more than $500 a year for hospital or home care and no more than $250 in doctor's bills.[11] The president first announced this program in January 1976, but it met with general opposition on Capitol Hill. Senator Edward Kennedy was particularly critical, arguing that only 1 percent of the elderly would benefit and that the rebate would drain $2 billion out of Medicare.[12]

Although Ford claimed that 3 million seniors would benefit from insurance for catastrophic illnesses, he conflated the economics of healthcare with the actual healthcare needs of the elderly. President Reagan echoed this calculation in 1988 when he offered an injection of funds into Medicare to protect personal finances in the face of catastrophic illness with the Medicare Catastrophic Coverage Act.[13] However, by 1983 it was estimated that a third of seniors were receiving inadequate care, a fact that suggests that Ford's and Reagan's actions were too little too late. (The 1988 act was deeply unpopular and was repealed by Congress within sixteen months.)[14] This was certainly the opinion of Maggie Kuhn who, inspired by Simone de Beauvoir's recent book on public perceptions of the elderly, *The Coming of Age*, was raising awareness of aging as a universal condition and not the sole province of the old or infirm, as captured in the Gray Panthers' slogan "Age and Youth in Action."[15] This perspective echoed new research on the physiology and psychology of aging, such as the work at Duke University on the correlation between high blood pressure and senility and the effects of aging on the nervous system. Even preliminary research revealed that the health challenges the elderly faced could not be adequately addressed in simple policy terms.[16]

Unless a disease is of epidemic proportions—such as drug use in the early 1970s or the spread of AIDS during the 1980s—the federal government has rarely taken into full account the social impact of illness, rather than its economic impact. Perhaps because of this, President Carter argued that the previous nine years had been a time of "inaction" and an unwillingness to provide basic rights for the elderly, a tone that echoed Butler's conclusion in *Why Survive?* that "the tragedy of old age is reinforced by inaction."[17] This response to the half-hearted policies of the Nixon-Ford years was a major stimulus for Carter's Commission on Mental Health and for the revitalization of home care and halfway houses as alternatives to long-term hospitalization. Carter's healthcare plans went much farther than Ford's single campaign issue of insurance to cover catastrophic care, but Carter did not speak about the challenges seniors faced at a time when dementia was being touted as the fourth or fifth highest cause of mortality.[18] These estimates revealed that 1 million Americans were living with what was at the time called severe senile dementia and another 3 million had mild to moderate dementia. These startling statistics were presented in a 1978 study that suggested that research efforts needed to step up to address this looming health crisis.[19]

To explore how the politics of aging and medical research on age-related conditions intersected during the mid-1970s and in the following years, this chapter links three perspectives. First, I examine the federal response to age-related care and the expanding population over 65. Second, I discuss the neurological, medical, and psychiatric understanding of the complex etiology of dementia and Alzheimer's, which became the most visible form of dementia in the 1980s. Finally, I explore cultural texts that focus on debilitating conditions, profound memory loss, and the often-devastating effect of dementia on families and caregivers. In this way, I follow the pioneering work of sociologist Stephen Katz, who argued in the 1990s that only a multidisciplinary view of aging can do justice to the role of medicine and to broader sociocultural factors that inform gerontological knowledge.[20]

To address these factors, this chapter includes a consideration of two texts by famous writers: *Awakenings* (1973), Oliver Sacks's neurological account of a community of aging patients, and Philip Roth's *Patrimony* (1997), a personal exploration of Roth's midlife depression and his father's worsening condition because of a brain tumor. The early discussion focuses on age-related dementia, while later sections include three powerful yet contrasting evocations of Alzheimer's: Patti Davis's diary *The Long Goodbye* (2005), in which she wrestles with her father Ronald Reagan's Alzheimer's after it became public in 1994; Canadian writer Michael Ignatieff's *Scar Tissue* (1993), a semi-fictionalized account of his mother's Alzheimer's; and Amy Tan's 2001 transcultural novel *The Bonesetter's Daughter*, in which a daughter struggles to understand her mother's Chinese past as she learns to care for her in new ways. Instead of echoing Christopher Lasch's jeremiad on the superfluity of the elderly in the 1970s, these texts explore both the capacity and limitations of narrative for preserving (at times even reviving) chaotic and diminishing voices as well as the medical and interpersonal problems that ensue when language and memory lose coherence.[21] We have seen fissures in the war and drug narratives of the previous two chapters, but the ontological implications of the capacity to tell cohesive stories are weightier in cases of dementia.[22]

Aging and Mental Health

It is unfair to suggest that the Ford administration was interested only in the economics of healthcare. Ford's secretary of health, education, and welfare, Forrest David Mathews, was keen to focus on "the normal physiological changes occurring with age" and "the social, cultural, and economic environment in which the elderly live."[23] In line with Butler's claim that "good mental health in old age . . . means the capacity to thrive rather than simply survive" and Gail Sheehy's developmental view of the life cycle in her widely read 1976 book *Passages*, Matthews switched emphasis away from infirmity and toward physical fitness and self-care.[24] This view chimed with clinical trials in West Germany that suggested that physical training programs could slow aging, increase work performance, and reduce family medical costs, three factors that led to a 1975 reissue of the U.S. federal brochure *The Fitness Challenge . . . in the Later Years.*[25] In addition to commissioning further research on physical and dynamic fitness ("the resources to move vigorously, to do, to live energetically"), the aim of the newly formed National Institute on Aging was to look more holistically at the health issues seniors faced.[26]

The Ford administration gave little attention to mental health, though, perhaps because of the lack of research that could easily determine to what extent such issues were neurological or psychological. Geriatric initiatives at five dedicated university centers on aging were beginning to provide a more nuanced picture of the illnesses the elderly were susceptible to, but research was still moving slowly, particularly on dementia. Two pioneers of gerontology helped galvanize new projects in this field. Carl Eisdorfer, a New York-trained psychiatrist, had coordinated a project on blood pressure and senility at Duke University's Center for the Study of Aging and Human Development before moving in the mid-1980s to the Institute for the Study of Aging at Miami University, where his research turned to stress, dementia, and depression. In between these posts, Eisdorfer worked alongside the pioneering neurologist Robert Katzman at the Albert Einstein College of Medicine, part of Yeshiva University in the Bronx, which had opened in 1955 following President Truman commitment to expanding medical facilities (it was the first new medical school in New York since 1897). Eisdorfer's and Katzman's research into the hidden realities of aging did not extend far into the public sphere at the time (except for a January 1978 interview with Katzman on WNBC-TV), but it profoundly influenced medical research and social policy in the following decades. This helped raise the profile of Alzheimer's from a variant of senility to what Jesse Ballenger describes as a key facet of the "health politics of anguish."[27]

The third White House Conference on Aging, which was planned under the Carter administration and held in the winter of 1981, did little to increase public awareness of Alzheimer's.[28] Instead of profiling specific medical conditions, the conference focused on economic security and productivity, although there were differing views of what they meant. On the one side, the Leadership Council of Aging Organizations called loudly for a coordinated national health policy and Carl Eisdorfer argued that the system was failing 85 percent of seniors with mental health needs.[29] On the other side, Reagan's health secretary Richard Schweiker envisioned more private-public alliances and planned for the conference to be more interactive than the previous two, linking to both the National Institute of Aging plan *Toward an Independent Old Age* and to the goals of the World Health Organization in better supporting the elderly.[30] However, the event did not prove to be consequential. There was little discussion that directly addressed mental health beyond general stress factors, improving services, and the promotion of self-help and mutual help groups, even though the conference briefing notes stressed that aging "is urgent and will become critical in the coming years."[31] More influential was the advocacy work of the Alzheimer's Disease Society (founded in 1978) and the Alzheimer's Association (founded in 1981) and research on ethical issues relating to aging at the Harvard Medical School (which informed second-wave feminist Betty Friedan's 1993 book *The Fountain of Age*). But perhaps most significant in terms of public awareness was the Alzheimer's-related death of movie star Rita Hayworth in May 1987 after six years in her daughter's care and Ronald Reagan's dramatic announcement of his illness in 1994, which led to the founding of the Ronald and Nancy Reagan Research Institute as an affiliate of the Alzheimer's Association.[32]

Media coverage of the disease started to pick up in the mid-1980s, but the first national conference on Alzheimer's had been held as early as 1977 in Bethesda, Maryland, with the intention of profiling the disease as "the major cause of dementia in the elderly in developed countries" and as something that was distinct from the normal aging process.[33] Alzheimer's disease had first been identified by the German psychiatrist Alois Alzheimer seventy years earlier yet had fallen out of medical parlance, mainly because of confusion about whether plaque in the brain was part of the normal process of aging or a symptom of pathology.[34] Psychiatric nomenclature did not help, at least not until the third edition of *DSM* in 1980, when dementia became a category in its own right, succeeding the broad neurogenerative category "organic brain syndrome" of the first edition in 1952.[35] The decline of psychoanalysis in the late 1970s and the rise of neurological and genetic research into organic brain structures helps explain this shift, which led to a more systematic approach to dementia based on autopsies, drug research, and a series of clinical trials. By 1978, the National Institute on Aging had accepted Alzheimer's as a disease in its own right, even if it was aligned with metabolic changes and was sometimes confused with depression.

Two theories of Alzheimer's were still nascent in the 1970s. Following Alois Alzheimer's early research, neurologists saw the disease as stemming from neuropathology in the brain, whereas the group that later became known as "entanglement theorists" thought it was inflected by biological, psychological, and sociological processes that lent unique qualities to the experience of each sufferer.[36] Both groups of theorists focused on the amyloid plaques and neurofibrillary tangles that distinguished Alzheimer's from other types of dementia, but the second group looked beyond neuropathology, partly because the provenance of the abnormalities and their effect on behavior and cognition was far from clear. It was generally agreed that the aging brain tends to lose its flexibility, but this was accompanied by a realization that separating out the "aging process from the diseases and other environmental factors that accompany it" was a tricky matter.[37]

Of particular importance was communication between patients and medical researchers, both for understanding dementia from the inside and for providing data for longitudinal studies. Although partial memory loss was a common feature, this was not unique to Alzheimer's or to other forms of dementia. The patchiness of case histories did not help researchers identify unique neurological patterns, while the speed and intensity that marked many cases meant that it was difficult to look beyond specifics, apart from noting the presence of plaques and neurofibrillary tangles. Contributory factors—"occupational exposures, family history, diet, cigarette or alcohol use, and history of infectious diseases"—could not be reliably gleaned from speaking to the patient, particularly as many elderly patients of the 1970s had been children or teenagers when medical recording keeping was in its infancy.[38] Meaningful dialogue was easier in cases where dementia was detected early, yet it was quite often undiagnosed until a significant change in functionality identified the patient as needing medical or palliative attention.[39] Deinstitutionalization in the late 1960s and 1970s meant that fewer long-term inpatients could be closely observed, and the chances of early detection among individuals in rural and minority communities remained slim.

The trope of the diminished voice returns us to the primary theme of this book and points to the paradox that dementia was an intensely private disease that often had a public face. Patients are often unaware of their condition or their awareness is submerged in an inability to structure sentences or link short-term and long-term memories. Whereas narrative medicine offered a potential lifeline for veterans with war trauma and those whose egos had become distorted through sustained alcohol and drug use, it often proved ineffectual for patients for whom words and memories were disappearing. This was particularly true among the very elderly (towards whom Butler claimed that psychiatrists often displayed "a sense of futility and therapeutic nihilism") and for complex cases in which alcohol-related disease intersected with metabolic and neurological changes.[40] The quest for an authentic voice is very tangled when it comes to organic brain disease, especially (but not exclusively) among the elderly.

I will return to the macro-concepts touched on here: communication, voice, knowledge, and memory. But before looking at specific case studies, both neurological and literary, it is worth pausing to see how the mental health of the elderly was being dealt with in the cultural sphere. While Butler claimed in 1975 that the media often ignored the elderly, this began to change in the years following his book *Why Survive?*, albeit slowly.[41] Butler adamantly stated that all physicians should understand the natural process of aging instead of equating it with senescence or disintegration. Nevertheless, writers and filmmakers tend to be drawn to dementia because, as film historian Sally Chivers notes, it magnifies "what people fear most about how age could manifest itself—that is, in an apparent loss of sense and self."[42] This trend was more prominent in the 1990s, when Alzheimer's was becoming more widely recognized and postmodern writers such as Paul Auster were exploring themes of memory loss and unknowing. However, there are examples from the "pre-Alzheimer's period," such as Toni Morrison's *Sula* (1977), Canadian author Alice Munro's short story cycle *Who Do You Think You Are?* (1978), and Illinois writer Janet Majerus's 1976 novel *Grandpa and Joey*, which focuses on the emotional bond between an infirm grandparent with dementia and his high-spirited granddaughter. Written for a young readership, Majerus describes Grandpa's condition in simplistic terms (after a stroke "his whole left side quit working and he could only mumble") and tones down medical language ("the mind kind of wears out . . . he's not as sharp as he used to be, and he's slowing down").[43]

Predating by four years one of Henry Fonda's defining performances as a retired professor in the 1981 movie *On Golden Pond*, Fonda played Grandpa George McDermott in *Home to Stay*, a Canadian-financed film adaptation of Majerus's novel. The opening is set on a farm in rural Illinois and focuses on Grandpa's infirmity and his son's intention of sending him to a nursing home. Refusing to believe that her infirm Grandpa is mentally deficient, his granddaughter Sarah and her friend abduct him with the intention of driving to Chicago, where she is convinced that the family doctor will declare him to be in good psychological shape. Neither the book nor the film adaptation offer deep insights into the psychology or neurology of dementia, but they highlight the common experience that a family member often becomes the surrogate voice and memory of the aging parent or grandparent. This is the case in Rosalie Walsh Honel's *Journey with Grandpa* (1988), which documents her grandfather's decline from Alzheimer's over seven years and the profound effects on her family and home life. These texts also point to the value of listening to the aged—as a 1978 book on nursing described it, both "to learn about gerontology and geriatrics" in clinical terms and to understand the tangled language of aging from an intimate perspective.[44]

Another, more compelling, literary account of the trials of old age focuses on the mid-1980s, when the narrator is facing his own worries about growing old. Philip Roth's *Patrimony* links his depression at the age of 54 with the decline of his father, Herman Roth, who developed a brain tumor in 1987. Philip Roth mentioned his own depression as the stimulus for his first autobiographical account, *The Facts: A Novelist's Autobiography* (1988), and he refracted anxiety and pain through his fictional alter ego Nathan Zuckerman in the 1983 novel *The Anatomy Lesson*. His second autobiography, *Patrimony*, has a different primary focus: Roth's challenging and tragicomic relationship with his aging father, which Roth tells through memories, stories, and family encounters. The account centers on the hearing loss and partial paralysis of the face that Herman experiences when they decide he is too frail to undergo brain surgery.[45] The anguish that Roth detects in his father reflects his own struggle with middle age, exacerbated by fears that Herman might become like a zombie and lose the power of expression.[46] Although the role of primary caregiver places a significant strain on Roth, it also keeps alive his father's spirit more effectively than consigning him to a care home would have done.

This fear that identity is in danger of collapsing or being hollowed out in the face of dementia is expressed beautifully in the opening pages of Robert Gard's semi-fictional book *Beyond the Thin Line* (1992). Gard explores the diminishing lifeworld of a World War II veteran, Harry McDare, whose memories of war blur with the realities of being an inpatient with dementia after he has been referred to a nursing home by the Veterans Administration. Whereas Herman Roth and George McDermott retain their mobility, at least until the latter stages of their lives, Harry's internment in a German POW camp as a young man is replayed through his hospitalized incarceration many years later. The narrator worries that seniors like Harry are often "left to find their own way through the perplexity of places from which they will not escape." Harry tries hard to prevent his identity from disintegrating into a series of temporal fragments.[47]

Beyond the Thin Line strives to recreate a lost life through a form of "assisted identity."[48] The narrator is encouraged that Harry seems to derive pleasure from talking and sees his role as a co-investigator, supplying an imaginative element that has been lost amid Harry's plaques and tangles. He tries to be as faithful as possible to the old man's past and is sensitive to the ontological implications of Alzheimer's—confusion, frustration, entrapment, a longing for home—yet he also realizes that his narrative re-creation might be "utterly wrong" and that communication is fraught and sometimes meaningless. The reconstructed story of Harry's life demonstrates a sensitivity to both the benefits and restrictions of being a long-term inpatient. The book hovers between recognizing the patient's helplessness in the face of worsening dementia and taking heart from the flashes of insight and vitality that punctuate Harry's day-to-day existence. It is to this situated sense of the trials of old age and the challenges of long-term institutionalization that I now turn, before returning to intimate portrayals of Alzheimer's later in the chapter.

A Brief Awakening

One of the most dramatic descriptions of elderly patients experiencing a renewed sense of hope is *Awakenings*, British émigré neurologist Oliver Sacks's account of an experimental procedure for treating severe cases of Parkinson's disease and another example of the tangle of neurological, physiological, and psychological issues. The story came to light early in 1972 with the publication of Sacks's article "The Great Awakening" in the British magazine *The Listener*, which was followed by the full text the next year. The encounter begins in the mid-1960s, when Sacks was working as a chronic-care consultant at Beth Abraham Hospital in the Bronx and as an instructor at the Albert Einstein College of Medicine. His clinical work focused on a group of elderly patients, all of whom had developed a form of encephalitis lethargica in the late 1910s and early 1920s as a result of the influenza pandemic that caused devastation on both sides of the Atlantic. Many recovered and returned to regular working lives but developed profound neurological difficulties later in life. *Awakenings* was Sacks's attempt to document the case histories—or, as he calls them, "clinical tales"—of twenty of his patients as he grappled with a set of neurological and psychiatric symptoms that defied conventional forms of rehabilitative treatment.

Although the patients shared similar illness experiences in early life, they tended to polarize around the spasms, tics and states of high animation associated with Parkinson's at one extreme and an almost catatonic state of non-animation at the other. Both poles concerned Sacks, but the torpid patients affected him most because they seemed to be ontologically bereft, "insubstantial as ghosts, and as passive as zombies."[49] As a clinician who was critical of the taut medical formats that had been designed to record patients' symptoms, he thought that storytelling was a necessary complement to an experimental procedure involving the psychoactive drug L-DOPA that had the potential to compensate for a natural deficiency in the neurotransmitter dopamine. The procedure was risky, but such was the catatonic state of the patients that Sacks thought it was a risk worth taking. The central section of *Awakenings* centers on the physiological and psychological reactions of the patients to the course of L-DOPA. When it was first administered in summer 1969, this seemed to be the kind of wonder drug that harked back to the pharmaceutical breakthroughs of the 1950s. Sacks's case studies illustrate both the health-giving properties of L-DOPA and its side effects, meaning that these are drug narratives as well as accounts of an experimental medical procedure.

The book is remarkable for combining a close empirical study of a group of elderly patients with differing symptoms of Parkinson's and its attention to personal stories. Written a decade before the journal *Literature and Medicine* started to explore the interface between medical inquiry and storytelling, Sacks adopts a "double approach" of narrative and reflection, mixed with a "proliferation of images and metaphors . . . remarks, repetitions, asides and footnotes."[50] Taking his cue from existential psychology, Sacks avoided viewing his patients simply as biophysical systems in favor of discerning and representing their "landscapes of being."[51] His work embodies the ethical imperative of approaching the patient with what literary critic Amelia DeFalco calls the "careful balance of empathy and respect," especially those who have lost command of their life stories.[52]

Sacks includes the patients' own accounts in the narrative whenever possible, but he also raises ontological questions about their state of being and epistemological questions about how a physician can know the condition of those who lack an obvious voice. This makes the case studies twice-told tales, in which the patient's and clinician's accounts complement each other. Sacks was aware that a straightforward empirical account of the patients would be insufficient for understanding how a spectrum of Parkinson's symptoms had developed or for recording the patients' responses to L-DOPA. For this reason, he treats their stories as open accounts and avoids overly clinical language. He was aware, too, that this is not what was expected of a neurologist, as his approach had more in common with psychoanalyst Roy Schafer's techniques (as discussed in the introduction) than a medical account of neurological dysfunction. In his 1983 and 1992 books *The Analytic Attitude* and *Retelling a Life*, Schafer argues that the Freudian endeavor to reconstitute a forgotten or repressed past can often be a wild goose chase because a life history has multiple strands and cannot easily be resolved into a singular account. This quest is even more acute for patients who find speaking difficult or are experiencing profound memory loss. Lacunae and lapses do not mean that those narrative strands have been extinguished, though: Sacks and Schafer agreed that the analyst and patient must together construct a history whenever possible, but in a "more provisional" manner than the typical medical account.[53]

The previous chapters have shown the difficulty of retrieving the authentic voice of traumatized war veterans and drug addicts from a mass of psychological and physiological factors. This difficulty is more acute in *Awakenings* as the elderly patients are unable to sustain a narrative perspective even within the window of self-awareness that L-DOPA stimulates, when to the doctor's surprise they burst back into life after years of virtual silence. What Sacks provides is the means of linking scraps of autobiographical information and incomplete memories with case-study documentation. It is important that these are not isolated patients' stories: the book highlights the hospitalized community and takes pains to recount twenty stories of the fifty individuals who emerged "from the decades-long isolation their illness had imposed on them."[54] Sacks emphasizes the limited methods by which the patients can remain "alive and human in a Total Institution."[55]

The first case study in *Awakenings* focuses on Frances D., who had contracted encephalitis in 1919 while in high school. She recovered with some lingering respiratory and oculogyric problems but then developed post-encephalitic symptoms in the 1950s that caused her to both freeze and hurry in her movements and her speech. By the time Frances was admitted to the hospital in 1969 in her mid-60s, her condition had worsened to the extent that she was unable to walk or hold her body upright and had a tendency to flail her limbs. Sacks realized that Frances's restlessness could be quelled only by occupying her hands. This was not so easily achieved, though, particularly as her handwriting varied between extremes of pulsion and festination, resulting either in chaotic scrawl or writing that became "smaller and slower and stickier until it became a motionless point."[56] Her face took on a mask-like expression too, but Sacks balanced this observation by pointing out that she was always punctual and could empathize with others on the ward who had similar conditions.

Once L-DOPA was administered to Frances, Sacks found that she was able to channel her kinetic energy into pedal movement, had more coherent speech patterns, and possessed a greater sense of well-being. The drug hastened further respiratory crises, though, and quickly became both a regulator and a lifeline. Symptoms of addiction led Sacks to consider discontinuing the medication, but when Frances protested, he agreed to a half-way dose. The scientific reasons for doing so were in tension with the ethical imperative because Sacks realized that the drug stimulated "releases or exposures or disclosures or confessions of very deep and ancient parts of herself," as if latent parts of Frances's personality sprang to life in virtually uncontrollable ways.[57] Although Frances's story was one of a remarkable awakening, it was also a "labyrinth" of complex and bewildering factors from which there often seemed to be "no exit."[58]

Perhaps realizing that he was in danger of becoming lost in the labyrinth himself, in the final section of the account, "Summer 1972," Sacks retreated to a point of professional concern, noting that the struggle of 1969 had served to "temper" Frances rather than break her. He administered a lower dose of L-DOPA, which caused a milder version of the sequence of "improvement–exacerbation–withdrawal symptoms." By that time, Frances was able to predict the approaching stages.[59] He also realized that non-invasive techniques could help her regain composure, particularly "shapely" and "legato" music that enabled her to channel excessive energy and coordinate movement. This was not exactly what Arthur Frank in his 1995 book *The Wounded Storyteller* calls a "restitution narrative," but the account is upbeat in its suggestion that Frances found a healthier balance than she had for many years.[60]

The most famous patient narrative of *Awakenings* is that of Leonard L., partly because it was recreated in a 1990 film in which Robert De Niro plays the patient to Robin Williams's character study of Sacks (the film renames him Dr. Sayer).

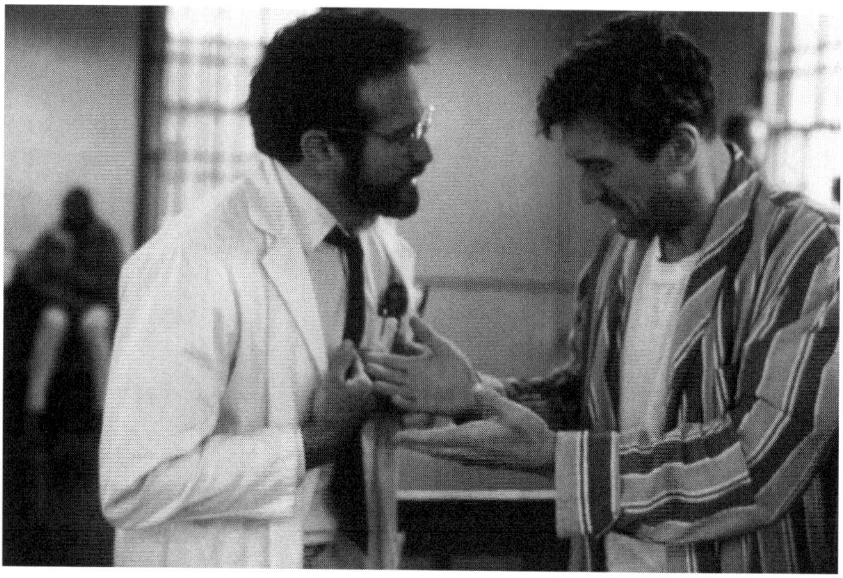

Figure 4.2 Dr. Sayer (Robin Williams) resorts to personal and drug interventions to rouse Leonard (Robert De Niro) from his catatonia in *Awakenings* (dir. Penny Marshall, 1990). Columbia / The Kobal Collection / Louis Goldman.

As was the case with Frances, L-DOPA opened up Leonard's ability to articulate his inner world after fifteen years of silence. Leonard was only 46 when Sacks started treating him in 1966, but he was more mummified than Frances: his rigidity was severe, his face was masked, and his voice was toneless. His only means of communication was a letter board on which he painfully tapped out phrases in "an abbreviated, telegraphic, and sometimes cryptic form," whereas L-DOPA stimulated his voice and a new sense of life.[61] But there is was downside. He displayed symptoms of what Sacks terms "over-abundance" that become more exaggerated once the initial benefits of L-DOPA wore off, leading to a "pathological driving and fragmentation," messianic delusions, and a promiscuous sexual drive.[62] Sacks commented that Leonard soon became "completely decomposed," and only his autobiography, which he tapped out on his writing machine, gave a pattern to his excessive energy. Just as music gave Frances moments of coordination, so the letter board presented Leonard with a creative channel for expressing his "floods of sexual phantasy, jokes, [and] pseudo-reminiscences."[63]

Whereas the side effects Frances experienced on L-DOPA were simply worrying, Leonard's side effects were violent and potentially dangerous, and Sacks sometimes had to use restraining measures. Eventually he resolved to discontinue the drug and found that Leonard returns to a "cool" state of composure that he seemed to accept as more manageable than uncontainable feelings of overexuberance. Both the doctor and patient realized that the drug was both an elixir and a poison and that the therapeutic benefits were sometimes overwhelmed by deleterious side effects. Leonard managed to convey this through his writing board, and although he was profoundly saddened by the fact that the awakening could not be sustained, his narrative ended in triumphant self-affirmation: "I've broken through barriers which I had all my life. And now, I'll stay myself, and you can keep your L-DOPA."[64] Once again a wonder drug proved to be inadequate in and of itself, but the interpersonal contact between Sacks and Leonard and the use of a cultural outlet (Leonard's writing board, Frances's music) for releasing expressive energies means that the patients' voices can be heard strongly amid the medical and institutional detail.

The other case studies in *Awakenings* have common themes, yet they are all marked by the individuality of response to both the post-encephalitic symptoms and to the L-DOPA treatment. It is this variation of response that makes *Awakenings* a multivocal text, even though Sacks sometimes had to supply more of his voice than he would have liked, especially when the patients built up a tolerance to the drug and found that their awakening was only a briefly expressive moment. The importance of *Awakenings* is that it overlays the patient's narrative with the humanistic belief that the individual survives despite the ravages of illness and that reality persists for them even if it cannot be expressed. In *Awakenings*, Sacks tested his belief that scientific and imaginative elements are equally essential in medical research with a group of patients who are highly unlikely to reach a point where they can regain a stable version of their former lives. This does not diminish the significance of their briefly reactivated voices, in terms both of neurological enquiry and within their own life stories.

By way of a coda to this section, it is worth pausing on Sacks's best-known text, *The Man Who Mistook His Wife for a Hat* (1985) and its important contribution to narrative medicine. In this series of clinical tales, Sacks relied on metaphors and imagery to bring to life a range of conditions marked by excess, deficiency, and altered perceptions. The most interesting are those that deal with the effects of memory loss. These include Jimmy G. ("The Lost Mariner"), who suffers from "alcoholic degeneration" of his brain's limbic system and cannot sustain a conversation, and William Thompson ("A Matter of Identity") who is diagnosed with Korsakoff syndrome (which was reclassified as "alcohol amnestic disorder" in *DSM-III*) to such a degree that he lives in a continual present. In William's case, overexuberance does not manifest itself in aggression or overt forms of sexuality but through "ceaseless tales, his confabulations, his mythomania."[65] The neurologist detects both "quasi-coherence" in the patient's "confabulations" and a loss of self, as William is seemingly unaware of how fractured his narratives have become.[66] Discerning "ceaseless inner pressure" hovering beneath William's proliferation of stories, Sacks senses that he is tacitly aware of the "meaninglessness, the chaos that yawns continually beneath him."[67] In this way, William embodies the paradox of a patient who has both too much and too little voice. But the two cases also raise fundamental questions about chaos and meaning that go well beyond the sphere of health and were reflected in Alzheimer's narratives of the mid-1990s, a time when Sacks published another set of clinical tales as *The Anthropologist on Mars*.

The Private Life of a President

The highest-profile case of Alzheimer's was, of course, that of President Reagan. Signs of memory loss were arguably evident in Reagan's first term in the White House and became more obvious in his second term. There were two health scares during his eight years in office: a punctured lung from the bullet shot by John Hinckley Jr. in March 1981 and an operation on his colon in 1985, when Vice-President Bush was given presidential powers for nearly eight hours during and immediately after the operation. On the campaign trail five years earlier, Reagan had announced that he would not remain in office if his relatively illness-free life caught up with him, and, apart from these incidents, he stayed physically fit while he was in Washington. It is significant that Reagan's Alzheimer's was not diagnosed until late 1993, and his family was keen to maintain that it had had no deleterious effects on his presidential decisions. His 1990 autobiography *An American Life* even credits his memory as one of his strengths, describing how in public speeches he would shorten words on prompt cards and that he only needed to write three or four words to be able to remember an anecdote or a joke.[68] His single admission was that he feels he was not "very good at remembering faces and names" during public speaking engagements and while interacting with White House employees.[69] This, of course, is endemic to public life, but Reagan's hearing loss (an issue he did not mention in his autobiography) was a hindrance and he was forced to adopt avoidance strategies to circumvent the embarrassment of having to ask someone's name or of getting it wrong.

He mentioned his health only once, saying that at 65 he did not feel his age, which led him to accept the swell of opinion in his nearly successful run for the Republican Party nomination in 1976. Nancy Reagan's autobiography *My Turn* (1989) also largely avoids the issue of her husband's health but instead criticizes gossip in the press and the knee-jerk reaction of the stock market to empty rumors about the president's age.[70] Incidents where Reagan made public gaffes or appeared disoriented when asked complex questions fueled rumors that he had a feed in his ear, as satirized by Robin Williams on *Saturday Night Live* in 1986. In Williams's skit, the messages coming through to him through his earpiece during a press conference get scrambled. Ronald Reagan Jr. later claimed that early signs of dementia were evident in his father's floundering response during the first presidential debate with Walter Mondale on 7 October 1984, when he was "uncharacteristically lost for words," particularly during his closing statement.[71] However, if Alzheimer's affected Reagan's ability in office, it probably was not until late in his second term, in 1987–88. The family believed that the onset of his dementia stemmed from a fall from a horse in 1989, when he sustained moderately severe head injuries. This date is significant because it preserves the Reagan presidency and coincides with the year that George H. W. Bush was stressing that the nation needed to renew its "moral contract with our senior citizens" and "those in the shadow of life."[72]

Reagan disappeared from public life after Richard Nixon's funeral in June 1994. In November of that year, he wrote an open letter announcing that "I am one of the millions of Americans who will be afflicted with Alzheimer's disease" and reminding the nation that the disease weighs heavily on a family perhaps more than the individual.[73] Signing off with the line "I now begin the journey that will lead me into the sunset of my life" but affirming that the country had a "bright dawn ahead," Reagan's voice went silent. Consequently, we have no first-person account of his later years. The publication of the correspondence between Ronald and Nancy in 2000, *I Love You Ronnie*, does not offer many insights into the ways onset dementia in the 1980s or full Alzheimer's in the 1990s affected Reagan's memories, moods, and daily functioning. Nancy writes about her initial ignorance of the disease and how she quickly learned to cope, but she also emphasizes that this was a physical disease and did not warrant the stigma that still surrounded mental illness, a year after the White House held its first conference on that topic. She clearly wrote the book so the public would remember the warmth and charisma of the fortieth president as he entered a terminal stage that led to his death four years later at age 93.

The most important insight into the development of Reagan's dementia and those four silent years was by his daughter Patricia, who was a controversial figure throughout the White House years. Patti Davis had already published *Home Front* in 1986, a lightly fictionalized account of her life as the eldest of Ronald and Nancy's two children, and the controversial *The Way I See It* in 1992, a year before her father's Alzheimer's was confirmed. She had been outspoken about her father's conservative politics, and she returned to the subject in her haunting reflection on his later years, *The Long Goodbye*.

The book spans eighteen months, from April 1995 to October 1996, plus a single entry for February 1997 and a few final thoughts added during the week of her father's death in June 2004, prior to publication late that summer. The journal is partly a document of the emotional journey of a father-daughter relationship that had become strained by Davis's outspoken comments, but it is also an account of her delving deep to rescue something lost in childhood and an attempt to "come together lovingly, peacefully, and sadly" with Nancy Reagan after "many years of a chilly, dispiriting war," in which she had accused her mother of cruel treatment and of taking tranquillizers regularly, even into the 1980s, when the First Lady was the face of the Just Say No campaign.[74] Davis saw the campaign as hypocritical because her mother closed her eyes to prescription drug dependency; she hears behind her mother's anti-drug slogan "the soft voice of a victim and the louder voice of denial."[75]

The Long Goodbye is a book driven by an impulse to put differences aside in the face of a devastating disease about which there were few narratives when Davis began her journal entries. Written with enough tenderness and honest reflection to suggest that she was not just cashing in on her father's death, the book is a meditation of time stretching ahead and time running out: she comments in the preface that "Alzheimer's disease locks all the doors and exits. There is no reprieve, no escape. Time becomes the enemy, and it seemed to stretch out in front of us like miles of fallow land."[76] Compared to the narrative trajectories discussed in the previous two chapters, where loss, trauma, unreliability, and deception characterize war and drug stories, this is an encounter, at least from the family's perspective, of "long stretches of waiting—waiting for things to get worse, or end." In the arc of Alzheimer's disease, the patient tends to plateau but then suddenly sinks to another slightly less capable level that demands an ever-increasing level of care.

For a daughter who remembers her active father swimming and horse riding, this is a strange kind of grieving process in which she is forced to deal with the slow diminishment of a life. As she looks around his beloved ranch north of Santa Barbara, she muses that her father is both present and absent. In the later stages of the illness he was incapable of even registering the national trauma of 9/11. However, Davis believed that although Alzheimer's attacks almost all aspects of an individual's higher and lower functioning, it "can never cross the boundaries of the soul." She sees his spirit everywhere on the ranch and describes wordless conversation between them, yet the journal forces her to keep faith in a life that is not yet over. She quickly dismisses the possibility that this is wish fulfilment, even though she plays the little girl at times, seeking her father's attention when she knows he cannot give it. Perhaps her decision to break off the journal was an acceptance of reality, or an inability to face the lower level to which her father was sinking, or a realization that the moments of mutual recognition that gave Sacks joy when he saw life return to his patients were no more.

The element of reconciliation in the journal is very strong. As a teenager of the 1960s, Davis's personal beliefs were very different from those of her parents. She reflects on one incident at the Peace Sunday anti-nuclear rally of 6 June 1982 in Pasadena. Because Davis went on stage soon after Rev. Jesse Jackson made personal criticisms of her father, many concert-goers and the press saw her short speech as an assault on her father's presidency. These tensions continued into the 1990s, and Davis began her journal only three years after the controversial publication of *The Way I See It*, with its accusation that her mother had been abusive and her father neglectful.[77] She recognizes that her journal cannot undo her past conflict with her parents, which she admits was fueled "by my arrogance and my youth" as much as her liberal political convictions.[78] Now, in place of the "rigid silences" between parents and daughter, her father's eyes "frequently look beyond us" through no fault of his own and she realizes that "my penance is the words left unsaid."[79]

The journal does not try to grapple with the clinical details of Alzheimer's. In fact, Davis states that she does not want "my thoughts to be cluttered with other people's impressions, or with medical predictions and evaluations."[80] She swings away from a medical account toward the more ontological orientation of *Awakenings*, using her journal to meditate on language, love, and loss and to evoke what she calls the "mysterious choreography" of Alzheimer's.[81] These themes push her writing in two directions: an attempt to make sense of the present and a reanimation of her father's voice that leads her to examine the dynamics of time, which becomes paradoxically elongated and compressed. She tries to look at the world from his perspective, but the loss nags at her and she feels she is in a state of limbo in which time "might just be standing still, stalling, lurching forward unevenly, or not at all."[82]

The chief technique for making sense of temporal disorientation is the act of storytelling: sometimes these are small stories that crouch in the corners of daily life or are triggered by photographs, and other times larger stories encompassing a whole life or a generation. One of Davis's cherished memories is of her father as a storyteller who combined folk wisdom (she associates this with his family's Irish ancestry), an affinity with nature, and an eye for a choice phrase that contributed to his reputation as the Great Communicator. The conversations about "life lessons," nature, and folklore that enraptured her as a child have been usurped by more mundane conversations with her mother about arrangements and how to handle the media.[83] Memories are not always comforting as she winces at her outspoken behavior and recalls being strung out on drugs and contemplating suicide as a 19-year-old. However, a palpable sense of nostalgia runs through the entries, not just for a carefree world of childhood but of a simpler time before the 1970s, when even the Los Angeles air seemed cleaner. Davis's grasp of making sense through words, images, and stories stems from her instinct to write as a child, when she learned to hide her compositions from a mother she found to be prying and dismissive of her inner world. In her 1990s journal entries, she reflects that once again "writing became my lifeline, something beyond choice, something vital, but at times destructive," yet she also claims, perhaps surprisingly, that she is writing for both herself and her mother.[84]

The most evocative element of the journal is Davis's meditation on voice and words. She finds both supreme irony and profound sadness in a phrase her father used in his speech at the 1988 Republican National Convention: "as long as words don't leave me."[85] The line was intended to convey undying loyalty to the nation, but it played out cruelly over the next decade in his enforced retreat from public life. Words are often profound and indelible for Davis. Reflecting on her public criticisms of her father's policies in the 1980s, she recognizes that words can also be loud and hurtful. Yet at other times they are flimsy and inadequate, reminiscent of the "Popsicle-stick forts I used to build as a child—they're good until a wind blows in." While she finds comfort in the meaningful silences she shares with her father, there is also a groping for words that can give meaning or "words we were just about to say but couldn't, because we got there too late."[86] The themes of helplessness and belatedness run through the journal, yet so too does a belief in an emotional language that lies beyond words and taps into a deeper reality. Even when her father's voice is completely silent and he gulps for air in his last few days, Davis hangs on to her faith in an untarnished spirit, which she believes is vindicated when her father meets her mother's gaze just seconds before dying.

Given the private nature of Davis's reflections, this is also a public testimony in which she reminds the world that her father's humanity cannot be defined by what many liberals of Davis's generation saw as a backward lurch to the Right in the 1980s. She encloses the story within the family circle, wanting the media and well-wishers to leave them alone, and is critical of her mother's plan to give everything, both personal and public, to the Ronald Reagan Presidential Library that had opened in Simi Valley in November 1991, midway between the fall from the horse and the confirmation of the Alzheimer's diagnosis. Davis turns to the press clamor and the pageantry of the funeral in her final entries of 2004, but this public side does not shut out the tugging simplicity of the moments that bring her father back to her. This veracity is echoed in Davis's eulogy: she juxtaposes a grand evocation of her father's voice through Alfred Tennyson's 1889 elegiac poem "Crossing the Bar" (lines her father had adapted) with a childhood memory of his comforting words on the death of her goldfish and a mental picture of the lakes of Illinois where Reagan swam strongly as a boy.[87]

This, then, is as romantic a narrative as Sacks's *Awakenings*. It is more intensely personal, though, both in re-remembering her father and in reforging the maternal bond. Many sentences begin "My mother" or "My mother and I," and Davis is relieved to learn and to value her mother's voice, especially as she realizes that "I might have been too late. I might have been left with only silence and distance."[88] Significantly, the book's title is taken from a phrase that her mother uses in *I Love You Ronnie*, in which the "truly long, long goodbye" refers to "the way Alzheimer's slowly steals a person away."[89] In *The Way I See It*, Davis writes about their relationship as a "story that needed to be told—for myself, and for others who might be motivated to turn inward to their *own* stories."[90] While we might be cynical about the opportunistic moment of publication of these two books, the urge to give expression to feelings of abandonment seems to be her primary motivation. The two images that do most to connect father and daughter are simple and genuine: Ronald encouraging the young Patricia to look for new shoots of life in the soil after a fire and teaching her how to find her way home by the location of the North Star.

Voice and No Voice

Despite its primary subject matter, *The Long Goodbye* may be read as the fulfilment for the wish of a paternal relationship that never was or an early middle-age narrative in which Davis recognizes traits in her mother that she had previously dismissed. However we approach the text, it sits alongside other accounts of dementia in the early to mid-1990s in which a son or daughter deals with the reality of a parent who will never return to themselves or ever evade the degenerative disease. There were a few first-person accounts of Alzheimer's in the 1990s, including *Living in the Labyrinth* (1993), by Diana Friel McGowin, and *Show Me the Way to Go Home* (1996), by Larry Rose, two authors who were in their mid-50s when they were diagnosed with Alzheimer's. Another account is Dutch author J. Bernlef's remarkable first-person novel *Out of Mind* (1988), which explores the taxing reality and fading memory of the retired Boston-based maritime consultant Maarten Klein, who was living with his wife and dog on the coast in Gloucester, Massachusetts.[91] More often, in this period, the story is told by a family member. This trend follows novelist Jonathan Franzen's insight that although Alzheimer's is the parent's story, it is often the son or daughter who must tell it as they grapple with family memories in order to prevent silence from usurping a slowly diminishing voice.[92] This section returns to Philip Roth's autobiography *Patrimony* before focusing on Michael Ignatieff's 1993 novel *Scar Tissue*, a fascinating literary exploration of Alzheimer's.

Philip Roth's father, Herman, does not experience the same type of neurological degeneration as Reagan or as the mother in *Scar Tissue*, but remembering is nevertheless a major theme of *Patrimony*. The book is also a meditation on mortality as Roth contemplates his roles as son and caregiver when a tumor starts to affect Herman's basic functions. Once Herman has decided against brain surgery, memories and stories become increasingly important to him. In one scene, we see Herman regaling Roth's partner with stories that everyone has heard many times before: Roth muses that these were both "tedious" and "pointless" stories that recounted familiar material with no development or elaboration.[93] He suspects that the stories are "tremendously repetitive" even to Herman but takes heart from the "freshness" and "urgency" with which his father retells family anecdotes night after night. Roth half-recognizes that Herman's emotional investment is more important than the stories themselves for keeping his mind alive. Whereas Roth is stuck in the narrow channel of his father's decline, the 87-year-old Herman prepares himself for an operation to help correct his fading sight by telling a "meandering saga" in which the strands of the immigrant family's history have an animating effect on him.[94]

Herman's decline comes both slowly and in fits and starts; he suffers rectal bleeding after a biopsy and eventually becomes incontinent. In one scene, Herman collapses abjectly when he soils himself, but this episode affects his son profoundly as well; flecks of feces remain in the grouting between the bathroom tiles even after Roth has scrubbed at length, leading him to reflect that scrubbing feces is "like writing a book. . . . I have no idea where to begin."[95] The flecks of feces become indelible traces of both lives. However, the gaps in the story are as important as such markers, the most significant being when Roth is forced to recuperate for six weeks from an unexpected heart attack. Missing Herman's eighty-eighth birthday distresses him so much that during his convalescence time elongates and six weeks seem like a year. He barely recognizes his father on his next visit; age has become "incalculable" and has left the old man as "little more than a shrunken thing, with a crushed face, wearing a black patch and completely inert, almost unrecognizable now, even to me."[96] Herman's inability to walk and swallow does more than just erode his self-respect; it also creates a chasm for Philip Roth, who struggles to reconcile a happy photograph of his 36-year-old father with his two young sons and the stark reality of his aging father's "ruined face" that has had the life stripped from it.[97] When he finally finds a spark that allows him to bridge the fifty years between the two versions of his father, he experiences a strange simultaneity of time. This is a fragile and passing moment, but it prompts Roth to reflect that this connectedness might just be a form of wish fulfilment (rather than an expression of "the facts") in which he is compelled to remember as a means of preserving his own identity.

Herman Roth's death three weeks later, in October 1989, offers both father and son a sense of closure and prevents more indignity. Philip Roth ultimately makes the decision to relieve his father of the "agonizing battle" to breathe on a respirator, the tumor having made it impossible for him to survive off the machine.[98] Despite these graphic images of suffering, the narrative does not end tragically and the stories keep coming through dreams and memories. Roth recalls a dream after Herman's second brain scan in which the arrival of a ghostly boat in Newark Harbor reminds Roth of both his father's immigrant narrative and the death of President Roosevelt forty years earlier, thereby linking family and national stories. Following another dream in which his father's spirit visits him to complain that he should have been buried in a suit rather than a shroud, Roth has an epiphany that he had half-acknowledged many pages earlier: "to be alive, to him, is to be made of memory . . . if a man's not made of memory, he's made of nothing." Although death does not resolve ambiguity or uncertainty for the author, ultimately Herman is preserved through his own stories and in his dreams, making memory both a willed act and an involuntary impulse. This is a major theme of *Patrimony*, inflected in the final solitary line: "You must not forget anything."[99]

Michael Ignatieff's novel reflects some of the themes of *Patrimony* by focusing on the onset and development of his mother's Alzheimer's. Whereas Herman Roth retains self-awareness for much of *Patrimony*, within the first fifty pages of *Scar Tissue*, the protagonist's mother begins to lose her short-term memory and an ability to perform daily functions. It is important that this is a novel rather than a memoir; the trajectory echoes the experience of Ignatieff's mother Alison Grant, but the narrator-protagonist plays a different role, balancing a career as an academic philosopher with that of primary caregiver, particularly after his father dies suddenly. In actual life, this role of caregiver was played by Ignatieff's younger brother, Andrew, who is transformed into a geneticist at a remove from the emotional drama that grips the family (none of the characters are given names). Central to the drama is a moment when the narrator witnesses his mother hitting his father and then scrabbling on the floor to "frantically" recover the beads that have broken off a necklace given to her by her granddaughter. Startled by the obvious symbolism of the dispersed beads and the ugly domestic scene, the narrator looks down from the top of the stairs, like a small child "sobbing on all fours in the dark."[100]

Although *Scar Tissue* was written in England, it is a distinctly North American text. We are not given an exact location, but the proximity to Boston and Alton, New Hampshire, makes this both a New England story and one that is resonant of an immigrant family; the family comes from Scotland on the narrator's maternal side and from Russia on his father's side. This is a variation of Ignatieff's own family history, but the suggestion that Alzheimer's is carried through his mother's bloodline gives the narrator's early memories a bleak cast. Early onset dementia was particularly hard on the family because the mother had been self-sufficient, living with "the ease of a born swimmer" and with the imagination of a dedicated painter. Speaking meaningfully becomes increasingly difficult for her, yet the narrator reflects that for many years her spoken sentences "would begin and stutter to a halt. Words spilled out of her in a jumble . . . as if her thoughts came too fast to be fixed down in words."[101] This is perhaps why painting is so important; it allows her to express herself in a nonverbal form. After she is transferred to a nursing home following the death of her husband, she manages to sketch a likeness of her son, as if the relationship between hand, charcoal, and canvas bypasses the buildup of plaque. Late in the text the narrator compares his mother's decline to that of abstract expressionist artist Willem de Kooning, whose dementia pushed his late paintings toward the edge of chaos but also, from another aesthetic perspective, gave him a "surer line and firmer grasp of colour."[102]

It is not just the mother's memory and the ability to articulate herself that diminish, but also the capacity to exist outside habitual routines. Even before she loses the ability to read, the narrator is convinced that she cannot understand written words: she reads a paragraph of a murder mystery novel "in a childlike singsong, without inflection, unaware that the words are forming into meanings."[103] However, despite the diminishment of her language and the loss of her self-awareness, the narrator is convinced that she retains a sense of herself deep down. In some of the most moving passages, the narrator searches for small signs that his mother is still there, with a kind of somatic language that compensates for the loss of voice:

> Every morning she wakes up a little farther away from us. Yet she still manages to convey something, if only with a glance, of the world she is entering. Beyond the fear and the loss, she seems to say, there is life of a sort here, at the dark edge where everything is crumbling, falling away, becoming indistinct. Occasionally her pacing ceases . . . and she sits on the porch, watching the sunlight stream through all the trees they planted over twenty-five years, and I see something pass over her face that I might call serenity, if I believed there was such a thing.

Like the description of the aging Ronald Reagan and Sacks's patient William Thompson, the natural world lends the mother a serenity that her domestic habitat cannot. It certainly gives the narrator pause for thought as he muses on memories that lie beyond words, "a trapped neural impulse, an infinitesimal synaptic spark in the circuitry of her mind." This might derive from his emotional need to believe that his mother continues to exist despite her neurological degeneration, but he tries to understand his mother's world on her terms despite the widening ontological fissure between them. When she is in the nursing home he holds the belief that her illness still allows her "a small margin of manoeuvre" (what the doctor called "prosodic variation" in her gestures), even though in the same breath he also acknowledges that "I couldn't tell the least thing about my mother's state of mind."[104]

The drama is heightened as the narrator's marriage crumbles around him and he strips back his life to near zero in order to better empathize with his mother. He intuits this, yet seems incapable of halting a process that accelerates when he is drawn into an affair with a nurse. After confessing the affair to his wife, he moves into a shabby flat overlooking the nursing home, where he abjects himself in an act of maternal devotion, leading the critic John Wiltshire to read the text as a "pathography" in which the psychic boundaries between the narrator and his mother start to collapse.[105] This is exacerbated by the gulf between the two sons: the narrator is emotionally bound to his mother and drawn to abstract art and self-help philosophy, whereas his younger brother sees Alzheimer's from a strictly neurological perspective. But even though the brother reduces her condition to a laboratory experiment, scientific distance does not mean he has a full understanding of the disease, nor can he detach himself entirely from the human drama. When the pair take their mother to a French art film, they are surprised that she asks to leave; only afterward does the brother draw from his anthropological understanding of primitive tribes to realize that she had no way of separating her chaotic sense-impressions from the film's disorienting cinematography. Whereas art is a means by which she is able to maintain a tacit understanding of the relationship between subject and object and of controlling a relatively static environment, the zooming camera work takes her into a world of perplexing sense impressions in which there was "no membrane of knowing between her and the screen."[106]

Despite the filial and professional differences between the two brothers, the narrator wants to understand his mother from both emotional and scientific perspectives. In pursuing this double vision, he becomes fascinated by the brains of patients with dementia, in which "the dark blotches with long curving tails" of neural tangles take on the beauty of a "galactic storm, a starburst from an extinguished universe."[107] But this scientific engagement does not lessen the impact of his mother's decline and eventual death. Engaging in conversation with another fragile patient reinforces the narrator's sense that his mother retains a locked-in sense of self—a concern that predated a substantial amount of medical writing on Alzheimer's from the late 1990s onward.[108] His mother's art is evidence that she still exists on a subterranean level, even though her hand seems to be "disconnected from intentions and feelings." The narrator searches for vocabulary to describe her state: science is sometimes helpful, but he draws on extraterrestrial imagery too ("some piece of satellite debris tumbling over and over in space") as he grasps for words that do justice to his mother's fading selfhood. However, when she convinces him to paint over several of her carefully composed canvases, he becomes complicit in his mother's neurological degeneration. This "scene of mutilation" arouses deeper emotions in his usually calm brother, perhaps because it is an act that distorts or overwrites the past in graphic form.[109]

Nancy Davis in *The Long Goodbye* and the narrator of *Scar Tissue* struggle harder to maintain their parental relationships than Philip Roth does in *Patrimony*, largely because Herman holds on to his sense of self and voice until his last few days. We see the decline most visibly in *Scar Tissue*, but in some ways this softens the impact of the mother's deathbed scene in which her breath is "slow and agonising and rasping, and her cheeks had collapsed on her gums" before becoming more "terrifying" and violent as she nears the end.[110] The fact that her primary mode of expression is painting, rather than the stories that define Ronald Reagan and Herman Roth, arguably lessens the impact of her last breath, however painful it is to describe. Ironically, perhaps, it is the narrator who is left to struggle with words and metaphors while pondering the possibility that Alzheimer's might strip away his identity too. This may be the fears of a middle-aged man who has been through the most difficult phase of his life—or an intuition that a genetic fate awaits him where, in time, his own voice will stutter and cease.

Memory, Family, and Ethnicity

The narratives discussed in this chapter explore the complex medical, social, and familial factors that contribute to an understanding of dementia. They deal with isolation, the loss of selfhood, and the search for techniques for coping with a decline in memory and linguistic competency. Yet none of these accounts fully examine the ways cultural forces shape different illness experiences. This is implicitly dealt with in *Patrimony* and early on in *Scar Tissue*, when the narrator traces the genetic line back to his European ancestors, but even in these two texts—and especially in *Awakenings*, given that many of the community of patients were Jewish—cultural identity is underplayed. This can be attributed to the paucity of research on the ethnic variations of dementia. In October 1978, President Carter recognized this and also that resources needed to target "low-income and minority elderly."[111] There were hints of movement: the Administration on Aging brought together a coalition of voices to address specific ethnic health needs, and racial representation was better at the 1981 White House Conference on Aging than it had been at the previous two conferences. However, despite President Reagan's twin announcements in 1983 that November would be National Alzheimer's Disease Month and that funding for Alzheimer's research would increase significantly (it rose from $11 million in 1983 to $300 million in 1994), an understanding of the dementia experience within minority communities remained poor.[112]

A new emphasis on cultural plurality during the Clinton years began to push medical research projects to focus more closely on the socioeconomic factors that shaped experience of dementia and the effects of Alzheimer's on families.[113] The family had a pronounced role in the care of elderly relatives in African American, Asian American, and Hispanic communities, not only because of the costs of institutionalization, although these costs weighed heavily on groups with high unemployment rates.[114] That some of these communities associated mental illness with a curse or fate meant that they were unlikely to seek formal medical help except as a last resort or to accept medical wisdom in the face of their culture's own spiritual beliefs. Given the dearth of hard data, this often led to advanced states of undiagnosed dementia and a significant strain on primary caregivers, especially where dedicated bilingual care facilities were in short supply.[115] For many Asian American and Latino families in the 1980s, the aging parent often spoke a different primary language than their children, a communication gulf that widened when the parent's short-term memory began to fade.

An illuminating example of familial obligations and the cultural language of dementia is Amy Tan's transcultural 2001 novel *The Bonesetter's Daughter*. Published the same year as Jonathan Franzen's *The Corrections*—which addresses how dementia widens the gulf between family members who already find it difficult to communicate—Tan's novel explores a complex mother-daughter bond and a vanishing cultural horizon in the face of advancing dementia. All of Tan's novels explore memory and language, shaped both by her cultural heritage as a child of Chinese immigrants and her work in the late 1970s as a language-development specialist for training programs designed for young children with developmental disabilities. Although *The Bonesetter's Daughter* is specifically a Chinese American novel, it raises broader questions about the status of dementia in some minority communities at a time when medical authority was often treated with skepticism.

The Bonesetter's Daughter presents a complex narrative in which dementia is woven into a family drama that links the living and the dead, a theme that amplifies an aspect of Maxine Hong Kingston's *The Woman Warrior* (1975), in which Kingston's mother has to speak for her newly arrived sister, whose inability to assimilate is exacerbated by possible psychosis or dementia. Developing Kingston's idea of a "talk story" as a method of transmitting beliefs and messages across generations, Tan's novel, set in San Francisco in 1998, revolves around Ruth Young's attempt to rescue a Chinese past that her widowed mother, 82-year-old LuLing Young, remembers only in snatches. Like many Asian Americans and Pacific Americans of her generation, LuLing was born outside the United States and has only partly assimilated. At a young age, Ruth had become her mother's "mouthpiece," but LuLing's advancing dementia makes it more difficult for each of them to reach beyond their own cultural limitations and, importantly for Tan's narrative, for Ruth to distinguish truth from embellishment in her mother's anecdotes.[116]

The diagnosis of LuLing's dementia occurs early in the novel in a comic scene set in a doctor's office. It is impossible to ascertain if she is toying with the doctor, being obstreperous, or losing her functionality. Given that relatively few elderly Asian Americans used conventional medical services at that time (even though the number of Chinese American psychiatrists in San Francisco was on the rise during the 1980s), it is probably a mixture of all these factors. But the scene also raises questions about the socio-emotional stressors Asian Americans commonly faced that the medical establishment often underestimated or ignored.[117] Tan's narrative uses LuLing's dementia to complicate Ruth's search for a meaningful past that already seems culturally and linguistically distant to her. The multiple meanings of Chinese ideographs had always both perplexed and fascinated Ruth, and she painfully tries to decipher a document that appears to offer a key to understanding the family's maternal line. Evoking Maxine Hong Kingston's exploration of ghosts, the mystery of the novel centers on LuLing's biological mother, who turns out not to be her sister's mother, but her nursemaid, Precious Auntie. Once beautiful, Precious Auntie is badly disfigured and rendered mute when she swallows hot ink resin in an extreme state of grief after her father and fiancé are killed by bandits on her wedding day. Her real mother is a source of wisdom and instruction in LuLing's early life, using the medium of sign language as an alternative to speech. Yet LuLing does not come to know the truth of her maternal line until much later, nor does she understand the meaning of the secret dragon bones in a local cave that give the novel its name and link to a much broader ancestral story.

Her mantra "these are the things I must not forget" runs through the novel and is almost an exact echo of Roth's line in *Patrimony* "you must not forget anything." This mantra also helps orient Ruth toward her ancestral past in China, and she realizes that she needs to listen to LuLing patiently, resolving "to be here as her mother told her about her life, taking her through all the detours of the past, explaining the multiple meanings of Chinese words, how to translate her heart."[118] The emphasis on cultural translation becomes an important theme on three levels: Precious Auntie has to translate her knowledge into sign language and into a letter that LuLing does not read until much later; LuLing's life story is slowly disappearing through her dementia, but she retains the ability to translate her past in fragmented and embellished form; and Ruth must learn to translate a language system that she barely knows. LuLing holds a long-standing belief that Ruth possesses a special mystical power that subliminally connects with Precious Auntie and that takes them beyond words to a deeper biological and spiritual core that resonates with the image of bones in the novel's title. The reader might hope for a sustained meditation on Alzheimer's or a reflection of culturally sensitive community facilities (such as the Chinese Hospital in Chinatown that was developing an active community health plan in the mid-1980s), yet the medical story is just one element in an epic narrative of family genealogy and cross-cultural translation in which language and memory prove vital yet elusive.[119]

These themes are by no means restricted to literature dealing with dementia, as they touch on much broader social issues of identity, assimilation, generational change, and competing conceptions of mental health. It would be an assertion of a version of cultural separatism (a trend of which Amy Tan was wary) to suggest that the medical burden among some minority communities was greater than others, but studies in the late 1980s and early 1990s in New York City and Washington, DC, revealed that feelings of stress and depression among African American and Hispanic caregivers were more acute than the norm. Clearly the importance of close interpersonal contact that we have seen in this chapter in the examples of Oliver Sacks, Philip Roth, Patti Davis, and Amy Tan is likely to suffer when the caregiver feels overwhelmed by a domestic situation over which they have little control. In these narratives, informal support from other family members often falls short of adequately supporting the primary caregiver, whose own health often suffers as the demands on them grow. These studies also suggest that within certain demographics, counseling and mental health facilities (that might help caregivers work around the limited language of their dependents) were underused or ignored because of the tendency in the community to somatize mental illness.[120]

With this in mind, it is helpful to conclude this chapter by returning to the broader political and medical context of the 1990s, a time when Alzheimer's research during the Clinton years was making significant advances in understanding the neuropathology of the disease. In a major boost to the credibility struggles of the Gray Panthers and other health advocates, the 1995 White House Conference on Aging, which took place fourteen years after the previous conference, resolved to inject $50 million of federal funds immediately and to increase funding on

Alzheimer's research by over 35 percent over five years.[121] Donna Shalala, Clinton's secretary of health and human services, commended the final report, *The Road to an Aging Policy for the 21st Century*, as a "successful example of grass-roots involvement and democracy in action." She also praised the 1995 conference for being more coordinated about establishing a holistic healthcare plan for the elderly than the previous three White House conferences had been.[122]

By the time the multidisciplinary *Journal of Alzheimer's Disease* was launched in the spring of 2000, the research community had a better understanding of the genetics of the disease, but its cultural variations were only starting to be recognized as late as 2011, when President Obama signed the National Alzheimer's Project Act into law as part of another wave of research, treatment, and consciousness raising. The rise of Age Studies among humanities scholars in the mid-1990s had helped in this respect, especially in illuminating the ideologies and gender implications of middle age and old age, and public awareness of Alzheimer's at the millennium was certainly much sharper than the moment when President Reagan made his dramatic announcement of 1994.[123] But the slow pace of age research in the years that followed Robert Butler's wake-up call *Why Survive?* meant that the voices of many seniors suffering from dementia were prematurely silenced.

PART TWO

Health Voices of the 1980s and 1990s

5 *Developmental Disabilities beyond the Empty Fortress*

On 29 March 1977, at the inaugural gathering of the President's Commission on Mental Health at the White House, the twenty-member planning group set out their ambitions. President Carter joined the meeting briefly, stressing the national importance of the project and promising that it would not "lie on a shelf gathering dust and would be implemented in the most direct manner possible."[1] Child psychiatrist George Tarjan followed up by proposing that the group focus on specifics, one of which should be to help change public attitudes about health needs. As the Director of the Mental Retardation and Child Psychiatry Division of UCLA's Neuropsychiatric Institute, Tarjan was concerned about the fact that the complex relationship between disability and mental health remained underresearched and underdiscussed. This was being corrected to an extent with the help of two recent workshops organized by the American Medical Association's Council on Mental Health, but Tarjan believed that public advocacy should be prioritized over the accumulation of empirical data.[2] Commission chair Thomas Bryant agreed that the project could not "remedy all social and economic problems," but he believed that it should be "both pragmatic and idealistic" and equally about healthcare provision and health advocacy.[3]

As the first half of the book discussed, the 1977 President's Commission set the tone for a number of intersecting health initiatives that tried to redress the lack of focus during the Nixon-Ford years. Given the fact that many large state facilities had closed during the 1960s, Carter and his advisors believed that the delivery of effective outpatient and aftercare services was a key to rectifying the "nonsystem" that he identified when he took office in 1977. Six years later, President Reagan agreed that the "patchwork quilt of existing politics and programs" needed simplifying, but for very different reasons. The Reagan administration was keen to help individuals with disabilities secure economic independence, but under the aegis of a scaled-back federalism that stressed self-reliance and home help instead of patient services for all but the very needy. Whereas Carter thought that the federal government was ultimately accountable for failures in healthcare provision, Reagan believed that individual states should be primarily responsible for health services.[4] This ideological shift could be interpreted either (positively) as a recognition that federal programs can never guarantee effective local provision or (negatively) as an evasion of responsibility, especially as the block grant system that the Omnibus Budget Reconciliation Act of 1981 brought in represented a 21 percent cut in funding to state healthcare programs.[5] The three topics discussed in the first half of this book—veterans' health, addiction, and dementia—all received increased attention in the 1980s and 1990s, but preventive care suffered the most from these budget cuts and planning was often reactionary after years of underinvestment, as Surgeon General C. Everett Koop noted in his 1988 report *The Future of Public Health*.[6]

Instead of focusing primarily on healthcare policy, the second half of *Voices of Mental Health* assesses how the health legacy of the 1970s played out across a range of experiences—developmental disabilities, anorexia and body image disorders, mood and personality disorders, and clinical depression—all of which saw a dramatic rise in reported cases during the 1980s and 1990s. Silence at the federal level could politicize a health issue as much as active engagement. For example, on the few occasions that President Reagan addressed disability, he did not acknowledge the healthcare needs of those with cognitive and developmental disabilities and did not differentiate below the level of "mental problems."[7] The book's second half retains the focus on political and moral responsibility for mental health provision, but this and the next three chapters also explore the cultural politics of health at a time when the rise of consumerism, the influence of the mass media, and an increasingly technologized health industry pushed the spheres of politics, medicine, and culture closer together.

Focusing on the connections between these three spheres enables us to assess how the experience and knowledge of mental health conditions was constructed in the late twentieth century, at a time when skepticism and relativism seemed more prevalent than ever. This tallies with what the 2000 volume *Pathology and the Postmodern* describes as an "anti-foundational approach to meaning and linguistic boundaries" that challenges "naturalized dichotomies between subject and object and knower and known."[8] This is primarily an epistemological point but it has therapeutic implications, propelling mental health beyond the spheres of medicine and health policy into what Dwight Fee, the editor of *Pathology and the Postmodern*, calls "a new world of contingency, flux, and thus of profound possibility."[9] This sense of possibility offsets the bleak view of some late-century cultural theorists that selfhood and reality were in jeopardy or were even being erased.

In order to frame the convergence of and tensions between the spheres of politics, medicine, and culture, this chapter focuses on the evolving experiences of and changing nomenclature of developmental disabilities, a term that began slowly to replace "mental retardation" during the late 1980s. As we have seen, the Carter years were the most active phase of mental health reform. We have to go further back, though, to the Developmental Disabilities Services and Facilities Construction Act, signed by Richard Nixon in 1970, to gauge efforts to improve health services and training for children and young adults. The act established a legislative framework for understanding the healthcare needs of children with cognitive and intellectual disabilities and was the first time that conditions such as autism, cerebral palsy, Down syndrome, and epilepsy had been recognized in federal legislation. This move echoed the emphasis in *Action against Mental Disability*, a publication of the President's Task Force on the Mentally Handicapped, on socio-environmental factors. The task force recommended a Joint Council on Disabilities that could span advocacy for the mentally retarded, the mentally ill, and those with physical disabilities.[10] The Nixon administration went further: in 1971, it released a fact sheet that pledged to halve the occurrences of mental retardation by the end of the century and promised to help a third of those with related disabilities in public institutions "return to useful lives in the community."[11]

The rise in activism around disability rights in the 1970s provided a framework for a better understanding of cognitive and developmental disabilities, but when disability was discussed in the 1980s it tended to be in physical terms.[12] Even the extension of basic civil rights for those with disabilities was hard won, as evidenced by the Section 504 controversy. This clause in the 1973 Rehabilitation Act, which was intended to guarantee rights related to education, training, and work for those with disabilities, was not signed until 1977 when pressure was placed on Carter's secretary of health, education, and welfare, Joseph Califano, and it remained contested until the mid-1980s. In response to protests against federal cutbacks, President Reagan announced a "National Decade of Disabled People" in November 1982 and charged Vice-President Bush with the task of reviewing Section 504 and looking for ways to create new job opportunities and tackling public perceptions of the disabled as "dependent and sickly."[13] Despite these positive noises, lobby groups such as the American Coalition of Citizens with Disabilities struggled to be heard and misunderstandings about the relationship between mental health and disabilities persisted.

The emphasis on refining definitions was a distinct legacy of the period. A 1980 World Health Organization report claimed that mental retardation was "losing the stigma of hopelessness which over centuries has been attached to it."[14] This was partly because the overlapping fields of biomedics, psychology, education, and sociology were starting to be understood better, including research that revealed a possible correlation between autism and a fragile X chromosome. 1980 was also the year the third edition of *DSM* was published, following six years of drafting. Melvin Sabshin, the medical director of the American Psychiatric Association, wanted to shift focus away from a grand classificatory system based on psychopathology toward a nuanced multi-axial evaluation model. The creator of *DSM-III*, Columbia University psychiatrist Robert Spitzer, was also eager for a precise nosology, partly to advance research and partly to counter the claims of "anti-psychiatry" figures who were arguing that mental disorders were a myth and cannot be medically verified. In her account of the writing of *DSM-III*, Hannah Decker identifies the June 1976 Midstream Conference in St. Louis, Missouri, as a crucial moment in this refinement of psychiatric terminology, instigated by a group of "diagnostic purists" at the Washington University School of Medicine.[15]

Marking the attempt to shift from psychoanalytically informed concepts to precise empirical classification, *DSM-III* offered a more detailed account of developmental and cognitive disorders than its predecessor, even though its emphasis on "disorders" did not move far away from the language of pathology. Some of the subcategories were discrete, such as some distinctions among disorders (for example, cerebral palsy or Down syndrome), but general categories like "unspecified mental retardation" or "pervasive developmental disorder" tended to be used when more exact definitions did not fit.[16] Sub-average intellectual functioning, impairments in adaptive behavior, and onset before the age of 18 were three features of the *DSM-III* section on "mental retardation." This terminology was reflected in the name change of the American Association on Mental Deficiency: the 90-year-old non-profit organization adopted "Mental Retardation" in its title in 1987, then changed its name again in 2007 to encompass intellectual and developmental disabilities.[17]

Even though a 1980 World Health Organization report was calling for urgent investment in research, training, public engagement, and an explicit national policy, U.S. federal engagement was limited to the President's Committee on Mental Retardation, which was marking its twentieth year in 1986.[18] Chaired in turn by Reagan's three secretaries of health and human services, the committee tended to focus on legal regulations and barriers to employment rather than on educating the public.[19] When issues of definition arose, they tended to be about disability claims that stemmed from the combination of a physical injury and an underlying cognitive condition.

Two such cases from 1982 and 1987 are instructive examples. The first of these was filed by a 36-year-old Vermont man, Elmer Berry, against Reagan's first secretary of health and human services, Richard Schweiker, after five years of failed claims for Social Security disability benefits (*Berry v. Schweiker*). After an initial suit in 1977, Berry returned to court in 1979, citing problems with his foot, a "constant headache," and "brain damage." A psychiatrist concluded that he had "impairments of inadequate personality and borderline intelligence," but as none of these disabilities was thought to be severe, the claim was not upheld in January 1982, when it went to a final decision. A similar case came to the U.S. Court of Appeals in November 1987, when night watchman John Rawlins submitted a claim against Reagan's third secretary, Otis Bowen (*Rawlins v. Bowen*). Rawlins's claim for disability benefits was based on a broken ankle, a back injury, long-standing "mental retardation," and "nervousness." A psychologist concluded that Rawlins, who had an IQ of 73, was "mildly retarded" and was dealing with mild depression and "dependent personality traits." Again, the claim was denied, with the judgment that he was capable of doing unskilled work even though he did not, in fact, have the numeracy and literacy skills required to perform the tasks of a night watchman in the first place. Even though the courts ruled against the plaintiffs in these two cases, they raised questions about the status of multiple cognitive and physical conditions and the dangers of accident or injury for individuals with very limited vocational options.

In order to assess the politics of developmental disability, this chapter begins by returning to the late 1960s, when research, particularly into autism, established a fixed conceptual horizon that was slow to recede in the 1970s and 1980s.[20] The middle parts of the chapters look at alternative therapies for congenital and early onset conditions, the importance of Barry Levinson's 1988 film *Rain Man* for stimulating public awareness of autism, and how later written accounts explored the autistic spectrum in more subtle ways. These accounts coincided with heightened awareness of disability that both helped bring about and was stimulated by the Americans with Disabilities Act of July 1990, which promoted a shift toward the social model of disability (with its emphasis on environmental factors) as a challenge to the medical model (with its focus on diagnosis and treatment).[21] The medical model has been widely criticized by theorists and activists since the millennium, following earlier critiques such as Ralph Nader's 1974 Study Group Report *The Madness Establishment*. However, it is difficult to adequately understand the interface of genetics, environment, and behavior without adopting a perspective that incorporates elements of both models.[22] This dual outlook is an important theme of earlier chapters, but it becomes more explicit in the second half of this book in order to emphasize how the field of mental health was both more nuanced and more fiercely contested as the century drew to a close.

Early Accounts: *The Empty Fortress* and *The Siege*

The work of Austrian émigré Bruno Bettelheim is often taken as a starting point for understanding the etiology and diagnosis of infantile autism. The Sonia Shankman Orthogenic School in Chicago, a residential facility where Bettelheim served as director from the mid-1940s, provided the educational context for what became his most notorious book on autism, *The Empty Fortress* (1967), which followed his National Institute of Mental Health-sponsored publications on child care, *Love Is Not Enough* (1950) and *Truants from Life* (1955). Bettelheim's training in psychology and art history at the University of Vienna gave him a particular perspective on emotional and behavioral disturbance, which he thought needed to be treated by innovative educational means. Because parents can unintentionally cause their children harm by being overprotective, inattentive, or erratic, he was keen to ensure that the staff at his school remained free of psychological conflict and could create a safe environment for the residents. Bettelheim encouraged his staff to provide a consistent level of support in an effort to stimulate a new "inner attitude to life" by encouraging their charges to be active learners—as he tried to do with two Austrian children with autism who he said had lived with him during the 1930s.[23] However, the language of damage still creeps into his writing at times, as if therapeutic and educational techniques are the only means of correcting something that is broken or absent.[24]

The observational work that led to *The Empty Fortress* began in the mid-1950s and followed Austrian American psychiatrist Leo Kanner's emphasis on the tendency among autistic infants to withdraw. Kanner discussed this tendency in a number of papers published in the 1940s and in the updated version of his pioneering 1935 study *Child Psychiatry*. Bettelheim notes that Kanner's subjects tended to be quiet or pensive in the face of interpersonal contact, often "giving the impression of silent wisdom."[25] His language also mirrors Kanner's use of symbolism to describe what often seems to be an inaccessible and unrepresentable condition. Quoting a passage from Kanner's "Case Nine," including the line "he walks as if he is in a shadow, lives in a world of his own where he cannot be reached," Bettelheim adopted a similar metaphor for his opening chapter, "In the Region of Shadows."

Noting that the understanding of autism was very hazy, early in *The Empty Fortress* Bettelheim associated the dehumanization he had experienced in Nazi concentration camps in Dachau and Buchenwald (which he documented in his 1960 study *The Informed Heart*) with what he saw as the autistic child's dehumanizing withdrawal "from the world before their humanity ever really develops."[26] Although Bettelheim was generally more optimistic than Kanner, the book outlines an "inescapable" condition that differentiates the autistic child from normal children and unhelpfully blurs infantile experiences with imprisonment.

Bettelheim is often upheld as a figure who not only prolonged the stigma associated with autism but whose work confused a range of conditions—genetic, medical, psychological, developmental, and mythical—and perpetuated ingrained stereotypes about feral children and savants.[27] This is not an entirely fair assessment, particularly as he insisted that infantile autism should be distinguished from discourses of the "feeble-minded or brain-damaged," and that it should be seen as a functional disturbance "which we know to be reversible in many cases."[28] The controversy pivots on Bettelheim's emphasis on unhealthy maternal relationships. This view stemmed from Kanner's claim that autism or "childhood schizophrenia" (terms he used interchangeably) was often determined by the mother-child relationship. The hypothesis was widely promulgated as the "refrigerator mother theory." In a 1960 *Time* interview, Kanner claimed that mothers of autistic children were described as "just happening to defrost enough to produce a child." Although Kanner scaled back his view on parental blame by 1969 (a year after *DSM-II* had categorized autism as a form of "childhood schizophrenia"), his theory led Bettelheim to focus on abnormal parent-child relations.[29] Bettelheim fused moral judgements about bad parenting with the mythical elements of *The Empty Fortress*, placing shadows, fortresses, and pathology in the way of scientific clarity and interpersonal understanding.

Although other practitioners in the late 1960s and early 1970s, such as the controversial child neuropsychiatrist Lauretta Bender (who had used electroconvulsive therapy in her tests on autistic children in the 1950s), were arguing that autism had a biological underpinning, Bettelheim's study set the stage for understanding autism as an intellectual and behavioral disorder that centered on the maternal relationship. Bettelheim's mythical language was echoed in a very different type of study of autism, New York English professor Clara Claiborne Park's book *The Siege*, which was first published in 1967 and reissued as a mass market paperback in 1972. Park's account focused on her daughter Elly, who displayed autistic behavior at a very early age. The account is tenderly written and sharpened with an analytic eye that Park says was gained from reading Benjamin Spock's manual *Baby and Child Care*, which she found just as applicable "to the disturbed and defective" as to "ordinary parents of normal children."[30] It is noticeable that *The Siege* uses Bettelheim's metaphorical language, particularly the title image, "the mysterious self-absorbed delight" of the autistic infant and the "solitary citadel, compelling and self-made, complete and valid" in which she see her daughter.[31] Park even uses the word "fortress" to describe Elly's world, which she was determined to breach by "every stratagem we could invent . . . to beguile, entice, seduce her into the human condition."[32]

The Siege was an important text because it was the first to convey a dual perspective; it tempered parental concern for a child's development with an academic viewpoint that renders description and analysis indistinguishable at times. Given the fact that autism was three times more common in boys in the late 1960s, the book was ground-breaking in its portrayal of a young girl who seemed ontologically remote from her parents and unresponsive to a range of engagement techniques.[33] Park had meager educational models to draw upon, but her concern with Elly's language development led her to closely document her vocabulary and expression. This was not too taxing an empirical study, given that Elly had only spoken thirty-one words by age four and only five to six words at any one time, many of them sporadic and decoupled from real-world objects. When Elly used words, they did not signify in any conventional sense but were part of her sealed play world, leading Park to conclude that "Elly's words were things-in-themselves that led to nowhere and nobody."[34] She understood that Elly needed active parenting and that too much chatter was distracting because she needed to hear words above background noise. Park realized that the pitch and rhythm of words was often more important than their meaning and that this was often better conveyed through music, particularly if linked to rocking movements. Just as we saw in chapter 4 in the case of the post-encephalitic patient Frances, music could provide an "avenue to words" when conventional lexis could not. Believing that Elly was refusing to escape from her "walled fortress," Park reflected that music was a way of lowering "the barrier that Elly maintained against words."[35]

Much of the middle section of *The Siege* explores the ways Park believed that her daughter was willfully refusing to participate in an interpersonal world. This section is full of perceptive descriptions of Elly's behavior and her mother's efforts to ensure that activities are reciprocal, but the question of how to tap into Elly's motivation gnaws at Park. Nevertheless, with perseverance and sustained interaction, Elly's slow developmental curve leads her away from total isolation, and by the age of four she is able to add human features to a stick drawing. Elly completes this figure with "faint yet certain strokes," and although Park detects elements of her behavior that "remained strange," she feels that her daughter is starting to "live more nearly among us than ever before."[36] Even though at times maternal feelings push the account away from analysis into the emotive realm, Park checks herself after she responds angrily to what she initially takes to be willful disobedience.

The author is as much concerned with Elly's mental health as her developmental challenges, which she sees as a continuum that does not categorically separate "sick children" from well ones.[37] She agrees with Bettelheim that "love is not enough" but argues that love is a unique resource and that parents can be trained to become co-workers to prevent scientific analysis from being the only criterion for determining a child's training. To ensure that loving does not distort her relationship with Elly, she thinks carefully about discipline, routine, and the benefits of outside help, which becomes a necessity when she takes a job in a local community college. Park is convinced that the more interaction they have, the more at ease with the world Elly will feel and the more likely she will be to develop capacities that emerge only sporadically. It is important that Elly's story is told in domestic terms before any psychiatrists are introduced; this places the diagnosis of schizophrenia and autism in the context of a human story and tests Kanner's theories against lived reality. A visit to a psychiatrist, a report from a local children's institute, and a trip to London's Hampstead Clinic bridge an account of Elly's first four years, her "long, slow" journey toward speech, and a more stable identity between ages five and eight.

There are glimmers of Elly's visual and spatial intelligence toward the end of the book that sit alongside her limited manual dexterity and her struggle to adapt to new social interactions. *The Siege* was part of a growing trend toward examining the relationship between parenting and developmental disabilities, possibly triggered by climbing divorce rates and fragmenting family units. Books such as Joan Beck's *How to Raise a Brighter Child*, which first appeared in 1967 and was republished a number of times into the 1980s, argued that the right kind of stimulation and training could help young children develop their intelligence by increasing opportunities to think, imagine, and create. Beck's widely read book does not deal specifically with autism or children like Elly whose intelligence cannot easily be expressed in the classroom. Instead of looking at atypical cases, Beck gave advice to mothers on how to protect children from learning difficulties in order to minimize the chances that a child would develop brain damage. The book claimed that bright children were "more self-sufficient and self-directing" than their peers, they could adjust to "problems and stress," and that they "cause fewer discipline problems" and "are less likely to have undesirable personality traits."[38] However, behind Beck's progressive language was an inclination to normalize "brightness" and to criticize parents and schools that did not create a stimulating environment. Beck warned that an unchallenging school or a disruptive family can turn gifted children into "troublemakers or unhappy introverts."[39]

Despite the positive language of Joan Beck and her belief that brightness takes different forms, her philosophy was still very much defined by regular school learning instead of recognizing the kind of artistic talents that children such as Elly displayed.[40] The tendency to scapegoat mothers for their children's psychogenic or behavioral disturbances was being challenged in the 1970s in the context of a growing recognition that autism has a biological component and that autistic behavior is not simply a child's reaction to an unsettling environment.[41] Kanner's refrigerator mother theory had been discredited by 1974, but with the recognition that "inadequate human interaction in infancy" can exacerbate underlying organic conditions and, in extreme cases, have a profoundly detrimental effect on cognition and language.[42] Evidence that autism occurs even among children in stable and loving homes did not banish the specter of neglectful parents. As the number of cases of hyperactivity and attention deficit disorder increased, it was clear that disruptive homes often had an adverse effect on the growing child. When President Nixon threw a football at the White House with six-year-old Kevin Heald from

Cedar Rapids, Iowa, the National Association for Retarded Children's 1972 Poster Child, it was as much to emphasize the supportive role of Kevin's parents as the importance of specialist education for helping Kevin learn within the limitations of his IQ of 50.[43]

Evolving Horizons, New Programs

When Dorothy J. Beavers, president of the Rochester, New York, chapter of the National Society for Autistic Children, wrote to the White House in 1970, it seemed that the following decade would fare little better for autistic children: "Trapped in the world of the living dead, mentally ill children continue to be completely ignored and forgotten in our enlightened society of the seventies."[44] Beavers pointed to environmental and educational factors rather than pathological origins and argued that developmental disability was complex and should not be reduced to a single cause. Her letter was bleak and angry and did not meet with more than a cursory response from the Nixon administration. However, while the coupling of pathology and infantile autism lingered into the 1980s—even after *DSM-III* offered more precise diagnostic language—the trend was offset by positive accounts of children who benefited from educational programs and learned ways of compensating for limitations.

Most of Bettelheim's analysis in his case studies of autism did not advance beyond fairly low expectations, and experimental drug procedures in the 1960s aimed at treating childhood schizophrenia also proved to be largely unsuccessful. But starting in 1976, AMA workshops on the complementary roles of physicians, parents, and healthcare workers offered a more contextually sensitive approach to developmental disabilities. Mega-doses of vitamin B6 and magnesium were thought to help cognitive development and improve eye contact, often accompanied by the belief that children who were diagnosed early had the capacity to develop within a supportive environment.[45] The Bill of Rights for the Mentally Retarded (which Senators Ted Kennedy and Jennings Randolph introduced to Congress in January 1973) reinforced the need for a variety of health workers beyond psychiatrists and child psychologists, and the Developmentally Disabled Assistance and Bill of Rights Act of 1975 promoted treatments that are "least restrictive of the person's liberty."[46] Yet this legislation proved to be no more a panacea than megavitamins were. Despite high-level advocacy, the Bill of Rights was effectively dismantled when the Supreme Court ruled in April 1981 that it was simply advisory and did not guarantee any substantive rights at the state level for those with developmental disabilities.[47]

This chapter will return to the politics of developmental disability, but here I want to analyze two examples from the late 1970s and early 1980s of how nontraditional educational training might be beneficial when conventional forms of medicine and psychiatry fall short. The first of these deals with two cases of severe autism. The second focuses on the learning needs of a child with cerebral palsy and introduces a broader educational context that attends to more diffuse developmental needs. Neither of these cases was without controversy. The first is documented in two books by Massachusetts psychotherapist and self-styled autism trainer Barry Neil Kaufman, *Son-Rise* (1976) and *A Miracle to Believe In* (1981), which document his professional interactions with his son Raun and an autistic Mexican boy Robertito. The second involves a rehabilitative training regime singer-songwriter Neil Young and his wife Pegi adopted to help their son Ben. These cases offer positive instances of the child's potential that offset the earlier bleak cases, but the techniques were not easy to sustain outside controlled environments, at least without significant effort from the parents.

The first example links Raun Kaufman's struggle to communicate and the case of Robertito Soto, who was placed under the Kaufmans' care after his parents had concluded that there was little they could do to advance his education and sociability. Barry Kaufman begins *A Miracle to Believe In* with a joyful run through the Massachusetts countryside, then switches to reflect on his third child, Raun, who had been diagnosed in his first year (in 1974) as "severely impaired developmentally, neurologically and cognitively." This condition was possibly linked to an adverse reaction to antibiotics to treat an ear infection that was administered when Raun was four weeks old.[48] His son's autistic behavior posed a dilemma for Kaufman and his wife: should they see him as an "opportunity to be either diminished, saddened and defeated by our own unhappiness or to thrive, explore and be enriched by our encounter with this special human being?"[49] The book is full of the new age flourishes that informed Kaufman's Son-Rise program (as featured in a 1979 NBC movie of that name), which emphasized personal growth and the capacity to overcome psychological and even organic hurdles. Kaufman developed the Son-Rise program in the mid-1970s specifically to help his son, who in his second year "slipped behind an invisible, impenetrable wall" in which he "spent endless hours immersed in self-stimulating rituals" and showed no signs of language development. Moving beyond echoes of Bettelheim's fortress and Park's siege, Kaufman sees a rare intelligence and a very real world behind Raun's compulsive behavior and a capacity for "sheer joy" that Washington, DC, educator Sally Smith detected in many "learning disabled" children, as she discussed in her 1978 book *No Easy Answers*.[50] In contrast to Bettelheim's idea that love is not enough, Kaufman outlined a philosophy of acceptance that upholds play as a guiding star for severe cases of infantile autism, especially when other methods have failed.

Detecting that the young Raun is alive in his own world (Kaufman described him as "a seventeen-month-old Buddha contemplating another dimension"), Kaufman began play therapy with his infant son. Kaufman, his wife, and their two elder daughters started mimicking Raun's behavior, "rocking when he rocked, spinning when he spun, flapping when he flapped."[51] Frustrated by early diagnoses and Bettelheim's judgmental categories, Kaufman refused to see his son as "just another dismal statistic." Instead, he and his wife Suzi started to develop a customized educational program that, over the course of three years, drew Raun out of his solitude and helped transform him from a "withdrawn, mute, self-stimulating, functionally retarded, autistic and 'hopeless' little boy" into a "social, highly verbal, affectionate and loving human being displaying capabilities far beyond his years."[52]

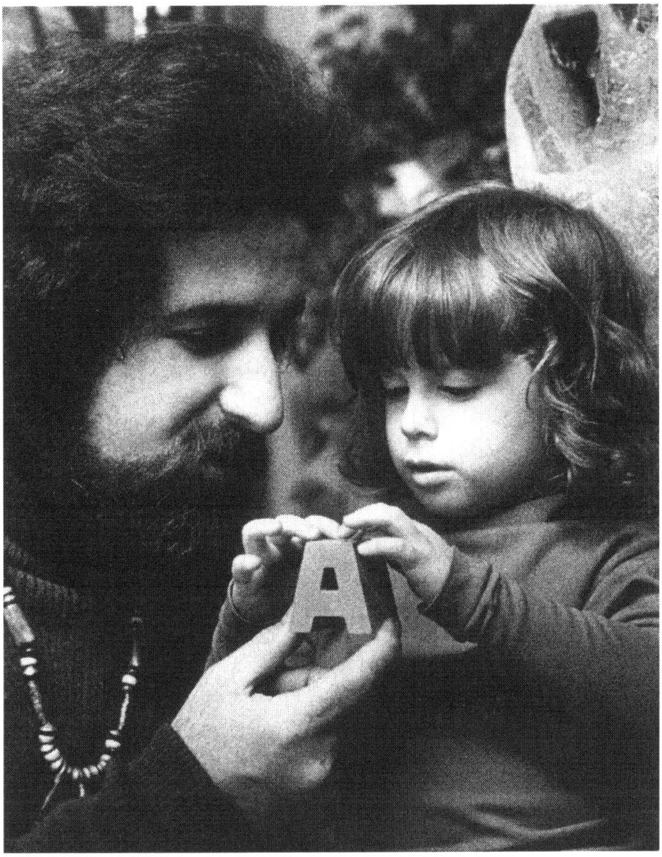

Figure 5.1 Barry and Raun Kaufman, as originally published in *Son-Rise* (1976). Courtesy of Raun Kaufman at the Autism Treatment Center of America®.

Although Raun was not a savant, the sense that he was exceptional, albeit not in a conventional or cerebral way, echoes Joan Beck's notion that a bright children can develop through an appropriately stimulating environment. Kaufman realized that the environment should be conducive to building a bridge between Raun's sealed realm and the sociable world of others. This belief in the possibility of "evolving horizons," as Kaufman terms it on the final page of *Son-Rise*, was even more of a test for Robertito, about whom his parents had all but abandoned hope.[53]

The opening chapter of *A Miracle to Believe In* shows a marked development in the interaction between five-year-old Robertito and his parents and the wider family that Barry Kaufman, his wife Suzi, son Raun, and interpreter Jaime become to him. Instead of showering him with affection, as his Spanish-speaking parents had done, they learn to be gentler in their approach, which enabled him to relax a little in their company. His therapist was initially confronted by a perpetually moving boy who clicked his tongue and refused to let anyone through his impenetrable wall. Diagnoses suggested that Robertito was "severely retarded," possibly schizophrenic, "complicated by unknown bio-chemical irregularities," and probably "uneducable."[54] Kaufman was unhappy that these abstract accounts failed to capture the contours of the boy's behavior or identify an appropriate treatment program. Instead of trying to prevent his hand flapping or his grunting, Kaufman extended techniques that he had developed with Raun, mimicking Robertito's actions in the hope that he could build a bridge to his play world. Noting that one of his symptoms was unresponsiveness to sound, Kaufman tried different pitches and volumes, noting that the boy was particularly responsive to soft sounds, including the recording of a Chopin nocturne.

These techniques, according to Kaufman, were ways of respecting Robertito's lifeworld without imposing rigid expectations. He believes that they managed to stimulate a new will to live in Robertito within just a few days, based on the evidence that the boy's level of eye contact and tolerance for physical contact improved. He continued to make clicking sounds, but they now seemed to express happiness, or at least Robertito's parents were trained to hear them as such instead of the "weird, unearthly noises" that had pushed his mother into a state of bewilderment and panic. Kaufman attempts to reeducate the Sotos, encouraging them to accept their son and to interact patiently on his terms instead of wishing that he was something different or that he could attain a normative educational level. The Sotos took these lessons back with them to Mexico. There they found that Robertito showed signs of development, but they also returned to a frantic anxiety that undermined the progress their son was making in formal therapy.

A Miracle to Believe In is a meditation on the difficulties Robertito's parents faced and Kaufman's personal engagement in a scenario that closely mirrored the one he had faced with his own son a few years before. While the Sotos learned to be nonjudgmental, their own anxieties had a deleterious effect on their son. When Kaufman saw Robertito a year later, the boy had partially retreated "behind the impenetrable wall" and the positive attitude he had gained in formal therapy had been eroded.[55] His therapist occasionally reached for language that was similar to Bettelheim's, describing the boy as "deviant, alien, a perplexing enigma," a view that is underlined when Robertito fails to develop any meaningful vocabulary or indeed "any specific, recognizable sounds in either Spanish or English."[56] A psychologist assessed that the five-and-a-half year old had an IQ of between 7 and 14, placing his general development at lower than two months and his intellectual development at nine months, and consultants believed that if Kaufman could improve his interpersonal contact and language abilities, it would be miraculous.

In the cases of Raun and Robertito, Kaufman portrays the ability to tap into hidden potential as a miracle, and he projects therapy as a kind of pilgrimage that trainers, parents, and the child take together. He argues that formal classrooms where the child was likely to remain marooned would fall short of what a creative, loving community could achieve. After documenting their 75-hour-per-week intervention program and the various interactions between family members, at the end of *Son-Rise*, Kaufman writes that the whole family was feeling "energized" and that

"Raun was working puzzles with great rapidity," increasing his language capacity, and appreciating his own accomplishments.[57]

The challenge with Robertito was greater because of cultural barriers and the fact that his training started at a later age than Raun's did. However, Kaufman claimed that within seven months, Robertito's IQ had increased to over 45 and his language abilities were catching up with his actual age.[58] The presence of Raun also seemed to help the Mexican boy, although their often-silent communication is filtered through the eyes of a father who believes that his son possesses a rare spiritual presence. For Kaufman, Raun plays an important role in Robertito's "rebirth," in which he travels from a "mute, blank-faced, staring, self-stimulating" little boy to one who "could talk, love his parents, share his affection, even play basketball . . . a responsive, participating and loving human being."[59] The language of miracles sits uncomfortably with the medical and social models of disability, but the fact that Raun went on to complete a degree in biomedical ethics at Brown University and became director of the Autism Treatment Center of America in Sheffield, Massachusetts (which Barry and Suzi Kaufman established in 1983), offers a strong counterexample to the lost cases of *The Empty Fortress*.

My other example is that of Ben Young, who was born with cerebral palsy to Canadian singer Neil Young and his wife Pegi in 1978. Ben had a severe form of cerebral palsy, a congenital condition that Young's first son Zeke experienced in milder form. Because Ben could not easily speak due to a high degree of muscular spasticity from birth (he was quadriplegic and had very limited coordination), his parents worked hard with him on alternatives to vocal articulation. They instituted a strict regime from an early age, inspired by the Philadelphia-based Institutes for the Achievement of Human Potential, in order to help Ben navigate through particular developmental stages. The neurophysiological training regime was very demanding on both the parents and the child and required almost constant attention for twelve hours each day. The institute began treating "injured" and "hurt" children in the 1960s with the belief that such children can develop much further through a combination of physical therapy, receptive stimulation, and expressive activities designed to expand the range of movement than they can with other training programs. The validity of the program, particularly "patterning"—in which parents rock the child's head to and fro rhythmically to stimulate functional and neural development—had been questioned by a number of medical journals and associations since the late 1960s, and after eighteen months the Youngs too began to believe that Glenn Doman's claims that his institute could make paralyzed and speechless children "totally well" outstripped reality.[60]

Ben's repetitious activities were captured in Neil Young's 1980 album *Re-ac-tor*, as was a father's sense of disappointment that the course of therapy did not match the grand claims of the institute.[61] But the Youngs found hope in computers, which they believed might make a difference for Ben when they realized that the interventionist activities of Doman's institute could only go so far and were placing undue pressure on all three of them. The advent of home computers was the stimulus for this breakthrough, as is featured in Young's 1982 song "Transformer Man." The most personal of the tracks on his experimental electronic album *Trans*, "Transformer Man" explores how computers generate alternative expressive possibilities for his son. The song's themes are both worldly and imaginative: a push button allows the boy to gain a mastery over his environment that is imaged in his shining and electrifying eyes. And a transformer turns disability into agency, as symbolized on the reverse of the album cover, which depicts the cross-section of a fully functioning heart, but with circuitry added.

Neil and Pegi Young's work with Ben led to the creation of the Bridge School based in Hillsborough, California, which has worked developmentally and collaboratively with children with a range of physical, cognitive, and speech-related conditions since it opened in 1987. The school offers specially designed education programs for children between the ages of three and fourteen who have "such severe communication and physical disabilities that they don't use speech to meet the majority of their communication needs."[62] In 1986, the Youngs also launched an annual all-acoustic Bridge School Benefit Concert to raise awareness of and funds to support treatment of developmental disabilities. They believed that stripped-down acoustic music can offer a bridge for children, revealing a path between repetitive rigidity on the one hand and what postmodern theorist Fredric Jameson called a chaotic "rubble of distinct and unrelated signifiers" on the other.[63] Neil and Pegi Young also thought that exposure to accomplished musicians can go some way toward preventing the child from feeling marooned outside mainstream culture.

These two examples are at odds in many ways: the Son-Rise program makes room for children to express themselves in ways that caregivers follow through mimicry, whereas the Human Potential model imposes an exacting regime that can be taxing for both parents and child. Structured classrooms may help by establishing enabling systems of behavior, but so, too, can adults' active participation in the child's play world, thereby countering Bettelheim's idea that parents damage their children. This was a point Sylvester Stallone emphasized in a 1985 interview for *People* magazine when he reflected on his autistic son Seargeoh: Stallone's crumbling marriage and film acting commitments meant that his son did not receive sustained attention from either parent over a crucial three-year developmental period and his autistic behavior consequently worsened.[64] Given the demise of the family unit that so concerned Christopher Lasch, Seargeoh Stallone's case was far from unique. Determining the correct level of stimuli remained a contested topic, though, into the 1990s, a period when applied behavior analysis was being widely adopted as an effective immersive technique for aiding children with mild and moderate forms of autism.[65] More broadly, the examples of Raun Kaufman and Ben Young both emphasize creative engagement with the object world, equal attention to cognitive and motor functions, the importance of integrating empathic therapy into home life, and recognizing unique elements among typical symptoms. Not only can play create new patterns of meaning but it also has the capacity to alleviate feelings of isolation through a culture of participation in which children, adults, and therapists are active co-creators.

Rain Man: Subjects and Objects

The cases considered so far in this chapter have focused on children. Psychologist Robert Coles brought attention to their plight in "Children of Crisis," a five-volume series of field studies, beginning with *A Study in Courage and Fear* in 1967 and running through the 1970s, in which he tried to get to know young Americans from different regions and backgrounds from a developmental rather than a medical perspective. By the early 1980s, genetic research was beginning to explore the possible correlation between a fragile X chromosome and occurrences of autism, but its neurobiology and the effects of neuroregulators were only dimly understood, leading some writers to expand the category to take into account a number of symptoms that might otherwise be seen as childhood idiosyncrasies.[66] Although it was thought that such conditions affected less than 1 percent of the country's population, films such as *Taxi Driver*, in which Travis Bickle (Robert De Niro) displays adaptive and expressive problems as an adult, and *Being There* (1981), which focuses on an enigmatic yet educationally challenged Chauncy Gardener (Peter Sellers), are evidence of a general awareness of the effects of childhood conditions on adult life. The protagonists in these cinematic portrayals combine adult and childlike traits, preserving an aura of innocence despite the political and social corruption that surrounds them. That does not mean that the characters are tabula rasa onto which the frustrations and fantasies of others are projected, but both struggle to find meaning in urban spaces that are especially challenging to people uprooted from family structures. Neither film indulges in nostalgia for a halcyon moment that might have rescued them; rather, they hint at underlying neurobiological conditions (Travis's case is complicated by war trauma) that are exacerbated by the loneliness that define their adult stories.

The tendency to expand the categories of developmental and intellectual disabilities in these and other portrayals meant that the strict diagnostics of *DSM-III* were at odds with cultural representations. However, the one event that changed public perception of autism more than any other was the release of Barry Levinson's film *Rain Man* in December 1988.[67] Dustin Hoffman's portrayal of the adult savant Raymond Babbitt was partly based on the Utah-born Kim Peek, who had an amazing gift of recall alongside developmental challenges that affected his childhood and schooling. It was Peek's savant qualities that interested screenwriter Barry Morrow when they met in 1984. Morrow had previously written a screenplay about Bill Sackter, the Minnesotan son of Russian immigrants who had overcome mild intellectual disabilities and years of institutionalization to lead a relatively conventional life. Morrow carried his interest in individuals who are misdiagnosed and misunderstood into Hoffman's portrayal of Raymond Babbitt, which hinges on the relationship with his arrogant younger brother Charlie, played by Tom Cruise. Sackter was already in the public eye when Mickey Rooney embodied him in the 1981 CBS film *Bill*; this followed Sackter's Handicapped Iowan of the Year award in 1976 and a reception at the White House three years later. In contrast, Kim Peek's condition did not come to public attention until *Rain Man*, when Peek was 37, just a little younger than the fictional Raymond.

As a method actor, Dustin Hoffman interacted with Peek at length to ensure that his mannerisms were authentic. Raymond's ability to recall facts and to quickly digest large quantities of data was taken straight from Peek, but Hoffman's portrayal develops Morrow's original treatment of 1986, making him more contemplative than the extroverted Peek.[68] Arguably Peek's enlarged head (a condition called macrocephaly), his savant traits, his limited social skills, and his difficulty in carrying out daily tasks were too diverse for a character whom his brother and the viewer come to feel strongly about, even though Raymond speaks in a monotone and shows his emotions only in stressful situations. Although Peek receives a special mention in the closing credits, his condition was probably too complex for a Hollywood film and his savant skills too cerebral for a character with whom the viewer is encouraged to empathize despite his limited emotional range.[69] Echoing Peter Sellers's performance in *Being There*, there is something wondrous in Hoffman's performance. It creates a complex fraternal dynamic with Raymond's streetwise yet naive brother Charlie and arguably conjures a movie version of autism that molds to the narrative intent of the film.

The film does not easily fit the paradigm of Martin Norden's "cinema of isolation," the dominant concept of an insightful 1994 book on film characters with physical disabilities, in which Norden argues that such characters tend to be visually segregated from other characters on screen. The brothers' interaction (instead of Raymond's isolation) is an important aspect of Morrow's original treatment and is conveyed strongly through the acting skills of Hoffman and Cruise who based the relationship of Raymond and Charlie Babbitt on that of two New Jersey brothers, Peter and Kevin Guthrie. While Kevin lived a conventional life and became a Princeton football star, Peter was partially cut off from the outside world, even though he was able to live alone (with a roommate) and found employment in a Princeton library. Peter tended to use stock phrases and relied on statistics about individuals, dates, and songs instead of being able to conduct a meaningful dialogue. These traits of Peter's are reflected in Raymond's use of repetitive phrase such as "I'm an excellent driver," his recall of days and dates, and his tendency to verbally spell out the names. Hoffman also mentioned another autistic savant in his February 1990 Oscar acceptance speech: Joseph Sullivan, the son of one of the film's consultants, Ruth Sullivan, the founder (in 1979) of the non-profit Autism Services Center in West Virginia. This genealogy is important because it suggests that Raymond is a composite character and connects the feature film to two documentaries made by the UCLA Neuropsychiatric Institute and Hospital that focus on Sullivan as a child and in his mid-twenties. The first of these, *Infantile Autism: The Invisible Wall* (1967), showed Sullivan's withdrawal from the world at the age of seven. Hoffman carefully studied the second, *Portrait of an Autistic Young Man* (1985), a follow-up study showing Joseph's partial integration into an adult world.[70]

This notion of a composite is at odds with Fran Peek's claim that his son was the original rain man. However, the shift toward an exploration of autism within the framework of Raymond's personal journey from the Midwest care home Wallbrook (its name combining images of entrapment and possibility) to the

West Coast is a stronger aspect of the film than an exploration of his savantism. Stuart Murray notes that Raymond's savant skills are rare because he can recall both words and numbers with amazing precision but cannot repeat his feats of memorization when applied to real-life situations, such as the cost of food items.[71] Although he is unable to cope with even a mild deviation from his dietary regime, Raymond can calculate the number of toothpicks on the floor and recall a phone number after systematically reading the phonebook from A to G. His doctor, who is the trustee of his estate, labels him as autistic from the outset (a diagnostic term that Charlie initially finds difficult to comprehend), but the film deliberately limits interaction with medical officials to a check-up in a Nebraska town at a pivotal halfway point in their transcontinental road trip, at which point Charlie is just beginning to understand his brother.

Charlie's language is littered with insults and misconceptions early on; he impatiently tells Raymond to "stop acting like an idiot" and arrogantly announces "I know what's good for him." In the novelization of the film, this is more overt: Charlie tests out Raymond's special abilities as he would a dog and ridicules him when he recites the beginning of *Twelfth Night* with no understanding of the meaning or the story.[72] Early in the film, Charlie's body language is harsh and angular, yet subtle changes to his posture and vocal tone show that his interactions with Raymond positively influence his value system and educate him about autism. Just as Charlie starts to learn about the condition of autism from a zero base, so the film experience is a learning curve for the average viewer to such an extent that Hoffman's portrayal has become a baseline for future autistic representations. This seems progressive, given Hoffman's nuanced performance and the paucity of comparable cinematic roles outside an institutional setting, but it set a vanishing point for future portrayals, so much so that "Rain Man" became an identity label that was hard to shift.[73] Although it offers insights into the distinctive talents and social limitations of a savant, the film implies that savant syndrome and autism are always linked, which is not the case; only 10 percent of autistic individuals display savant tendencies. This does not mean that high-functioning cases are statistically insignificant, as Wisconsin psychiatrist Darold Treffert (a technical consultant on the film) discussed in his 1989 book *Extraordinary People*, but that these are the cases where the individual has most capacity to "introspect and report."[74] Nonetheless, the mental health aspect of *Rain Man* relates less to savant syndrome and more to questions of care, with a straight either-or choice between Raymond returning to Wallbrook and living with his brother.

The human dimension of the story captured the attention of influential reviewers such as Roger Ebert, who claimed that Charlie's "significant learning moment" provides the momentum of the film, particularly as Charlie slowly realizes that in some respects Raymond has more potential than he himself has.[75] In this respect, the road trip from Cincinnati to Los Angeles becomes symbolic of the voyage of discovery Charlie undergoes. Tom Cruise has commented in interview that Charlie is "emotionally autistic" when the movie begins. Paradoxically, the fact that Raymond cannot step outside himself means that Charlie has to work

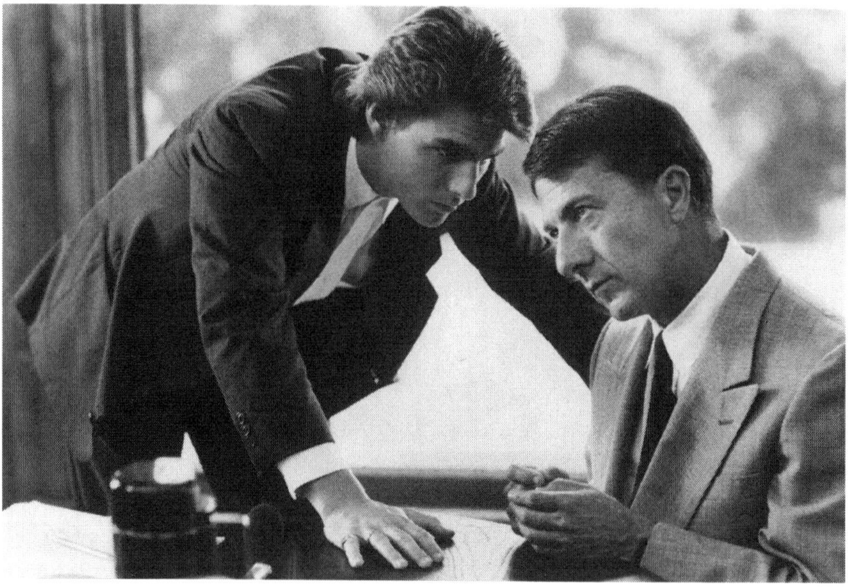

Figure 5.2 Charlie and Raymond Babbitt (Tom Cruise and Dustin Hoffman) interact in *Rain Man* (dir. Barry Levinson, 1988) as Charlie makes the case for Raymond not to return to Wallbrook. United Artists/The Kobal Collection.

harder to connect with a world that he feels has done him wrong, given that his mother died when he was very young, leaving him with an unloving father and a world of hard deals. His bond with Raymond grows in the aftermath of their father's funeral and against the backdrop of Charlie's failing business, but it takes a long time for Charlie to respect not only what Treffert calls Raymond's "islands of intelligence" (possibly due to a compensatory growth in the right hemisphere of the brain to offset a deficiency in the left hemisphere) but also the idiosyncratic lifeworld of his brother. During the course of the film, Charlie undergoes a sharp learning curve that takes him from a con man to a brother Raymond can trust and a man who is able to value people over material things.[76]

The learning curve is not just one way, however. Raymond does change to a certain extent and he moves, at least to a degree, from a world populated by objects, statistics, and schedules. This enables him to connect with others, albeit briefly, such as when he dances in the lift with Charlie's girlfriend and when the two brothers touch heads in one of the closing scenes after the attorney decides that Raymond should return to his care home. The film is as much about objects as it is about subjects, though. The opening image shows the shell of a sports car being lowered by machinery into Charlie's car yard, while Raymond is attached to his pens and drawing paper, his baseball cards, and food items. Raymond also takes photographs of shapes, shadows, and signs as he attempts to capture the new world outside Wallbrook. We see a series of out-of-focus and partial objects in the snapshots at the end credits; while the photographs are not artful, they are reminiscent of how Robert Frank's 1959 photo-travelogue *The Americans* exposed a hidden America that lies beyond the photographic frame. The psychological journey the brothers undertake helps them negotiate the object world in a more meaningful way. But it is easy to retreat into this world, as when Charlie exploits Raymond's savant memory in a Las Vegas casino to alleviate his debt and in the final scene when Raymond is absorbed in the glow of his portable television as he departs on a Cincinnati-bound train instead of reciprocating his brother's emotional good-bye.

Opinion on the importance of *Rain Man* for heightening awareness of autism was mixed. Bernard Rimland, a Californian psychologist who cofounded the Autism Society of America in 1965 (he also had a son with autism), argued that the film had "brought a great sense of relief to many autistics and their families," and the founder of the Central Florida chapter of the society claimed that it had "created more media attention than our national and local autistics organizations have been able to do in 25 years."[77] A 12-year-old boy, Brent Aden, received a confidence boost when he saw the film, prompting him to write to Hoffman to say that now "people say autism is OK. I'm free now."[78] However, others thought that the emphasis on Raymond's savant abilities was unrepresentative and many were negative about the return to Wallbrook; they argued that a third option of living in sheltered accommodation with a mentor would have been more progressive.[79] The belief that *Rain Man* relied on autistic stereotypes intensified in the 1990s, in the context of a growing recognition of the broad neurodiversity of autistic experiences. And despite the film's indisputable educational value, its mythic structure, the portrayal of a damaged hero, and the controversy over who is the "real rain man" could be seen as distractions from a more nuanced understanding.[80]

Closed Windows, Open Doors

Another text that arguably influenced the final shape of *Rain Man* exemplifies a comment that Clara Park made in *The Siege* about a mysterious will to live that is often missing in children on the severe end of the autistic spectrum but can be stimulated by a combination of internal and external factors. These factors came into play in the case of Temple Grandin, who in 1986 published an account of her life from the time she was diagnosed with autism at age two (in 1949) through to her considerable achievements as a professor of animal science at Colorado State University in the early 1990s. Grandin is not a savant, but after displaying slow language development in her early years, she developed an academic flair and attentiveness to animal behavior that enabled her to surpass the expectations of her parents and doctors. She recounts this journey in her co-written autobiography *Emergence: Labeled Autistic* with a direct style that does not strive for the reader's sympathy: for example, when she describes delayed language acquisition she writes simply that "screaming, peeping, humming were my means of communication."[81] The account is intended to show that autism does not necessarily lead to a limited horizon and that fortress-like behavioral traits can be "modified and controlled."[82] By confounding the expectations of doctors who believed that institutionalization was the best option, Grandin proves that individuals with autism can develop significantly and attain goals that seem out of reach.

Grandin has continued to write about her experiences, her work with animals, and the ways her visual imagination enables her to compensate for language limitations, but I will reserve my commentary to a pair of texts written in the 1980s and 1990s: *Emergence: Labeled Autistic* and *Thinking in Pictures*. The extraordinary nature of Grandin's story is often emphasized: for example, in the introduction to her 2011 book *The Way I See It*, Emily Gerson Saines (who produced the 2010 HBO biopic *Temple Grandin*) notes that the fact that she became "the most successful designer of humane livestock handling facilities" makes her story "remarkable."[83] That Grandin's story was exemplary does not mean she had innate exceptional abilities, just that supportive structures and a will to adapt meant she could tap into creative energies and visual thinking abilities that would have been overlooked in other circumstances. This resilience did not mean that she was averse to *Rain Man*. She thought that Hoffman's portrayal was subtle (he too displayed visual imagination through his interest in photography and drawing), yet she believed a better ending would have seen Raymond entering a partially residential group home, thereby channeling some of the energy he gains on the journey.[84]

The therapy that Grandin experienced as a child was a version of applied behavior analysis that involved repetition and reinforcement, but this was continuous with home life instead of distinct from it. Perhaps the most vital element was the fact that her mother and grandmother encouraged her to develop her painting skills. She found this to be a more creative outlet than language and later believed that it helped her learn flexibility, sequencing skills, and visual processing. Art also taught her to negotiate boundaries between subjects and objects without fear of anxiety or embarrassment. In *The Way I See It*, Grandin writes that the creative arts (particularly those that require care and attention over a significant time span, such as embroidery) can help build a sense of accomplishment and self-esteem that are vital for preventing the gloom and depression that sometimes envelop autistic children and for dissuading them from the belief that a fortress-like world is much safer than human interaction. The creative arts also help her see that children can develop "healthy self-esteem" and that hobbies can make a big difference, especially if encouragement and praise follow even small achievements.[85]

It is in her work with animals and her visual thinking that Grandin has contributed most to a fuller understanding of autism. Her discussion of these two topics include elements of storytelling, but in an unconventional way, using intuition and imagery as a bridge between herself and the world. More recently she has compared her mind to an Internet search engine that processes "photo-realistic pictures that pop up in my imagination." This is the method she used to design cattle equipment in her professional life. As a teenager, she managed to channel her capacity to visually associate images into a creative method that allows her to think around the edges of categories and to speed up her thinking processes to compensate for the difficulties she had as a child in assimilating data.[86] Although autistic children's drawings are often dismissed because they are seen as repetitive and as fixating on patterns, Grandin's interest in horses enabled her to focus on anatomical detail and to develop spatial skills that she later applied into designing equipment for livestock.[87] Drawing was not a solitary or escapist pursuit for Temple because it connected her with the outside world. After honing her skills at basic modeling, she designed a sophisticated dip vat for cattle, envisioning the experience through a cow's wide-angle vision to reduce the element of surprise that often panics cattle. This capacity for both pure and applied thinking allowed Grandin to work with psychological patterns instead of designing on a formulaic basis, thereby countering the idea that those with autism have an "empathic impairment."[88]

It is this empathic capacity that Oliver Sacks stressed when he dedicated one of his case studies to Grandin in his 1995 book *An Anthropologist on Mars*. He took his concept from a phrase of Grandin's. Yet instead of being a stigmatizing title (a charge that has been leveled at his earlier book *The Man Who Mistook His Wife for a Hat*), this phrase captures the subtlety of someone who often feels like a stranger in the midst of others but can see and imagine things from very different perspectives (as Sacks, a sufferer of prosopagnosia, or face blindness, tried himself to do). The best example of this is Grandin's rational thought process that led to the development of a human squeeze machine, which she based on a model she had seen deployed for cattle maintenance. Although she could not bear close physical contact, Grandin realized that pressure stimulation can be comforting for humans, just as it is for animals. With the encouragement of her science teacher, she devised a machine she could lie within where she could control the pressure against her body. After a session in the squeeze machine she felt relaxed and more empathic; she also found that her hypersensitivity was calmed in a safe environment. She realized, though, that the squeeze machine was not a miracle device and that medication such as Tofranil, Norpramin, and Prozac (at a lower dose than for depression) can also have a beneficial calming effect.[89]

Sacks's essay on Grandin, which was first published in the *New Yorker* in 1993, is a wonderfully sensitive account of a woman who combined strength and vulnerability in equal measure. Sacks is attentive to Grandin's environment: the wide open spaces and mountains of Colorado, her crowded office, the detailed instructions that Sacks receives about where they are to meet, and his sense that she was "a sturdy, no-nonsense cattlewoman" who would be hard to maintain in an eastern city.[90] Sacks is intrigued by Grandin's visual imagination, which enables her to approximate to the perspective of animals, and the squeeze machine, which reminds him of the calming pressure of a wet suit while deep-sea diving. He concludes that on a "primal, almost animal level . . . of the sensorimotor, the concrete, the unmediated Temple is enormously sensitive," but she finds it difficult to participate in games, visualize abstractions, or understand nuances of gesture and language. The latter difficulty dates back to her childhood, when pronouns, prepositions, and grammar confused her.[91] At the heart of the essay is an appreciation of the fine balances in Grandin's lifeworld that sometimes overwhelm her and other times makes her more adept than neurotypical people.

Grandin writes in straightforward sentences that move from a scientific reflection on her condition and an awareness of patterns that structure her mind.

Although she is often unsure about abstractions, she sometimes likens social discomfort to being trapped between windows (an actual experience in her teen years) and her ability to develop new lines of thought as a series of doors she is determined to open.[92] These developmental possibilities align with other accounts, such as the 1992 book *There's a Boy in Here* (which combines the retrospective perspectives of a mother and her autistic son) and, a year later, Catherine Maurice's *Let Me Hear Your Voice* (which promotes behavioral modification and is skeptical about Kaufman's Son-Rise program).[93] Grandin's writing also struck a chord with two new advocacy groups, the National Alliance for Autism Research and Defeat Autism Now! The latter group, which Bernard Rimland founded in 1995, looked to fund projects outside mainstream medicine at a time when the Internet was starting to offer a powerful tool for conveying new research and for helping families share stories.[94] The web was too much in its infancy for it to be considered an educational tool for those diagnosed with autism and it could spread misinformation based on unconfirmed data. Nevertheless, it offered a digitally augmented world that Neil Young had imagined a decade before and that chimed with Sherry Turkle's view that computers could help children navigate between subjects and objects and to "think in an active way about complex phenomena (some of them 'real life,' some of them not) as dynamic, evolving systems."[95]

Developmental Disabilities in the 1990s

In June 1997, newly elected Democrat representative Steven Rothman gave an impassioned speech in Congress. Reflecting on his nephew's autism, Rothman reminded his political allies and adversaries that one in five hundred American children is autistic and that 95 percent of that group would never be economically independent. He framed these statistics and a call for dedicated research by saying that the ways autism affects the lives of regular families "will not be learned from watching the movie *Rain Man*."[96] The film arguably contributed to the rise in reported cases of autism, although there is no hard data to confirm this and only a few related longitudinal studies.[97] More likely this spike of reported cases was due to a higher profile for disability rights and the introduction of the Institutional Development Award program in the early 1990s, which offered educational services to children with learning difficulties.

Rothman's speech was delivered three years after the fourth edition of *DSM* recognized that developmental disabilities encompassed a broader sphere of conditions, that diagnostics needed to be more nuanced, and that there were different versions of autism, such as Asperger's syndrome, which was included as a separate condition for the first time in *DSM-IV*. The development in terminology worked in tandem with the growing sense that it was harmful to use highly abstract categories or to lump together varying experiences across a developmental spectrum. Vaccine scares linked to mercury, such as Hib meningitis and hepatitis B (and the perceived dangers of the MMR vaccine in Britain in the late 1990s), might have been a possible cause of the increase in the cases of infantile autism. Although the panic in the United States was largely unfounded, by the time of Rothman's speech the number of reported cases of autism had risen twenty-fold over two decades.[98]

Despite President Bush's emphasis on employment awareness and his belief that all citizens should be able to participate in the "mainstream of life," the Americans with Disabilities Act of 1990 did not directly influence research on developmental disabilities. However, it did put pressure on employers to "open doors of opportunity," and by mid-decade new federal and state funds were dedicated to supporting the employment of people with disabilities.[99] More important in developmental terms was the Individuals with Disabilities Education Act of 1991, which built on the efforts of the National Center for Learning Difficulties to educate the public. This act embodied First Lady Barbara Bush's interest in special education needs and the transition from school learning to adulthood. It was expanded four years later to include assistive technology for those with cognitive and intellectual disabilities.[100]

In 1994, the NIMH began the Multi-Site Study of Mental Health Service Use to assess the types of mental health treatments and services used by a sample of 10,000 children and adolescents. The aims of this $45 million project were quite vague and it did not focus on children younger than four years old. However, it did mark a shift of priority to children's health during President Clinton's second term that led First Lady Hillary Clinton to become involved in a public discussion about the possible correlation between vaccination and autism. The Autism Society of America had lobbied Barbara Bush in the spring of 1993 to establish a task force on autism, but the topic was slow to appear on the federal radar despite Mrs. Bush's promise to speak to the new first lady about it.[101] By the mid-1990s, federal departments had begun to take the condition more seriously, signaled by an executive order in April 1997 that required deeper consideration of environmental health and safety risks on children and a bill that went to Congress in 1998 and again in 1999 that sought increased research on autism in the Department of Health and Human Services. The 1998 federal budget awarded the NIMH the highest increase of all the national health institutes to research the relationship between genetic and environmental factors in a range of childhood conditions. These initiatives, important as they were, were just a prelude to the Children's Health Act of 2000, which made autism research its highest priority in the fields of neurobiology, genetics, psychopharmacology, and epidemiology (other sections focused on Tourette syndrome, birth defects, and fragile X chromosomes), although worries about the overmedication of children persisted beyond the millennium.[102]

While historical reasons can be given for the increasing prevalence of autism and related developmental disabilities in the 1990s, a time when genetic research was offering a better understanding of the relationship between biology and environment, what remained dimly understood and usually undertreated was what Mohammad Ghaziuddin calls the "superadded conditions of autism," which include hyperactive behavior, depression, rage, and dissociation. The effective treatment of these conditions can lead to marked improvements in well-being and mental health.[103] Ghaziuddin argued that those older than 18 with autism were frequently lost in the system, making it more difficult to treat symptoms effectively in adult life unless there was a detailed case history from childhood.[104] Noting that psychiatric symptoms arise among individuals with autistic spectrum disorders at a higher rate than the mean, particularly those diagnosed with Asperger's, Ghaziuddin warned that untreated symptoms could sometimes lead to aggression or self-harm.[105] Concluding that those on the autistic spectrum are more vulnerable to environmental stressors that are sometimes exacerbated by genetic factors, he noted that the correlation between depression and autism was underresearched and that those without verbal competence could sometimes stay lost in their own isolated world.[106]

As philosophers such as Ian Hacking and writers such as Jean-Dominique Bauby were asking profound questions about the nature of insulated and isolated selves, the attempt to tell the story of developmental disabilities from the inside led to a number of films in the 1990s that tried to move beyond both the horizon of *The Empty Fortress* and the narrative limitations of *Rain Man*.[107] These films sometimes retain a medical framework, such as the 1999 film *Molly*, which echoes the narrative arc of *Awakenings* in depicting a young woman Molly McKay (played by Elizabeth Shue) who is released from long-term inpatient care when her institution is force to close. Under the care of her reluctant brother, Molly briefly experiences a functional return following an experimental drug procedure that at least does lip service to neurology. Healthy brain cells are implanted into her own in an unproven technique that gestures toward an experimental procedure performed on a multiple sclerosis patient through the transnational Myelin Project. The film mixes both optimism and loss into a trite account of "movie autism" that is played out through renewed contact between Molly and her estranged brother. This theme of emotional contact is taken further in the 2001 film *I Am Sam*, in which Sean Penn's portrayal of the autistic and childlike father Sam Dawson (who has the IQ of a seven-year-old) dominates a story about legal rights, caregiving, and literacy (the film strives for authenticity by including two actors from the Los Angeles developmental disabilities center L.A. Goal, which was pioneering acting therapy). Autistic behavior occasionally featured in other genres such as the 1998 neo-Cold War thriller *Mercury Rising*, based on Ryne Douglas Pearson's challenging novel *Simple Simon*, in which a nine-year-old boy plays the role of code cracker to decipher a national security code established during the Reagan years.

Quite often generic limitations constrain the health possibilities of protagonists or push actors toward the virtuoso styles of Penn's and Shue's performances that hide more pressing social or ideological issues behind emotive stories. Even the imperiled Simon Lynch in *Mercury Rising* and the abused autistic child Tim Warden in the 1994 mystery film *Silent Fall* do not move far beyond the clichés of the autistic savant.[108] Literary critic Mark Osteen points to the problem that authors face in trying to balance "narrative cohesion" and "the obligation to tell the truth" about autism. Like *Rain Man*, these tales sometimes descend into clichés about savantism or slip into focusing on the moral education of non-autistic characters.[109] Only when the autistic label is discarded or pushed into the background do narrative possibilities open up, such as in Jonathan Letham's account of the tourettic Lionel Essrog in his 1999 urban detective novel *Motherless Brooklyn*.[110] Because Lionel can "never leaves words unmolested," his verbal tics disrupt and reorder language patterns to open up what critic James Berger calls an alternative "symbolic landscape."[111] In exploring alterity, *Motherless Brooklyn* thus foreshadows the move to greater innovation in literary accounts written since the millennium that take into account neurodiversity and show evidence of heightened literacy about mental health.

Dubious claims about autism circulated in the mid-1990s, such as the controversy about facilitated communication (where the helper or therapist was thought to guide the writing hand of the individual) and claims that the diet pill Pondimin or the intestinal hormone secretin could have miraculous effects (the former was recalled in 1997 after being linked to severe side effects in cardiac functioning and the latter was debunked in 1999).[112] But I want to close this chapter by looking at two of the most interesting biographical accounts of autism at the turn of the century, both of them updates of books discussed earlier. Clara Claiborne Park revisited the story she had begun in the late 1960s with an evocative description of her now-adult daughter (this time given her real name of Jessica, or Jessy), and Raun Kaufman—who we see as an autistic child in Barry Kaufman's *Son-Rise* and as an affectionate child in *A Miracle to Believe In*—wrote a journal account of his interactions with the daughter of his elder sister. In both cases, the worlds of adults and children are bridged by the awareness that autism might just be another way of seeing and telling stories about the world instead of a radically different reality. Although the publication dates go beyond this book's historical parameters—Park's *Exiting Nirvana* was published in 2001 and Kaufman's *Autism Breakthrough* did not appear until 2014—the texts reflect on experiences in the 1990s and a more enlightened attitude toward a spectrum of behaviors.

Following the 1982 edition of *The Siege*, which included an epilogue updating Park's daughter's story fifteen years after the first publication of the book, *Exiting Nirvana* tries harder to give Jessy her own voice through frequent quotations that capture her unique intonation, the "strange systems" of her words, and the texture of her paintings.[113] The book is inspired by Grandin's accounts of her visual imagination and pivots on the idea that Jessy's life is both extraordinary and ordinary in equal measure: what Park calls "precious ordinariness."[114] This is best expressed in Jessy's art lessons, the only class that she could take at school alongside "normal children."[115] Park sees her painting technique as deeply autistic—"literal, repetitive, obsessively exact"—and yet "rich and strange" in its shapes and patterns.[116] Jessy has a "geometrizing eye" for detail and often paints in vivid colors, perhaps to overcompensate for a lack of shading and depth. It is not so much that painting transfigures her world, but it provides a technique to manage a world of objects and buildings that, even as an adult, is less threatening than a world of interpersonal interaction (her art rarely depicts people).

Raun Kaufman echoes the family contact of his father's *Son-Rise* book in his brief yet moving account of his niece Jade in the late 1990s whose language development was arrested at age two, when repetitive behavior and frequent crying and screaming also emerged. Kaufman's account of Jade is very personal: he feels compelled to make a transcontinental trip to work with her and describes the experience as one that helps awaken his caring and creative side. Instead of adopting a neutral descriptive voice, Kaufman's two brief vignettes of the five-year program are written in a poetic idiom. In the first extract, from September 1998, the play world of an imaginary ship becomes a real voyage of discovery for the pair, especially as he manages to prolong Jade's engagement in the activity for more than a few minutes. Kaufman uses a pair of *Sesame Street* toys, Ernie and Cookie Monster, to engage with Jade on her level. He mimics her behavior and makes a brief moment of contact before disappearing from her reality when he tries to introduce his own element of a capsized boat.

The second entry, from August 1999, reveals that Jade has developed a command of language and is able to tolerate the boat rocking on the water and physical proximity that she would not bear eleven months earlier. When he pretends to fall overboard this time, he is relieved and excited that Jade helps him back into the boat, an incident that reminds him of his own childhood journey from seclusion to participation. Kaufman uses these two accounts to illustrate the potential of the Son-Rise program, pointing out that although Jade's development was slower than his, she grew into a "social young adult" with a "great sense of humor."[117] He surprises the reader when he mentions that Jade was adopted by his sister, trying to dispel some genetic myths that would make developmental disabilities more firmly shaped by hereditary factors than he or his father would wish to believe. It is easy to be cynical about the account or point out that it ignores neurological and genetic research of the late 1990s. But in exploring the mental health implications of developmental disability, both *Autism Breakthrough* and *Exiting Nirvana* steer a course between science, therapy, and human interaction—and, in doing so, help banish the specter of Bettelheim's *The Empty Fortress*.

6 *Body Image, Anorexia, and the Mass Media*

When President Reagan's drug abuse policy advisor, Carlton Turner announced at the giant Health Care Expo '85 that "we are probably the most health-conscious people in the world," biochemical research into the benefits of vitamins and minerals for improving developmental disabilities was still in its infancy.[1] Turner's announcement followed a wave of interest in orthomolecular therapy and megavitamins as an effective dietary supplement for a spectrum of conditions that included schizophrenia, addiction recovery, attention deficit disorder, and autism.[2] The American Psychiatric Association had been trying since 1973 to temper the bold claims of such megavitamin exponents as chemist Linus Pauling, but this trend was just one facet of a growing medical and educational emphasis on nutrition and exercise. Concerns about balanced diets were most acute when linked to children's health, especially as obesity levels and public spending on fast food were increasing.[3] This helps explain why "vulnerable children" was a strong theme of President Clinton's second term and also why, in the surgeon general's 1996 report *Physical Activity and Health*, the Secretary of Health and Human Services Donna Shalala encouraged the 60 percent of Americans who were not regularly active to join a new "fitness movement."[4]

The health of children had become a hot topic in the 1980s, as exemplified by Nancy Reagan's Just Say No campaign and mounting worries among social workers about children of alcoholic parents and those at risk of sexual abuse.[5] There is no reliable data to pinpoint the moment when bodily dissatisfaction became normative for American women and girls, but the rapid growth of the mass media and the heightened visibility in the 1980s of the female body in advertising, fashion magazines, and music videos served to intensify self-scrutiny and dietary regulation. Feminist critic Naomi Wolf was less concerned about the vulnerability of certain social groups to "food oppression" (estimates suggested that food advertising doubled during the 1990s) and more how the beauty industry places undue pressure on the young to conform to unrealizable body images.[6] Whereas autism tended to lengthen childhood in terms of dependency on caregivers, Wolf argued in her widely read book *The Beauty Myth* (1990) that the pressure on American girls and teenagers to look a certain way was often so intense they risked having their childhood robbed from them prematurely.

Wolf's book was one of the highest-profile feminist publications of the 1990s. It linked a critique of the beauty industry to a belief that the new freedoms that women had recently gained were being undermined by "social limits" that were transposed onto their "faces and bodies."[7] Health was just one theme of Wolf's mission to reinvigorate feminism for a conservative era, contributing to a broader conversation about the politics of women's health that harked back to the early 1970s with the landmark publication of *Our Bodies, Ourselves*. *The Beauty Myth* can be criticized for its sketchy historical data. Yet behind Wolf's polemical stance is a perceptive account of teenage identity and eating.[8] Although her focus was on endangered young women, she acknowledged that in 1990—the year of the first study of eating disorders among males—men were also "being cast as a frontier market" and sold "the same half-truths" in the pursuit of beauty.[9]

The Beauty Myth leans heavily on the work of émigré psychoanalyst and anorexia expert Hilde Bruch, whose psychodynamic research, stretching from her 1957 book *The Problem of Overweight* to her posthumously published *Conversations with Anorexics*, explored the ways many girls and young women were struggling to maintain equilibrium between a balanced body image and food intake. Bruch's 1978 book *The Golden Cage* was her most important publication for raising public awareness of anorexia as a "new disease" of postwar America.[10]

There were a few earlier cases, such as that of the anorexic and suicidal patient Ellen West, as recorded in 1945 by Swiss psychiatrist Ludwig Binswanger. Forty years later, Ellen West was being discussed again at the autumn 1985 American Academy of Psychotherapists conference, following the publication of a poem about West by feminist poet Adrienne Rich, who saw Ellen as someone who was potentially transgressive in her hunger "for a forbidden life" but was entrapped by patriarchal language and treatment.[11] Despite popular interest in the politics of anorexia, a body of literature on the etiology and gender specificity of eating disturbances was slow to mature and its interrelations with other conditions were often hazy. Although there are profound diagnostic differences between autism and anorexia, both conditions pose radical questions about body boundaries and the individual's relationship with the object world. John Sours gave voice to this convergence in his 1980 book *Starving to Death in a Sea of Objects*, a title that evokes the difficulty anorexics often face in seeing their body image accurately and in fixating on food items through self-denial or a cycle of gorging and fasting. As a point of comparison, Temple Grandin also detected a blurring of subject-object relations for individuals with autistic traits, some of whom, she writes, "are unable to judge by feel where their body ends and the chair they are sitting on or the object they are holding begins."[12]

Although a fuller understanding of childhood autism made some advances in the 1960s, the rise of anorexia was only dimly felt in the following decade. Bruch began her research in the 1940s, at a time when Leo Kanner was studying autism, and she later concluded that anorexia was "a disorder involving extensive disturbances in personality development" and the anorexic individual's attempt to gain self-mastery.[13] However, she spent little time examining cultural pressures on the young. Such pressures were not discussed in much depth until the early 1980s, when bulimia nervosa first featured in *DSM-III* and the death of singer Karen Carpenter from self-starvation sparked public interest. In contrast, Wolf's chapter on eating disorders in *The Beauty Myth* begins against the backdrop of contemporary concerns by tacitly referencing fears about the spread of AIDS. Wolf might have been thinking more broadly about wasted bodies, yet there was a huge gulf in mortality rates between those with HIV/AIDS and those with anorexia.

Indeed, the turn of the 1990s was a moment for theoretical overstatements. French sociologist Jean Baudrillard explored the metaphor of anorexia in his 1989 essay "The Anorexic Ruins," at what he saw as an apocalyptic moment when individual agency was being put at risk by the cultural preoccupation with objects and surfaces. This was also a time of body distortions, exemplified by what President Clinton was to condemn in spring 1997 as "heroin chic" after the fatal overdose of Davide Sorrenti, whose fashion photography profiled the drug-addict look among extremely thin models.[14] Sorrenti's photographs can be read as symptomatic of what Baudrillard describes as "disgust for a world that is growing, accumulating, sprawling, sliding into hypertrophy."[15] On this level, food addiction might be seen as an obsessive-compulsive response to a world of object accumulation, where the body literally ingests the world. Conversely, anorexia—at least in its initial stages—may be an affirmative response to the ubiquity of consumption through denial or even an attempt to transcend the world through weightlessness. We might agree with British sociologist Morag MacSween that anorexia is "an attempt to articulate, at the level of the body, contradictory cultural expectations of women," but the danger is that the anorexic body merely ends up mirroring media obsession with slenderness and dietary control becomes just another form of addiction.[16]

Baudrillard's essay also marked a moment when the language of eating disorders had become unmoored from its medical specificity, where appetite, plenitude, denial, and emptiness were taking on more complex and sometimes contradictory cultural meanings. Just as the Slovenian theorist Slavoj Žižek tells us very little about autism when he calls it the "destruction of the symbolic universe," so Baudrillard's "Anorexic Ruins," despite its haunting title, does not offer much insight into the clinical manifestation of what *DSM-IV* called "body dysmorphic disorder" or the dramatic rise in recorded eating disturbances in the late 1970s.[17] The appropriation of the metaphors of anorexia by theorists does suggest, though, that it is risky to approach the subject without examining the confluence of clinical and cultural discourses on anorexia, bulimia, and body image disorder.[18] It is also important to recognize the ways this field became a focal point for feminist critics in the mid-1980s. This included writings by psychotherapist Susie Orbach, philosopher Susan Bordo, and psychiatrist and behavior specialist Katharine Phillips, each of whom explored "psychopathology and the crystallization of culture" (as Bordo described it in an important 1985 essay) and the interface between eating-related pathology and contradictory attitudes toward food at the cultural level.[19]

This chapter will reflect on these and related accounts that broadened the clinical focus of Hilde Bruch and anorexia specialist Steven Levenkron to assess body image and eating disorders as symptomatic of what Bordo calls "the multifaceted and heterogeneous distresses of our age."[20] Within this framework, Katharine Phillips warns us not to simply conflate body image conditions with anorexia but also to acknowledge that they share "compulsive behaviors such as mirror checking and body measuring" and "unusual eating or excessive dieting."[21] Bordo broadens the focus further to examine low self-esteem and "painfully self-critical standards" that are triggered by cultural expectations that individuals sometimes internalize because of pressures at home or from peers.[22] This does not mean the emphasis is transferred entirely onto the cultural sphere. However, from the early 1980s, when anorexia and bulimia were largely unknown to the public, through to the end of the 1990s, when Marya Hornbacher's autobiography *Wasted: A Memoir of Anorexia and Bulimia* placed the conditions firmly within the cultural mainstream, eating and body image disorders (alongside AIDS) arguably defined the medico-cultural landscape like no other.

The Case of Karen Carpenter

The moment when anorexia nervosa came of age in America was February 1983, when singer and drummer Karen Carpenter died at age 32 following more than a decade of health problems. She had begun dieting at 17 (in 1967), initially dropping twenty pounds on the Stillman water diet, and she increased her dietary regime following the success of The Carpenters' 1970 album *Close to You*. Although her family tried to cover up Karen's weight loss, it was plain from public appearances and interviews in the mid-1970s that she was suffering from extreme emaciation. Karen continued to play drums during performances, such as the brother-sister duo's performance at the White House on 1 May 1973, but her radio-friendly voice and patronage by President Nixon (he called The Carpenters "young America at its very best") meant that a dramatic rise to stardom, industry pressures, and shifting musical tastes took a toll on both Karen and Peter.[23] There are psychoanalytic theories for Karen's extreme dieting: she did not move far from home, she felt unloved, she experienced low self-esteem, and in 1980 she married an older father figure who betrayed her trust. These factors contributed to feelings of entrapment, leading Paula Saukko to claim that despite her "deep and sophisticated voice," Karen was "pathologized" by her parents and producer, who treated her "as an infantile woman with a regressive nonautonomous personality."[24] Whatever credence is placed on this quasi-clinical view, the reality was that her frail body dropped to 80 pounds in 1975 and she spent the next eight years at a dangerously low weight.

The control that Karen Carpenter sought over her body might be seen as the inverse of the excesses of the music industry, which saw Richard Carpenter addicted to Quaaludes by 1978 and as an inpatient at the Menninger Clinic in Topeka, Kansas in 1979. Whereas the death of Elvis Presley in August 1977 gave a very public face to alcohol and drug use, Karen's behavior was paradoxically both ascetic and excessive. Without an obvious specialist health center to visit for treatment, Karen no doubt felt isolated. Had more public health material on anorexia been available, she might have sought treatment earlier or have been pushed more strongly in that direction by her family and management. When her weight dropped to less than 80 pounds in late 1981, she began to consult New York psychoanalyst Steve Levenkron, encouraged by his 1978 book on anorexia *The Best Little Girl in the World*, which was turned into an ABC television adaptation in May

1981. Carpenter continued to see Levenkron up to the point when she was admitted to hospital in September 1982 with symptoms of arrhythmia and dehydration.

The fact that Karen Carpenter was taking thyroid medication on a daily basis (under a false name) to speed up her metabolism and laxatives to purge her body meant that she was active in the process instead of just restricting food intake. The topic of her weight sometimes arose in interviews, and she acknowledged that she was "sick" in 1975, the year that Richard claimed he first discovered Karen's eating disorder when he was forced to prematurely end a world tour.[25] This suggested that she was at an advanced stage of anorexic development that was starting to define her identity. However, not until Karen sought out Levenkron was she aware, it seems, that she was incapably thin and veering towards depression triggered by the breakup of her marriage. Levenkron practiced one-on-one therapy with Karen and held a group session with her parents and Richard, coming to the conclusion that the family dynamic was partly to blame, particularly Karen's mother Agnes, who, he assessed, was an "oppressive-dependent" presence who would not allow her daughter to grow up. In her final months, Karen regained some weight after being drip-fed in hospital, but this enforced feeding put a massive strain on her heart. Her death was triggered by cardiotoxicity stimulated by syrup of ipecac. After Karen died, Levenkron joined a campaign to ban over-the-counter sales of ipecac, a drug that bulimics were taking regularly to induce vomiting.[26]

Karen Carpenter's story spawned a mini-industry in 1983 and she became the celebrity face of eating disorders. That year the *Boston Globe* advice column received a letter from "Hating Myself in Calif." about a young women's inability to stop binging and using laxatives after she heard about Carpenter's death. The recommendation was to immediately call the Anorexia Self Help Group in Pasadena or seek referral from a doctor or mental health clinic.[27] *Chicago Tribune* journalist Joan Beck argued that Carpenter's demise "should focus some fresh concern on this bizarre and dangerous disorder that is now an epidemic among young women in this country."[28] Beck estimated that the death rate among women with eating disorders was around 10 percent, that 20 percent of college women were inducing vomiting, and that 70 percent of women were unhappy about their weight. Although Beck's "Self-Starvation in America" is a short piece, she understood media pressure, the dangers of semi-starvation, the psychodynamics of control and self-blame, and how innocent diets turn into dangerous habits for vulnerable young women. Her tone is slightly condescending when she describes anorexics as victims who in extreme cases "can no longer think clearly or understand the dangers they are creating for themselves." The piece is too brief to examine contemporary factors in any depth, such as what she calls "pervasive hyperactivity and competitiveness" that seemed to be prevalent in the United States in the early 1980s.[29] Overall, Beck's focus was on psychotherapy and family support, rather than on accessible support centers or deeper research into physical and psychological aspects of eating disorders.

The music industry had already moved through a cycle of disco, punk, and new wave by the date of Carpenter's death, but a young student at Bard College,

New York created an avant-garde film that kept her story fresh and gave it a new twist. *Superstar: The Karen Carpenter Story* is part Todd Haynes's homage to Karen Carpenter and part exploration of the cultural and familial pressures that pushed her to self-starvation. Co-written and co-produced with Cynthia Schneider, *Superstar* is an ironic film, using dolls in place of actors, a miniature set to emphasize the claustrophobia that Karen may have felt, and a soundtrack in which deep emotions are in danger of being lost in a wash of sentiment. Haynes's song choice highlights themes that were easily overlooked, such as the attempt to find everyday words for depression on their 1971 single "Rainy Days and Mondays" and the barely conscious desire for self-annihilation in many of their songs.[30] The ironic use of dolls and the fact that the duo's music was deeply unpopular by 1987 (the *Los Angeles Times* had described The Carpenters as "audio wallpaper" fifteen years earlier) meant that Haynes could play with audience expectations and test if the viewer would succumb "to an ensemble of plastic" in which objects replace human subjects.[31] This differentiates *Superstar* from the first film Haynes made as a high school student that also explores the uncomfortable dividing line between childhood innocence and sexual experience. His 22-minute montage from 1978, *The Suicide*, juxtaposes an uncomfortable dialogue between a boy and his mother, scenes of alienation and bullying at school, the boy's attempt to vocalize his pain, and a bathroom scene in which he cuts his torso deeply and fatally. The shift into a plastic world does not make *Superstar* an unfeeling film, though. It is as much a meditation on space, style, and the object world as it is a sensitive retelling of Carpenter's story from musical and medical perspectives.[32]

The film begins with news of Carpenter's death, before returning to a "doll-sized miniature" of Karen's teenage world in 1968.[33] The viewer remains in this doll world, except for explanatory captions and "a series of brief, generic images of human hands and objects against bright color backdrops engaged in various tasks."[34] Sometimes these hands are ominous; in one sequence we see the hands of a record company producer who encourages Karen to trust him, then a cut to a monochrome "Holocaust image of an emaciated female carcass being thrown into a pit" and a scream that emphasizes the perils of the music industry. It is clear from the caption that Haynes interprets Carpenter's story as the intensification of "certain difficulties many women experience in relation to their bodies" before a montage takes us into the euphoria of their early hit "We've Only Just Begun." Foreshadowing Jean Baudrillard's connection between "anorexic ruins" and apocalypse, the film interweaves fantasy and reality: footage from 1970 of bombs dropping over Cambodia, a stump speech by California governor Ronald Reagan, and images of the May shootings at Kent State University are juxtaposed with a fantasy scene of Richard and Karen's wedding and a shot of President Nixon at the real wedding of his eldest daughter Tricia.[35]

The narrative then focuses on the pressures Karen feels from all sides, the limited vocabulary she has at her disposal ("I'm really flubbing it up today"; "I don't know what's the matter with me"), and the medical story dominated by food and laxatives.[36] At this point, the frame is broken with a slow zoom into the text of the

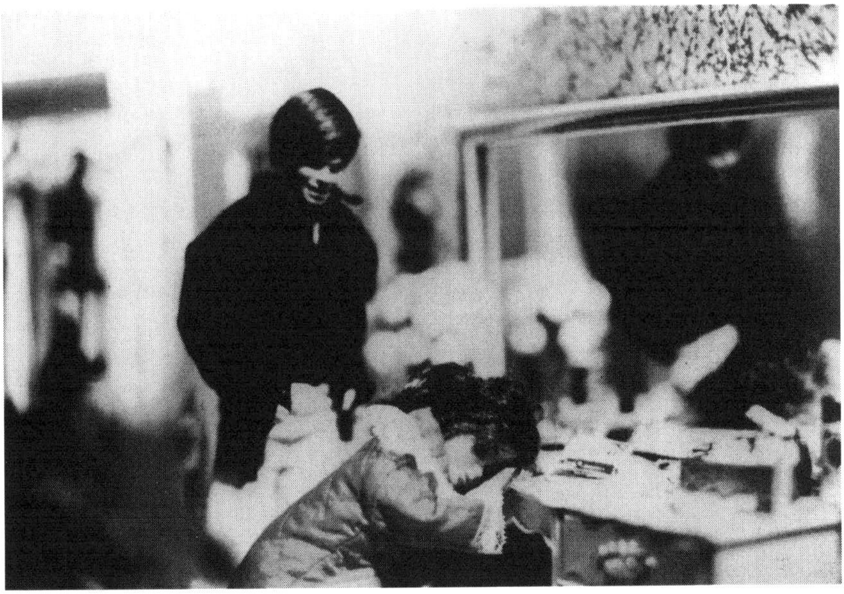

Figure 6.1 Richard Carpenter challenges Karen Carpenter (as represented by dolls) about her weight loss in *Superstar: The Karen Carpenter Story* (dir. Todd Haynes, 1987). Iced Tea Productions/The Kobal Collection.

clinical description of anorexia nervosa and an image of a stylized copy of *DSM-III* with a bright green backdrop. The film then cuts to a street scene, a sign for "'Slim-Way' Family Restaurant," and a "large 'baby' doll arm beside a tiny 'Barbie' doll body" to emphasize the distortion of body size in an anorexic's world.[37] The middle section contrasts Karen's food story with The Carpenters' songs and their growing international celebrity, including their 1973 White House performance. This section has two dimensions: the tight control Karen exerts over her body contrasts starkly with a broader postwar story about consumerist plenty, thereby reinforcing the view that anorexia is a response to the "epidemic of affluence," as a 1986 book on diets described it.[38]

The final phase of the film is increasingly bleak as we see Karen collapsing onstage, her hospitalization, Richard's discovery of an empty box of laxatives, and Karen's face dissolving into "a flow of sounds and images" as she stares at an oversize television in her condominium. A montage of violence follows: a reprise of the Holocaust scene, dolls being spanked, a plate of food falling to the ground, and Mrs. Carpenter's harsh voice. Karen's marital breakup sharpens her self-awareness: "I know I'm sick. I—I know something's wrong, and that I need help," she says, the carved lines in her cheeks conveying her worsening condition. Interventions by the recovered anorexic Cherry Boone O'Neill (singer Pat Boone's daughter, who had recently published her evangelical eating memoir *Starving for Attention*) and therapy with Levenkron do not arrest her falling weight.[39] Following a final visit to a hospital, the camera lingers in close-up on a drawer full of ipecac.

We see Karen downing two bottles and then a fast montage sequence: "a woman vomiting, Karen's body on the closet floor, the Holocaust carcass and, finally, the real KAREN CARPENTER, caught in a flash of light."[40] This flash of recognition is short lived. The coda returns musically to the beginning, this time with an emotional twist as the melancholy of Karen singing Burt Bacharach's song "Close to You" is juxtaposed with the headlines of her death.

Although the 43-minute film was not released commercially because the family did not grant Haynes the rights to The Carpenters' songs, *Superstar* developed an underground presence even though it has been out of legal circulation since 1990. Haynes's film is both a critique of stardom and an indulgent look at a decade that he believed was free of the cynicism of the 1980s; he saw the duo's music as one of the final embodiments of "earnest sentimental times."[41] The silencing of Haynes's film occurred at the same time that a sanitized, family-endorsed 1989 biopic, *The Karen Carpenter Story*, was aired on television. Barry Morrow, who wrote the screenplay for the biopic on the back of his *Rain Man* script, brushed over the details of Karen's anorexia, which were often reduced to horrified reaction shots of family members.[42] Mary Desjardins shows how both of these Karen Carpenter films investigate the maternal relationship and argues that for all its cultural disruption and identification with Karen, *Superstar* perpetuates the myth of the monstrous mother, especially because Haynes uses a burned doll's face and ominous low-angle shots to portray Agnes Carpenter.[43]

The American public's love-hate relationship with Barbie dolls and a weakening of the cause of second-wave feminists in the late 1980s add to the tangled gender politics of *Superstar* and the questions it poses about the relationship between individuals and objects in late capitalist culture. The film arguably plays the victim card rather too forcibly, and it reminds music historian Mitchell Morris of the victimized addicts of the 1967 film *Valley of the Dolls*, sucked in and then abandoned by the fame industry once they are hooked on pills and alcohol.[44] Perhaps Haynes's key message was a simple one: anorexia has intersecting causes (family, gender, biology, culture, class) and cannot be traced to a single source.

Anorexic and Bulimic Selves

After Karen Carpenter's death, a number of other female public figures disclosed that they had eating disorders. The most high profile of these was actress Jane Fonda, who admitted that she had become bulimic as a twelve-year-old in 1959 (the year her mother committed suicide) and remained so during her years at Vassar College, through the 1960s, and into her mid-30s. Fonda disclosed her "twenty-three years of agony" to *Cosmopolitan* magazine in 1985, inspired by her heightened political consciousness (she viewed the women she met on her controversial trip to North Vietnam in 1972 as "victims of the same *Playboy* culture that had played havoc with me") and with a sharper awareness of "bulimia nervosa" after it came into parlance in 1979 (the year the Center for the Study of Anorexia and Bulimia was established in Manhattan).[45] Fonda made her admission partly to disclose her "endless pattern of gorging food, vomiting, and gorging" and partly to promote her book *Women Coming of Age*, her *Prime Time Workout* video, and her new movie roles.[46] Instead of exploring her troubled family life (her mentally unstable mother Frances, her controlling father Henry, her wayward brother Peter), Jane Fonda spoke out because she believed that bulimia and anorexia were approaching "epic proportions" by the mid-1980s.[47]

The *Cosmopolitan* interview was published at a time when the press was reporting that the First Lady was losing weight and by 1983 was wearing a size 2 dress size. Nancy Reagan said that this was due to the stress of the assassination attempt on her husband, but the *Washington Post* speculated that she was depressed. In an interview with the *Los Angeles Times*, she made the bizarre claim that she kept cookies by the bed and planned "to keep nibbling" them "until I'm my normal size 6 again."[48] There was little speculation that the First Lady might be anorexic until her daughter, Patti Davis, published her revelatory autobiography *The Way I See It* in 1992 and spoke openly about her own teenage addiction to diet pills that she stole from her mother. Dieting enabled Patti to take control of her body in response to her mother's harsh treatment and she too veered close to being anorexic during her student days. This mother-daughter story of weight control and prescription drugs was one aspect of a much broader horizon of mental health issues that led Patti to abuse diet pills, Quaaludes, and cocaine; to face bouts of depression; and to contemplate suicide.[49]

It would be easy to rationalize the stories of Karen Carpenter, Patti Davis, and other cases at the time, such as that of singer Paula Abdul, who admitted to being bulimic for fifteen years, and teenage actress Tracey Gold (the star of ABC sitcom *Growing Pains*), who experienced anorexic tendencies from age 11.[50] We could assert that these eating disturbances were a reaction to the pressures of fame if it were not for two factors: when Carpenter and Davis started dieting neither were members of celebrity families yet (unless we count Ronald Reagan's career as film actor), and the increase in reported cases of anorexia and bulimia—as well as growing interest in the media—made these much more than isolated cases.

It is worth returning to *The Beauty Myth* to consider the voices of those encountering eating disorders before looking at a thinly fictionalized account of anorexia from the early 1980s. In the cases of Naomi Wolf and Susie Orbach (who described herself as a "compulsive eater"), their personal experiences authenticate their broader comments on anorexia.[51] We should remember, though, that the discussion of addiction in chapter 3 revealed that giving voice to health conditions does not always guarantee a truthful account, and we need to be suspicious, also, about the reliability of the anorexic or bulimic narrator. As we will see, deceiving others by hiding food or covering up an emaciated body can often spill into self-deception and an unjustified belief that a diet should go further or that bulimic purging is good for the body. But this does not undermine the importance of personal testimony that gives weight to Wolf's and Orbach's cultural commentary.

Labeling girls born after 1960 "the anorexic generation," Wolf discusses her own dieting experiences as a teenager. At age 13, in 1975 (the same year that Karen Carpenter was too weak to tour), Naomi felt confused by the fact that neither her teachers nor her parents confronted her about her weight loss, perhaps because there were "many starving girls" in her San Francisco junior high school.[52] Dieting had a deleterious effect on her speech, she remembers, almost as if an "alien voice" was taking over; she "lost expression and timbre and sank to a monotone." In a self-portrait, she envisaged herself as a small rodent in a "sort of burrow, surrounded by nesting materials," a trait which she now sees as a mechanism to protect herself from the beauty industry and overt forms of sexuality.[53] Using emotive language, Wolf describes self-starvation as being little different from the near-starvation diets of concentration camps. This analogy is far fetched, but she sees the invisible hand of the beauty industry giving her little option except to capitulate or to resist through extreme action. Anorexia "was the only choice that really looked like one," she claims, although the point at which choice becomes obsessive-compulsive behavior is underexplored, except tangentially when she describes Sally, a girl at school, who collapses in her arms as if "she had escaped gravity." Sally has no voice at all and Naomi comments that "there was nothing to her."[54]

Wolf worries that girls born around 1980 had even less chance of finding their way through the snares of the beauty industry, but she believes that her generation had similarly struggled to negotiate a world of illusory freedom. Wolf's commentary is powerful, yet she exaggerates statistics, lists a barrage of physical symptoms (as if all are inevitable), and does not really grapple with the psychology of a distorted body image beyond feelings of guilt and control. Hilde Bruch is her only reliable medical source for understanding the complex psychology of anorexia, particularly *The Golden Cage*, which was published in 1978, two years after the National Association of Anorexia Nervosa and Associated Disorders had formed. Wolf makes literal one of the opening comments of *The Golden Cage* when she likens dramatic weight loss to the experience of a concentration camp victim.[55] This analogy is reminiscent of the comparison Bruno Bettelheim makes between infantile autism and the dehumanizing forces of extreme incarceration in *The Empty Fortress*. It also amplifies a theme of an early fictional account of anorexia, Deborah Hautzig's 1981 teenage novel *Second Star to the Right*, a book that appeared the same year as the first issue of the *International Journal of Eating Disorders*, with a title that evokes the "Peter Pan complex" that Bruch identifies in *The Golden Cage*. Whereas Bruch might have been thinking of her native Germany when she made this comment about incarceration (she emigrated in 1934 before the extent of Nazi atrocities were known), Hautzig's anorexic character, Leslie Hiller, compares herself to "an inmate at Auschwitz" when her weight drops to 76 pounds.[56] In the case of the Hiller family there is a historical connection because Leslie's mother's cousin was killed in a concentration camp. Leslie identifies with and has a middle name in common with this relative, but the concentration camp image has broader currency with girls at her local school. In nearly all instances of comparing anorexia to the experience of being a prisoner it is the look of the emaciated body that is reminiscent of stark footage of incarceration.[57] However, in Leslie's case this analogy also links to her German Jewish identity, which (although it is underexplored in the novel) exacerbates her feelings of bodily discomfort.

There is often something formulaic about anorexia stories, and *Second Star to the Right* is no exception.[58] Written in straightforward language in the first person, it veers between Leslie's confessions of her eating regime and the family triangle: an emotionally intense mother, a distant father, a misunderstood daughter. She has only one friend at school, Cavett, who, perhaps because she lives in a less privileged area of Manhattan, accepts Leslie unconditionally whatever her weight is. The book is reminiscent of Sylvia Plath's 1963 novel *The Bell Jar* in places. However, the first-person narrative voice and the focus on anorexia is more persistent than in Plath's more varied text, in which Esther's breakdown and recovery is part of a broader story. *Second Star to the Right* starts uncertainly ("It's hard to know where to begin telling you about this") and Leslie states that when she changed schools at age 14 she "was in the middle of it all," although she "didn't even know it." Yet the beginning is fairly conventional, focusing on teenage anxieties about school, clothes, and boys before exploring the "contradictions and paradoxes" of anorexia as outlined in *The Golden Cage*.[59]

Leslie makes some references to films, but it is not the mass media or peer pressure that push her to believe that "if I were thin, my life would be perfect."[60] Rather it is a love-hate relationship with her mother and an internal compulsion that quickly becomes an obsession. Mirrors are often the symbol of discomfort for Leslie, as if she can never match up to the ideal image she has of herself. However, the novel does not strive for high symbolism in which occluded or distorted mirrors symbolize her pathology. As was the case with Karen Carpenter, Leslie's efforts to reduce her weight through diet and exercise start innocently enough; she decides to begin dieting in earnest after losing a few pounds during a bout of flu, as if she has a dictatorial voice within that pushes her into a strict starvation regimen. Leslie's is a different type of addiction narrative than those discussed in chapter 3; she experiences only a little of the euphoria associated with recreational drugs and does not suffer the same cycle of self-recrimination that we saw in *Go Ask Alice*. Leslie gains some satisfaction from jogging. She does not run to experience endorphin release, though, but as part of a self-punishment regime that gives her a degree of control mixed with elements of narcissism, hyperactivity, and food obsession. Leslie starts to hide her eating habits from her parents and keeps secret that she has stopped menstruating. Her worried mother encourages Leslie to see a doctor, but by that time she is under the sway of her inner dictator and unable to operate outside her self-imposed regime or take responsibility for her actions. She is hospitalized when her health worsens and is given a course of Stelazine to calm her anxiety. There she experiences solidarity with other emaciated inpatients, until the threat of force feeding pushes her to accept nourishment against her will. However, by this stage her logic has slipped into a state of semi-delirium and the dictator's voice inside her undermines a previously stable reality.

Eventually, the maturity that we see in the early sections of the novel evaporates entirely and we are left with a confused little girl taking out her frustrations on herself and her mother. She realizes that she has lost track of why she began her regime. However, when she exclaims toward the end of the narrative that "I want to be a skeleton—but I also want to be attractive. I want to die—but I also want to live. I don't deserve to feel good—but oh, I want to so much!" it is clear that she has regressed to an indecisive state in which the simple logic of charting her life by weight loss has crumbled.

When we learn from Hautzig's 1999 postscript that she finished writing the book at age 23 while suffering from extreme malnutrition and electrolyte imbalance, it is clear that Leslie's experiences reflect her own. Hautzig's weight did not drop quite as far as Leslie's, but her starvation cycle continued beyond the time frame of the novel and "the worst decade" of her life followed its publication, confirming the link between malnutrition and depression as the physical and psychological faces of extreme anorexia.[61] Hautzig admits that this was an active addiction over which she had little control. She finds professional help ineffectual and experiences severe medical problems, including stress fractures to her feet, extreme tooth decay, and arrhythmia. A mixture of the twelve-step Alcoholics Anonymous program, a course of cognitive behavioral therapy, and antidepressant medication eventually help Hautzig find the kind of stability in her early thirties that seemed a distant prospect a decade earlier. The 1999 reissue of *Second Star on the Right* closes with Hautzig's life back on track; she is married and has a daughter, she has a more balanced lifestyle, and she is pursuing a mode of therapy that keeps the specter of anorexia at bay without entirely banishing it.

Whereas Naomi Wolf relies on a feminist model to rationalize why teenage girls are drawn towards anorexia and Jane Fonda and Patti Davis position their experiences within the fabric of their turbulent lives, for Hautzig and her fictional character there is little outside the self to explain the condition. Therapy does not go deep enough to explore the relationship with her parents, and apart from subtle hints that her family has been persecuted for their ethnicity, we are not provided with enough sociological detail to place Leslie's narrative in a wider historical frame. Hautzig does not reveal a great deal about the status of Leslie's home, except that she has her own room and can secretly discard her food and hide her shrinking body in a way that might prove more difficult for a working-class girl. Giving some support to Bruch's idea that anorexia is a way of delaying puberty, the fact that Leslie's menstruation ceases at an early age also means that her dawning sexuality goes into abeyance and we are confronted with a desexualized being circumscribed by a world of childhood friendships. While Wolf positions anorexia and bulimia within the context of the historical rise of advertising, in *Second Star to the Right* we are given little evidence of any overriding factors that could explain Leslie's condition, except that her need for control and her skewed body image overwhelm her without her fully realizing that they have done so.

The Inner Life of Anorexia

It would be wrong to think that early depictions of anorexia focused unerringly on the individual while later texts are more sophisticated in taking into account caregivers and broader sociocultural pressures. Hautzig deliberately chooses a spare style to express Leslie's rather simplistic world view, her wasted body, her austere regime, and her narrow circle of interest. This style corresponds to a comment Levenkron makes in his popular 1982 book *Treating and Overcoming Anorexia Nervosa*, where he noted that the condition "has to be seen as a 'stylistic' breakdown resulting from cultural pressure, since it amounts to a pathological exaggeration of society's message to women."[62] Levenkron acknowledged the increased pressure of the fashion and diet industries and he warned feminists not to overlook "helpless, chaotic, and floundering children" in the name of a politicized cause.[63] Although he recognized that it is difficult to measure a precise point in the early years of a life cycle when food restriction becomes pathological, he details a number of symptoms (phobias, obsessional thinking, rituals, feeling of inferiority, splitting, passive-aggressive behavior, delusions, paranoia, depression, anxiety, and denial) that often emerge in cases where dieting goes too far.[64]

Not only was the etiology of anorexia often obscure but its wide range of symptoms and the fact that it is a self-imposed regime means that it is often difficult in its extreme form to treat without resorting to force feeding within an institution. While the trajectory of anorexia—from innocent dieting to body-image distortion—was typical, the actual precipitating factors were not. We can turn to two semi-fictional accounts published near the millennium that reflect on experiences from the late 1970s and 1980s and explore the inner life of the anorexic in the context of a sharper awareness of shaping cultural factors. The desire for self-control and feelings of self-annihilation in Lori Gottlieb's *Stick Figure: A Diary of My Former Self* (2000) and Marya Hornbacher's *Wasted: A Memoir of Anorexia and Bulimia* (1998) illustrate a loss of perspective and proportion that weighs even heavier than it does in texts published at the turn of the 1980s. The literary forms of diary and memoir suggest that these are private accounts made public, as if the slender body is a source of pride despite the debilitating process of emaciation. That both accounts signal their veracity—Hornbacher by reflecting on her body in an afterword and Gottlieb by including an epilogue in which she claims that she stumbled upon the diary of her 11-year-old self—reinforce their desire to be treated seriously as studies that are both intensely personal and representative of anorexia more generally. This is indicated by the two idiomatic titles—*Stick Figure* and *Wasted*—that hover between the desirable and the pathological. Moreover, the personal journeys are marked by a critical perspective that questions whether it is in fact a specific condition at all and whether a clear line can be drawn between anorexia and normalcy.[65]

Gottlieb's account begins with what we assume is a deliberately self-conscious style, but there is an element of doubt in what she tells us. If we believe her comments in the epilogue, then we approach the text as a public version of her preteenage diary written in 1978. However, if we do not believe that she stumbled across the diaries at age 34, then we must infer that she retrospectively recreated the voice of her 11-year-old-self. Why we might suspect that this is a retrospective account (or at least a combination of voices) is a passing reference to two singers, the anorexic Karen Carpenter and Andy Gibb (the younger brother of the three Gibbs who formed the Bee Gees), who led a self-destructive life and died of heart inflammation triggered by cocaine use over a long period. Although the narrative is set in 1978—five years before Carpenter's death and well before Gibb was undergoing depression and rehabilitation for cocaine addiction at the Betty Ford Center—their presence works spectrally through the text. Young Lori, who is suffering from an advanced state of emaciation, also identifies with the tragic nineteenth-century fictional heroine Emma Bovary of Gustave Flaubert's *Madame Bovary*, who, believing that the world is against her, commits suicide by taking arsenic. In *The Culture of Narcissism*, Christopher Lasch describes Emma Bovary as a "prototypical consumer of mass culture," especially when her agency vanishes into the illusory world of self-deception. Lori's logic by this point has become so distorted, though, that the passing comparison to *Madame Bovary* is just another refraction of her attempt to cling to the vanishing "stick figure" she has become.[66] The title image first emerges when Lori draws a self-portrait at her analyst's request; when she shows him a stick figure he asks that she draw herself again, but this time with more realism. Later in the text, the "stick figure" emerges more prosaically in Lori's lifeworld when she tries on a plain black dress that she considers to be suitable for her brother's graduation, only for her mother to convince her to wear a more feminine dress. Lori's mother thinks that more color will disguise her thin body, exclaiming that Lori "look[s] like a stick figure" in the first dress: "Your father and I will see a lot of people we know there. Please, Lori, do it for me."[67]

This expectation that Lori will conform to normative behavior displays the gulf between mother and daughter. Not only is Mrs. Gottlieb manipulative and unable to extract herself far enough from the central drama to really help her daughter, but Lori sees her secretly eating when no one is around, even though she presents a public face of denial and restraint. Lori depicts her mother as having her own obsession with food and a pinched attitude in public that Lori both kicks against and in some ways replicates. She points out the phoniness of adult behavior, yet she also develops an inferiority complex (she cannot find her cheekbone to apply blusher in the manner that her mother's *Redbook* magazine recommends) and an unhealthy attitude toward food that leads her into a fasting and exercise regime as she tries to impose order on her enclosed world. Lori is certainly not immune to social pressures, even though she can sometimes detect their phoniness. Midway through the diary she rejects Bruch's thesis in *The Golden Cage* that links anorexia to a Peter Pan complex in which the child does not wish to grow up (she decides that Bruch's view is "incredibly stupid"), yet she then gets seduced by self-help and diet books that suggest a "new you" can emerge out of self-denial.[68] This evokes an authenticity that Lori cannot otherwise discern around her, although she is not old enough to wrestle free from publications that see beauty as a saleable commodity.

There is one other subliminal literary reference point that seems to shape Lori's attitude toward fashion, makeup, and her relationship with her mother. We might detect echoes of Holden Caulfield's take on adult phoniness in Lori's reaction to her mother's generation (this is a major theme of J. D. Salinger's *The Catcher in the Rye*), but it is Plath's *The Bell Jar* that sets the psychological horizon of the diary. Both Plath's persona Esther Greenwood and Lori are high-achieving students born of anti-intellectual parents who display ambivalent attitudes toward a gendered milieu that places supreme emphasis on appearances. The arc of *Stick Figure*, from self-possession and control to breakdown and institutionalization, also follows the trajectory of *The Bell Jar*. It is not as rich in imagery as Plath's text, though, and, given Lori's pre-pubescent age, it is less concerned with sexual relationships, caught as Esther is between wanting to be virginal and sexually experienced at the same time. However, the two texts are closely linked by the inclusion of a hospitalized tragic figure—Joan in *The Bell Jar* and Nora in *Stick Figure*—who cannot cope with the rehabilitation regime. Whereas Joan commits suicide and thereby frees Esther to reenter the social order (albeit tentatively), Nora tells Lori that she wants to die when she is readmitted to hospital following a premature release. Joan and Nora become symbols of psychic freedom for Esther and Lori that enable them to survive in a threatening environment. However, *Stick Figure* moves beyond this survivalist phase: the penultimate chapter ends with the realization that Lori is "kind of happy that [she] was wrong" to think that she was the one destined to die in the hospital, and in the final chapter, she accepts her unique differences after months of struggle. This rite-of-passage moment might be a version of the false edification that Lori would otherwise reject, yet because of her young age—and a hint in the epilogue that her struggles are not yet over—we suspect that this is only a brief moment of realization before the pressures crowd in again.

Stick Figure recounts less than a year in Lori's pre-pubescent life. This is opened out in some respects in the epilogue, but we have to look to a more expansive text such as Marya Hornbacher's *Wasted* to see how the eating disorder arc develops through time. More overtly retrospective than *Stick Figure*, Hornbacher's memoir spreads over a decade. It charts her teenage years when she periodically veered between anorexia and bulimia and underwent so much treatment that she feels herself "poked and prodded and fed and weighed" like a "laboratory rat."[69] Whereas *Stick Figure* engages in the language of self-improvement and self-discipline, *Wasted* is a much more unruly and knowing text. Feeling at times like a "psychotic rabbit," Hornbacher struggles to match her own subjective experience with that of the clinical studies she consults while preparing her life story. Looking back from 1997 from the perspective of a 23-year-old, she acknowledges her eating disorder yet she refuses to be defined by it, seeing herself and her health condition as existing in an "uncomfortable state of mutual antagonism." This notion of something exterior to the self (food, diet pills, laxatives) in a fight with a more interiorized sense of self leads to a paradox where she feels that one's self-worth is "exponentially increased with one's incremental disappearance."[70] This "strange logic" spills into the prolix form of Hornbacher's memoir as an embodiment of what literary critic Sue Vice calls "anorexic ambivalence," in which the text twists between the protagonist's desire to be simultaneously sick and well, a trait that Vice reads into another anorexia narrative of the late 1990s, South African-born novelist Jenefer Shute's *Life-Size*.[71]

But instead of trying to resolve this paradox or locating a stable reference point by which to negotiate between these ethereal and corporeal states, Hornbacher's account takes in a wider circle of social, cultural, and personal interactions. *Wasted* positions the self-control associated with eating disorders as a significant yet not always primary element in a life full of "history, philosophy, society, personal strangeness, family fuck-ups, autoerotics, myth, mirrors, love and death and S&M, magazines and religion, the individual's blind-folded stumble-walk through an ever-stranger world."[72] The use of four hyphens in this list signals the complexity Hornbacher seeks to come to terms with. Much more eloquent a writer than Deborah Hautzig and Lori Gottlieb, Hornbacher strives for a middle ground between the belief that an eating disorder can be cured by therapy and that it is symptomatic of underlying instability. This makes *Wasted* one of the clearest American narratives of the 1990s to deal with the broader ambit of mental health in which addiction and protest, self-destruction and self-definition go hand in hand. Hornbacher might fit the stereotype of a white, middle-class, educated girl, but she refuses to tell her story within a narrow sociological ambit. She also uses the literary trope of the double to characterize different states of being and feelings of dissociation. Mirrors in *Wasted* are not so much symbols of self-reflection as facilitators of the deceptive gaze, beginning with Hornbacher's memory of her four-year-old self sitting in front of a mirror after liberally applying her mother's stage makeup. The feeling that she is "two girls, staring at each other through the glass of the mirror" defines her split self, the power of the gaze, and her feeling of disorientation and unreality.[73]

Although Hornbacher has the intelligence to be a high achiever, she is self-consciously wayward and has an exhibitionist streak that deters her from fulfilling her talents. She remembers her childhood as a happy one tinged with uneasiness and chaos that she realizes might actually be the figments of an adult memory. Recalling the Iran Crisis that came to define the final phase of the Carter administration, she has a nightmare that the Shah of Iran is hiding under her bed and fantasizes about being hatched out of an egg (reminiscent of the television show *Mork and Mindy*) and of living her life backward.[74] Hornbacher notes the contradictions of her childhood world, particularly when it comes to consumption: she describes her father as eating "like a horse," drinking "like a fish," and smoking "like a chimney," while her mother "stopped eating, grew thinner, sharper, more silent." The parental push-pull relationship of the "family dinner table" plays out in Marya's culinary association of her father with cheeseburgers and fries and her mother with cucumbers and cottage cheese, yet this association is sometimes reversed in her mother's desire for special treats and her father's periodic attempts to suppress his appetite. The young Marya describes this family drama as a "pantomime" in which she mirrors both sets of parental traits, but it soon settles into a resolve to prevent her body from "spilling out" by restricting her food intake.[75] Despite this resolution, she realizes that feelings of hunger and satiation are intricately linked to the loneliness and fear that she experiences even within the intimacy of the family unit.

It is unsurprising that Hornbacher draws from metaphors of performance given that her parents both work in the theater, and she is attracted to makeup and to trying out different hair colors and styles from an early age.[76] This fascination "with transformations, with mirage, smoke and mirrors" leads her to desire the theatrical "New Me" that could emerge from her mother's dressing room or come to life on stage.[77] Echoing two earlier texts, *The Art of Starvation* (1982) by the British author Sheila Macleod (which documents the life of an anorexic adolescent in mid-1950s London) and Franz Kafka's 1922 fable of emaciation "The Hunger Artist," the notion that self-starvation becomes a craft or technique of self-fashioning gives validity to Marya's actions. Experimenting with different looks leads her to a deeper awareness of selfhood, but at other times she realizes that theatricality is deceptive and can lead to the acting out or phoniness that the young Lori Gottlieb comes to despise. Marya pictures this as a series of Russian dolls without a center and anorexia itself as an "act of becoming invisible."[78] This sense of disorientation and emptiness is exacerbated when her parents begin fighting when Marya is around age six. This is followed by a new phase of growing up when the family moves from California to Minnesota.

Hornbacher's voice in *Wasted* is much more expressive than those in *Second Star to the Right* and *Stick Figure*, but it is also more unreliable. Hornbacher develops her theatrical metaphor by describing her acts of deception as a "seamless, smooth surface," as if it is a magician's endless scarf, "the slippery silk snaking on, and on, and on," and when she attends therapy she lies by confessing "a wide-eyed desire for health."[79] She is aware that she often has a "wheedling, delusional, lying voice" that undermines her perceptive insights.[80] She detects that the cultural seductions of her generation—"subliminal advertising, stupid television, slasher movies, insipid grocery-store literature, MTV, VCRs, fast food, infomercials, glossy ads, diet aids, plastic surgery"—are the "intellectual and emotional equivalent of eating nothing but candy bars." Although she often positions herself as a counterpoint to such a shallow world, she sometimes actively embraces surfaces and is only periodically aware of the health consequences of her actions.[81] For example, she is proud of the fine down that grows on her face and body when she is away at college, only dimly aware that this is her body's attempt to prevent her vital processes from shutting down. This form of psychic numbing was not out of keeping with the experiences of the young protagonists in novels of the late 1980s and 1990s who are able to perceive the problem of their generation yet are incapable of doing anything about it and at times are complicit in the environment they criticize, as is the case for Mary Gaitskill's "thin" character Justine Shade in her 1991 novel *Two Girls Fat and Thin*. While Hornbacher's voice is too expressive to be compared to the deliberate flatness of tone in the "blank generation" fiction of Gaitskill, Bret Easton Ellis, and Jay McInerney, as the next section discusses, this world of distortions brings together medical and cultural perspectives on eating and body image disorders.

In Search of an Embodied Voice

Stick Figure and *Wasted* are two examples of how personal stories that related to broader mythic patterns helped bring anorexia to public attention in the 1990s. Both narratives temper the tragic qualities of a wasted life with self-deprecating humor, just as they criticize the therapeutic machinery that often seems to make matters worse rather than better, particularly the coercive regime of force feeding during hospital stays. This perspective was also shared by one of the most visible accounts of institutionalized therapy of the period, Massachusetts writer Susanna Kaysen's 1993 memoir *Girl, Interrupted*.

Charting Kaysen's voluntary admission to McLean Hospital in the Boston suburb of Belmont in spring 1967 for a suspected borderline condition, a central chapter of *Girl, Interrupted* focuses on the tragic case of Daisy, a periodic inpatient with a food obsession that hints at a deeper source. In the 1999 film version, the story of Daisy (played by Brittany Murphy) is a clear turning point in the struggle Susanna faces in finding a therapeutic path forward within an institution that hides an oppressive regime behind a benign mask. Daisy's two passions are purgatives and food: she is desperate for laxatives and compulsively peels the skin off the roast chickens that her father brings her twice a week, hiding the carcasses under her bed after she eats the meat.[82] Some months after checking out, her former inpatients receive news that Daisy is dead. Her obsessive-compulsive behavior might be explained by the implied incestuous relationship with her father, a suggestion that is macabrely imaged through the carefully stripped chicken. The inpatients in Kaysen's book respond to news of Daisy's suicide with stunned silence, whereas in the film adaptation Susanna discovers the strangled body during a stress-inducing house call with her disruptive friend Lisa.

Daisy is not portrayed as an anorexic figure (although another patient who is losing significant weight is mentioned in the same chapter), nor is she a grotesque character despite her proclivity for collecting chicken carcasses. She is seemingly well enough to live semi-independently yet also fragile enough to require supervision and nursing. The fact that the relationship with her father is only implied is significant at a time when the correlation between sexual abuse and eating disorders was not well researched.[83] It is significant that Daisy's food obsession inflects the narrator's own response to meat. Susanna recalls the incident that precipitated her admittance to McLean: she took fifty aspirin before passing out at the meat counter of a nearby supermarket. Instead of reflecting on this episode or on the cause of Daisy's death, Kaysen suddenly associates animal flesh with suicide, recalling that the meat at the counter was "bruised, bleeding, and imprisoned in a tight wrapper."[84] Susanna's slender figure, particularly in the cinematic portrayal of her by Winona Ryder, contrasts with the appealing corporeality she associates with Daisy, despite the fact that the other girl smells of feces and chicken much of the time. This is an example of the confused subjective logic of *Girl, Interrupted* and reflects the shifting voice of anorexia narratives, in which food is sometimes a source of comfort and freedom and at other times is symptomatic of psychological troubles. The shock and remorse Susanna feels following Daisy's suicide fills her with new determination to rediscover herself. She finds an expressive voice through writing, talking, and art but then faces a major setback when the other girls punish her for candidly writing down her thoughts after Lisa steals her diary.[85]

This confusion between identity and expression epitomizes the connections between eating and mental illness in the 1990s. At the beginning of *Wasted*, for example, Hornbacher speaks of the ways that eating disorders hover in the background, "eroding the body in silence" and then strike at moments of vulnerability.[86] Yet she places this within a particular historical moment and social environment, which she describes as excessive, competitive, damaged, and narcissistic. *Wasted* is full of cultural reference points, signaled by chapter epigraphs from *Alice in Wonderland*, the suicidal poets Anne Sexton and Sylvia Plath, the minimalist selves of Samuel Beckett's *Waiting for Godot*, and the resurfacing imagery of Adrienne Rich. As a child, Marya is drawn to fairy tales that resonate with the escapist world Bruch outlined in *The Golden Cage*, but her distorted view of her body shape is countered by a realistic attitude about her corporeality and a sexual awareness (if not quite a sexual maturity) that is lacking in Gottleib, Hiller, and Carpenter. Surprisingly, given Hornbacher's age, there are no musical references in *Wasted*. Instead, her interest in literature—both imaginative and medical—preserves an imaginative inner life and (for the most part) keeps her at a remove from the lures of fast food and the mass media. She suffers most when her books are confiscated during a stay in hospital; she is told that this is so she can face herself instead of escaping into the imaginative worlds of Whitman, Emerson, and Thoreau.[87] She is aware that the attempt to preserve an inner life might be an escape, but at other times her body becomes a conduit for consumer culture, evidenced by the "system of 'markers'" that she deploys to ensure that her stomach is empty after vomiting. She eats brightly colored Doritos first so that she can see the food items egested in reverse order: "pizza, cookies, Ruffles, pretzels, Doritos, all swimming in dark swirls of Coke."[88]

None of the texts discussed here tackle the way the mass media peddles advertisements that depict idealized body shapes and the convenience and ubiquity of fast food. The Department of Health and Human Services, through its Public Health Service, realized that there was a need to promote exercise and balanced diets in the 1990s. However, despite its concerted effort to reduce obesity and increase physical activity, the plans for educating the public about diet lacked detail and tended to overlook the complex psychosocial roots of overeating.[89] Indeed, the press often polarized eating disorders, associating anorexia and bulimia with white middle-class girls and young women and obesity with working-class minorities who, it was often implied, lacked the education or the economic means to make better food choices.[90] Although the National Black Women's Health Project made efforts to reveal the multiple causes of eating disorders among black women, many of which were linked to prejudice and oppression, the mainstream media hardly ever covered these stories and published stories of anorexia were invariably from the perspective of young white women.[91] Instead, the media tended to collude in the cult of slenderness, particularly with the rise of supermodels in the 1990s and the spread of size zero for women's clothes, leading Susie Orbach to argue that many media outlets were recklessly promoting food deprivation, ignorant of the real-life consequences. Starting with her 1978 book *Fat Is a Feminist Issue* and the founding in Manhattan of the Women's Therapy Centre Institute in 1981, Orbach critiqued the late-twentieth-century obsession with food, and in her 1986 book *Hunger Strike*, she explored anorexia as "a metaphor for our time."[92]

The absence of a meaningful public voice politicized eating disorders for feminist critics of the 1980s and 1990s. In response, Carol Gilligan's *In a Different Voice* (1982) and the jointly written *Women's Ways of Knowing* (1986) were two key texts that emphasized speech and listening as forms of self-empowerment. The authors of *Women's Ways of Knowing* associated silence with isolation and disconnection from sources of knowledge. They argued that having the confidence to listen to others, to evaluate productive voices from background noise, and the ability to channel these voices after a period of self-reflection are markers of personal maturity and a willingness to cultivate an empathic environment in which others can develop their own voice.[93] This is in line with Gilligan's belief that women need a "different voice" through which they can mesh their experiences and thought processes. In her critique of a knowledge economy undergirded by patriarchal values, Gilligan does not deny that men can seek this "different voice" too, but she argues that women typically have more need to recognize "how these truths are carried by different modes of language and thought."[94] Gilligan believes that within this idealistic mode, an authentic voice that is both personally expressive and that acknowledges others can nurture an ethic of care and justice.

This path toward a public discourse might have helped early cases of anorexia, such as Karen Carpenter, who struggled to find helpful literature on the subject after many years of extreme dieting. It reflects the shift from an isolated individualistic lifestyle toward the public participation that Robert Bellah champions in his groundbreaking book *Habits of the Heart* (as discussed in the introduction), and carries through to *The Beauty Myth*, in which Naomi Wolf argues that women are likely to face media scrutiny when they speak out and that women's groups can become distracted by "aesthetics and personal style" instead of promoting differences of "agenda or worldview."[95] In 1983, Steven Levenkron warned feminists to keep their eye on particular cases of eating disorders instead of making grand gestures or treating these conditions as a metaphor for contemporary wrongs. Given that the statistics pointed toward anorexia as an eating disorder of white, middle-class, educated girls and young women, none of these feminist critics really tackled the relationship between race, ethnicity, socioeconomic status, and food, instead preferring to treat contemporary culture as a problem rather than as a resource for understanding the forces that shaped American women.[96]

This broader cultural focus does not to diminish the therapeutic importance of supportive communities, but the moral weight of these views is complicated in cases when the anorexic's voice proves to be untrustworthy. For example, in *Wasted*, Marya's voice at age 17 is far from stable. During a spell in hospital she finds she is beset with aggressive thoughts and internal voices (which are graphically represented by capital letters and italics, respectively) and she feels as if the austere regime is eroding her two primary identity anchors: her will to starve and her intellect. Without her books she enters a state of existential bewilderment and a sense that her "frantic scribbles" and "loud voice" are part of a tissue of lies.[97] Feeling "flat" and "two-dimensional" (rather like Gottlieb's stick figure) and believing that she is being pigeonholed in the hospital as someone who fears intimacy, she takes desperate measures: she shaves her hair in protest and then resorts to lying, claiming that she was sexually abused as a child.[98] Once again, she seeks theatrical imagery to describe her actions: "I lobbed a firebomb to the right, and while everyone was chasing the firebomb, I disappeared stage left. Absolved. I created a straw man and he took all the blame." Instead of seeing this false admission as a strategy for escaping the hospital, Hornbacher is haunted by the lie as "another in an endless series of manipulations that were designed to keep me, and my eating disorder, away from prying eyes."[99] Deception is not just outward for her: she deceives herself into believing that she is well again, only to fall into another cycle of self-deception soon after leaving the hospital.

We might say that the retrospective construction of *Wasted* means that Hornbacher has discovered a coherent and reliable voice that enables her to reconstruct her past from a perspective of relative stability. She comes to understand that her anorexic patterns are so "primal" that she has no healthy resources to fall back on. Instead, she has to relearn how to eat without the usual feelings of guilt and abjection that accompanied ingestion. This is in line with Jane Fonda's admission in her *Cosmopolitan* interview that she had to teach herself "to eat all over again, like a child" when she realizes that she had "lost all sense of what was normal or abnormal."[100] Fonda advises girls who begin extreme dieting or think that bulimic purging will keep down their weight not to delude themselves: "You don't know what you are starting; it will end up destroying you," she claimed, but from a point in her life at which she can appreciate a balanced diet and regular exercise. When the seventeen-year-old Hornbacher once again falls into bad eating habits, she lacks a support group (in fact, she ridicules group therapy while she is hospitalized) that could have helped her gain perspective during her teenage years. She eventually reaches a place where she realizes that active recovery has to come from within. Yet she also believes that cognitive behavioral therapy (to break negative cycles) and support groups (she becomes an advocate of the twelve steps of Alcoholics Anonymous) can reveal the underlying nature of the addiction and put her "on a path to recovery that involves spiritual and ethical change." This grants her the "permission to live" that Fonda spoke about.[101] Although her epilogue does not reflect the "different voice" that feminist critics were recommending, Hornbacher gestures toward a similar rising trajectory where she has to acquire a new language, "like moving to a country where you've never been."

The Perils of Idealization

While the accounts discussed so far explore the contested and ambivalent voices that are typical of anorexia narratives, they only weakly correlate with Naomi Wolf's thesis that the growth of the beauty industry explains the rise of eating disorders in the 1980s. However, we should not downplay the power of the media to promote ideal images or the seductive influences of these images on the young. Social science research in the early 1980s examined the shrinking waist and hip sizes of *Playboy* models. A follow-up study in 1992 detected that these models were 13 to 19 percent smaller than the average for their age group, and in the mid-1990s pressure groups challenged unrepresentative body shapes in the media.[102] While it is easy to pin the blame on an unregulated media, Sarah Grogan warns against thinking about the media as simply injecting consumer consciousness into unwitting citizens; she points out that individuals can choose or discard images and stories as they suit them. Although this notion of consumer agency is less likely among the vulnerable and impressionable, Grogan notes that a young woman draws upon a range of reference points (Susan Bordo calls them axes) "to construct her mental model of her present body image."[103] While the media, in all its multiplicity, undeniably played a significant role in the rise of eating and body image disturbances, family situation, sibling position, peer pressure, and other health and sociocultural factors also need to be taken into full consideration. *Wasted*, for example, introduces itself as Hornbacher's memoir of anorexia and bulimia, but its drama pivots on the parents' destructive relationship, Hornbacher's childhood interest in dressing up, her experimentation with drugs and alcohol, and the early signs of bipolar disorder (she dealt with these themes more explicitly in her sequel, *Madness: A Bipolar Life*, in 2008).

The notion of an idealized self also tends to provoke complex emotional responses. According to Emily Fox-Kales, this is especially the case in the fantasy ideals of what she calls "Hollywood media and beauty culture," which has widened the gap between "the culturally constructed ideal body a woman internalizes and that of her own biological template." Fox-Kales hypothesizes that even though it is broadly acknowledged that artifice, morphing, and body doubles are regularly deployed in Hollywood films, many consumers impose ever-harsher "regimens of body discipline and dietary restraint" in an attempt to close the gap between the cultural ideal and biological reality.[104] She worries that the "outliers"—the few women who are able to approximate to the ideal body shape—dictate norms that are then reinforced through advertising.[105] While Orbach asserts that "women are likely to use their bodies as their mouthpieces to express the forbidden and excluded feelings we carry inside," the vulnerable body can become the site of unrealistic ideals that undermine agency and health.[106]

This culture of "contemporary body management," as Susan Bordo calls it, links the commodity of food to diet pills and surgery, both of which became more prominent in the 1990s, despite attempts to regulate miracle diet cures and silicone breast implants.[107] It is unsurprising, then, that a culture that encourages both shrinkage and growth in equal measure should lead to a paradoxical logic among those who develop eating and body image disturbances. This shift toward a consumerist mentality both benefited the medical system in terms of profits and masked over the reasons—both personal and collective—that 400,000 Americans (87 percent of whom were female) underwent cosmetic surgery in 1994.[108] While diet pills, liposuction, and breast enhancement are in themselves fairly innocuous, the fact that surveys in 1994 and 1996 concluded that three-quarters of American women thought they were too fat and more than half would change their breast size if they could suggested that dissatisfaction had become the norm by the mid-1990s.[109] As early as 1992 second-wave feminist Gloria Steinem was calling unnecessary plastic surgery an epidemic.[110]

While there are usually multiple reasons that an individual seeks cosmetic surgery, the logic of diet pills offered a simpler method for bodily modification and for stimulating rapid weight loss.[111] Pills to speed up metabolism had been available since the 1960s, but amphetamine-style drugs such as Desoxyn and Ionamin were taken in increasing numbers for weight loss in the 1970s. Bulimics were particularly drawn toward diet pills because they meant that they could eat more without necessarily inducing vomiting, and amphetamines were just one option at a time when Dexatrim, Dietac, and Accutrim were available over the counter. A 1991 survey suggested that 65 percent of the population of bulimic outpatients had used diet pills (up from 50 percent in a similar survey three years earlier) and nearly 20 percent had taken pills for over a year, including a number who had used them in combination with laxatives, diuretics, and enemas.[112] By far the most popular of these brands was Dexatrim, which combined caffeine, green tea extract, and ginseng with two stimulants: the steroid hormone phenylpropanolamine (PPA) and the plant extract ephedra. Both ingredients came under the medical spotlight in the 1990s, when they were deemed to increase blood pressure to dangerous levels and heighten the risk of stroke. In 2000, the Food and Drug Administration warned the public to stop taking PPA, and in 2003, it banned ephedra. By far the most controversial diet medication was fen-phen, a combination of two drugs, fenfluramine and phentermine. Fen-phen was marketed as Pondimin and Redux in the mid-1990s. The Food and Drug Administration approved it for patients whose weight was 20 percent above the norm for their height and age, but it was more easily available at diet clinics.[113] The drugs were removed from the market in September 1997 when reports in the media suggested that the side effects of hypertension and heart damage could be fatal, while clinical studies revealed that up to 30 percent of patients who took Pondimin and Redux showed heart valve disturbances.[114] By then an estimated 18 million people had used the drugs, at a time when others such as the appetite suppressant Meridia were just coming on the market.

Within this context, Sara Goldfarb's story in Darren Aronofksy's disturbing 2000 film of Hubert Selby Jr.'s *Requiem for a Dream* makes salutary watching, particularly as it links the controversy of fen-phen to distortions of body image. Sara (played by Ellen Burstyn) is a lonely late middle-aged Brooklyn widow who clings to two hopes: that her son can make something of his life (she is unaware that he is a drug pusher) and that she will be invited as a guest contestant on her favorite television quiz show. When an unsolicited phone call suggests that she has won an appearance on the television show, she tries to lose weight by taking a combination of uppers and downers that her negligent doctor prescribes, seemingly unaware of or unconcerned about the effects on her behavior.

Alternatively wired and drowsy, she loses weight quickly, then starts grinding her teeth and hallucinating about snack food in the refrigerator. While the depiction of amphetamine psychosis in Aronofsky's film is true to Selby's 1978 novel, the symptoms of Sara's addiction in the film were probably prompted by the recent phen-fen controversy. The drug story plays out in *Requiem for a Dream* as a nightmarish one in which Sara loses her grip on reality while fantasizing about being

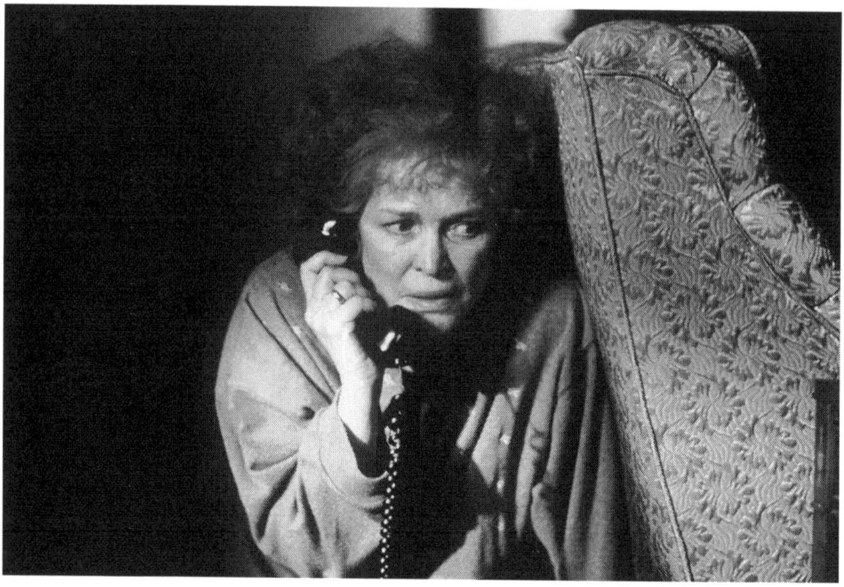

Figure 6.2 Sara Goldfarb (Ellen Burstyn) experiences both malnutrition and paranoia in the confinement of her Brooklyn home. *Requiem for a Dream* (dir. Darren Aronofsky, 2000). Artisan Pictures / The Kobal Collection / John Beer.

on the quiz show Sara's physical condition and psychological side effects rapidly worsen, though, and in a fragmented neo-gothic sequence she is committed to a state mental hospital, where she is given multiple drug treatments and electroconvulsive therapy. The end of the film is extremely bleak: Sara's dreams turn into psychotic ramblings, intercut by her son's heroin addiction, including the amputation of his arm when it becomes infected due to injection with contaminated needles. The film is self-consciously extreme, but it points to the fact that diet pills, addiction, weight loss, and delusions can often collide in life-threatening ways, even for relatively innocent individuals.

It is perhaps surprising that diet pills did not feature more strongly in feminist accounts of eating disorders in the 1990s, suggesting that the politics of eating and body image were tangled in the final decades of the century. This is particularly true of anorexia: a self-practice that often begins casually or as a deliberate protest against a world of diminishing options can quickly spiral into a loss of self and a regime of addiction. As we have seen, there is a moral undertow to many anorexia narratives, together with a realization on the part of the adult authors that their younger selves needed to learn habits that could both cultivate self-respect and embed their isolated voice in broader networks of care. This suggests that the act of sustained storytelling has the potential to therapeutically create a bridge between the voice of the enclosed self and a shared public voice.[115]

The danger, of course, is that in order to gain such perspective, the self becomes re-normalized and no longer strives for a new language that might more effectively speak to the contradictory logic of anorexia and thereby help broaden what philosopher Gail Weiss calls "our aesthetic ideals beyond the hegemony of the anticorporeal, fat-free body."[116] But the textual accounts discussed here rarely end up at a permanent point of resolution, suggesting that equilibrium is often only temporary. Instead of thinking of the anorexic narrative as generic, then, we need to see the portrayal of eating disorders in dystopian and apocalyptic worlds (as in the cases of *Superstar* and *Requiem of a Dream*) alongside domestic first-person narratives about eating, body image, and the quest for an authentic voice as divergent tendencies that cannot easily be reconciled. As Hornbacher says in her epilogue to *Wasted*, "we are not stories with narrative arcs, tidy plots."[117] Instead, the embodied self is unruly, contradictory, unreliable, and liable to break free of any label, be it clinical or cultural.

7 Disorders of Mood and Identity

In an August 1976 *New York* magazine feature, physicist, futurist, and former Rand Institute strategist Herman Kahn made some bold long-term predictions based on his new book, *The Next 200 Years*. Kahn focused mainly on trends in energy and economics, but he also spared some thought for future developments in the spheres of lifestyle, reproduction, and health. Raising probing questions about the ethics of genetic engineering and sex determination, he predicted that by 1985 it would "be possible for anyone to accurately manipulate his or her mood by taking the appropriate pills. One can become instantly introspective, extroverted, gregarious, buoyant, amorous, cool, calculating, quiet, etc."[1] Exaggerating for effect—or not quite understanding the nature of psychoactive drugs—Kahn questioned whether such "moods on demand" would be "freely permitted" without safeguards against self-diagnosis and self-medication. He was also worried that such a culture could lead to new forms of control in which exploitative bosses sought to modify employees' moods to serve their business interests.

Kahn was wrong in some respects and correct in others. In the 1970s concerns about psychotropic medication were increasing, especially when stories of Valium addiction came to light at mid-decade. However, some people saw drugs as more effective—and potentially more humane—than aggressive treatments. The nonstimulating antidepressant imipramine, for example, had been available since the late 1950s and, as Tofranil, was regularly prescribed for depression in the 1970s. In 1980, Temple Grandin asked to be put on Tofranil to control her panic attacks. However, the drug was far from a panacea: anxiety, mania, blurred vision, and constipation were common side effects, and it proved less effective than electroconvulsive therapy in treating cases of delusional depression.[2] In fact, its wide spectrum of often-unpredictable effects led Peter Kramer to call imipramine a dirty drug.[3]

This tricyclic antidepressant was not the drug that Kahn envisaged. Yet perhaps he had heard about early laboratory tests of fluoxetine, which a decade later was being hailed as a breakthrough drug for treating mood disorders and alleviating some symptoms of personality disorders. Released as Prozac in December 1987 by Eli Lilly, the same pharmaceutical company that had released methadone to the market forty years earlier, fluoxetine triggered specific effects by inhibiting serotonin uptake, leading Kramer to call it the first clean drug of its kind, "sleek and high-tech."[4] Perhaps Kahn's prediction was only two years premature, then, although it is debatable if a drug like Prozac could operate effectively as an "enhancement technology" for those who are already well.[5]

Kramer's widely read book *Listening to Prozac* (1993) was an important legitimation of the effectiveness of fluoxetine for treating mild depression and bipolar disorder. The book marked a moment when Prozac was seen not just as a low-risk treatment for depression but also as potentially transformative for obsessive-compulsive disorder, body image, and eating disorders, Tourette syndrome, and PTSD. Kramer's book was a chance to rescue antidepressants from the charge that they were impersonal therapy in disguise and facets of what controversial psychiatrist Peter Breggin called a "psychopharmaceutical complex" (echoing President Eisenhower's warning thirty-two years earlier of a "military-industrial complex"). Advertisements for psychoactive drugs increased in the early 1990s, as did fears that children were being overmedicated.[6] Prozac's visibility in advertisements marked it out and gave it the air of "a capitalist pill."[7] In 1990, it featured on the cover of *Newsweek* as a "breakthrough drug for depression," and in 1993 doctors administered 7.6 million new prescriptions for Prozac, leading Elizabeth Wurtzel to express astonishment in *Prozac Nation* (1994) that the drug had become a household name in only six years.[8] Wurtzel labels this broad cultural trend "the United States of Depression" and could barely believe that depression, "once considered tragic," had "become completely commonplace, even worthy of comedy."[9]

This chapter examines a spectrum of psychiatric conditions that a clean drug such as Prozac, either alone or in combination, was thought to alleviate more effectively than more established psychotropic drugs. In order to gear my discussion toward cultural texts and clinical research from the closing decades of the century, I have excluded the extensive scholarship on psychopharmaceuticals and anti-depressants that appeared in print after 2000.[10] Like the previous two chapters, chapter 7 aims to strike a balance between conditions categorized as "mood disorders" and "personality disorders" (two discrete sections of *DSM-III* that were significantly expanded for *DSM-IV* in 1994) and representations of lived experiences drawn from memoirs, case studies, fiction, and films that give narrative shape to conditions that often went beyond the diagnostic parameters of a "disorder."

This chapter is deliberately broad in scope, tracing lines from 1985, the year of Kahn's prediction, to the mid-1990s through a number of key publications: *DSM-IV*, Kramer's *Listening to Prozac*, Wurtzel's *Prozac Nation*, Joan Frances Casey's *The Flock*, and Chuck Palahniuk's novel of dissociating identities, *Fight Club*. There are moments when I return to the early 1970s—a backward look at *Sybil*, the famous 1973 account of multiple personality; the CBS television series *The Incredible Hulk*; and Christopher Lasch's 1978 treatise *The Culture of Narcissism*—and forward to Boston psychologist Lauren Slater's *Prozac Diary* of 1998, which brings together themes of medication and dissociation but also raises questions about medical, moral, and textual authority.

Language and voice are crucial concepts for this chapter because the diagnostic language of psychiatric conditions—bipolar, borderline, narcissistic, dissociative—shifted during the thirty years the form the historical spine of this book. Voice is also very important, particularly for patients on long-term medication and for those who shuttle between different identities. Sometimes these voices are difficult to reconcile into a meaningful whole, sometimes they are unreliable, and sometimes the effects of medication, including Prozac, means that self-expressive language sinks below the level of audibility. Lauren Slater, the director of AfterCare Services, an outpatient center for the treatment of mental illness and substance abuse in East Boston, noted in 1998 that Prozac can balance tensions and calm inner voices but can also lead to a loss of creativity: it "doesn't fill your mind so much as empty it of its contents and then leave you, like a pitcher, waiting to be filled."[11] Slater asked far-reaching questions about the authenticity of selfhood and she worried that the illness experience, despite the anguish that it brought, was potentially more real than the functional self that emerged when she began taking Prozac. Just as the literature on autism tends to focus on the theme of savantism, so the poles of creativity and violence are recurring themes in accounts of mood and identity disorder.

Mood Swings

The language of psychosis was more familiar in the 1970s than it had ever been before. That is not to say that psychosis had become an everyday phenomenon, but its symptoms could be identified in the increasingly common diagnosis of mood and borderline disorders, even though the media was drawn toward sensationalist stories of psychopathic behavior and gun violence. We see how psychosis is embedded in suburban experience in, for example, Robert Redford's Oscar-winning film adaptation of *Ordinary People*, based on Judith Guest's 1976 novel, which explores how depression and quiet conflict rends apart the lives of all four members of an average Illinois suburban family—a theme that the so-called dirty realist writers Raymond Carver and Richard Ford took further in the combination of metaphysical, psychological, and quotidian pressures their protagonists face.[12]

Such embedding in the everyday was partly attributable to the fact that psychiatric terminology was also becoming more familiar. Following a general description in *DSM-III* (and its revised version of 1987), *DSM-IV* subcategorized mood disorders into three types: episodes (of short or long duration); categories (including depressive and bipolar disorders); and specifiers (referring to a particular mood episode or a recurrent cycle). This taxonomy enabled practitioners to begin with symptomology and then proceed to diagnosis as a means of distinguishing between mild, moderate, and severe episodes; discerning whether psychotic, catatonic or melancholic features were typically present; and identifying specific triggers such as postpartum onset or seasonal patterns. In the first area of this tripartite system, *DSM-IV* lists four types of episodes. The first is major depressive episodes that span more than two weeks and are associated with additional symptoms such as erratic food intake, "feelings of worthlessness or guilt," irregular sleep patterns, loss of concentration, inability to make decisions, and suicidal tendencies. The other three episodes are described as manic, mixed, and hypomanic. Each one identifies a sustained phase with a set of related symptoms: manic episodes include "inflated self-esteem or grandiosity, decreased need for sleep, pressure of speech, flight of ideas, distractibility"; mixed episodes are characterized by oscillating moods; and hypomanic episodes are distinguished from their manic counterparts because they do not typically require time off work or hospitalization.[13]

DSM-IV differentiated bipolar disorder from major depressive disorder by specifying the presence of periodic mood swings. In turn, the two versions of bipolar disorder the manual described are divided by the severity of the manic stages, as distinct from the less severe form of hypomania and cyclothymic disorder for patients who do not meet the "major" criteria. The clinical entries emphasize that mood disorders need to be distinguished from schizophrenic conditions, medical disorders (such as hyperkinetic behavior as a result of orbitofrontal lesions), and substance-induced disorders that can be traced to recreational drugs, the side effects of prescription drugs (including dopamine, steroids, and antidepressants), alcohol intake, or exposure to toxins.

On the surface, this type of classification seems difficult to criticize. However, while the *DSM-IV* classification system makes it possible to gauge episodic intensity and duration and to distinguish between substance abuse disorders and major depressive disorders, it poses diagnostic problems when symptomology crosses over: for example, in cases of toxicity due to prescription drugs or for Vietnam-era veterans whose war psychosis might have been complicated by drug or alcohol use over a sustained period.[14] *DSM-IV* did more to recognize the variety of cultural experience than its 1980 version, outlining somatic symptoms in Hispanic cultures, imbalance in Chinese cultures, and "problems of the 'heart'" in Arabic cultures, plus it gave attention to the rise of major depressive episodes among women. (There is nothing, though, on high levels of suicide among Native American groups.)[15] Similarly, this taxonomy hints that there might be other atypical cases that cannot be given discrete labels, which psychopharmacological expert Stephen Stahl later described as "bipolar ¼" and "bipolar ½" on a broader spectrum that more easily accounts for substance use.[16]

DSM-IV clarifies some of the diagnostic issues that concerned the Mood Disorders Advisory Group, which had been established in the mid-1970s to prepare the ground for the tighter descriptions *DSM-III* offered.[17] Neither edition deals explicitly with treatment, but the authors of *DSM-IV* would not have been blind to drugs like Prozac that could alleviate the symptoms of milder disorders. While there were some Prozac scare stories, such as a 1994 *New York Times* story that reported that most of a town in Washington state had been prescribed the drug, there were other treatments for depression, including more established tricyclic antidepressants and cognitive behavioral theory, that could help the patient break cycles while accepting the pattern of their fluctuating moods.[18] Advocates of Prozac claimed that it was the first intelligent drug of its kind, yet there was good evidence by the early 1970s that lithium was also effective, not just for controlling manic episodes but also for balancing the extreme moods of those diagnosed with hypomania and manic depression.[19] Lithium worked for the actress Patty Duke, for example, after she experienced more than a decade of violent mood swings linked to excessive alcohol and drug use (reflecting the fate of her Judy Garland-like character Neely O'Hara in *Valley of the Dolls*). Duke started taking lithium in 1982 when she was undergoing psychotherapy. While expressions of bipolar illness can be identified in popular culture—in the manic stand-up performances of Robin Williams that seem shot through with melancholy and the extremes of "sadness and euphoria" of which Billy Joel sang in his 1976 track "Summer, Highland Falls"—it was not until Duke's 1987 autobiography *Call Me Anna* and her appearances on a daytime talk shows that year that the subject really opened up in the general public, particularly after Duke's personal account was adapted for television in 1990.

Duke found that lithium gave her balance and comfort. In this respect, she concurred with Ronald Fieve's speculation in his 1975 book that lithium not only helps recalibrate manic depression but also has a positive therapeutic effect on some schizophrenic disorders.[20] Instead of relying on protracted inpatient treatment or more aggressive therapies, Fieve champions the properties of lithium (overlooking the fact that a safe dose of lithium is actually very close to a toxic dose) and notes that influential public figures seemed to benefit from the creative energy that mood swings can bring. Duke claimed that lithium made her more creative, enabling her to "face life as a garden-variety neurotic, not a green, squirrely monster"—in essence, lithium made psychosis more of an everyday reality than a nightmarish aberration.[21] Fieve's book, which was published over a decade before Duke tackled the stigma of manic depression, can be read as a response to the crisis in leadership following Nixon's resignation (he speculates that Nixon covered up his depression during the Watergate hearings) and the stigma that led to the withdrawal of Senator Thomas Eagleton as George McGovern's vice-presidential running mate two years earlier (see chapter 1). Fieve argues that the stigma that Eagleton faced should not be tolerated. However, the danger of linking charismatic leadership to manic depression is that mania starts to be seen as a mode of desirable behavior that leads to exploitation by drug companies and advertisers.[22]

An instructive text that explores mood swings from a first-person perspective is clinical psychologist Kay Redfield Jamison's 1995 memoir *An Unquiet Mind*, which traces the development of her condition to her itinerant childhood in the 1950s. Redfield had already made a mark with two studies, a clinical account, *Manic-Depressive Illness* (1990), with National Institute of Mental Health psychiatrist Frederick K. Goodwin, and a more popular book, *Touched with Fire* (1993), that followed in Ronald Fieve's footsteps in assessing the creative benefits of conditions typically classified as debilitating.[23] Focusing on writers and painters whose creativity stemmed from their pain, *Touched with Fire* can be read, first, as an account of the pattern of "creative surges and creative blocks" that Jamison claims both manic depressives and artistic individuals experience and, second, her working through of a condition that in her twenties came to define her identity.[24] As a student drawn equally to science and poetry, Jamison experiences a pattern of manic energy and crashing lows; she could be productively creative and dangerously despondent in equal measure.

As with other psychological memoirs, *An Unquiet Mind* reaches into the past in an attempt to make meaningful patterns out of inchoate experiences. Critics hailed the text for skillfully linking clinical and autobiographical experiences, but Jamison sometimes uses dramatic language that does not always evade the stigma she strives to avoid.[25] She begins the text, for example, by claiming that "within a month" of being appointed assistant professor of psychiatry at UCLA "I was well on my way to madness" and that two months later she was "manic beyond recognition."[26] Despite the hyperbole, Jamison tries to maintain the double perspective of observer and experiencer throughout the text. Not quite as exuberant as Marya Hornbacher's turbulent *Wasted* or as dramatic as second-wave feminist Kate Millett's 1990 text *The Looney-Bin Trip* (which charted her attempts to withdraw from lithium in the 1980s), *An Unquiet Mind* works through Jamison's educational experiences and relationships in order to assess a condition that at times she can observe with a clinical eye and at other times she loses herself in.[27]

Jamison pinpoints one childhood memory as a touchstone for her bipolarity. Looking up one day from her schoolyard, she sees an airplane flying dangerously low to the ground, then crashing into a nearby copse of trees and exploding on impact. The fright that she felt that day takes on a different complexion when it becomes clear that the pilot might have saved himself but did not want to risk the plane crashing into the schoolyard. This spectacle and the pilot's bravery change Kay's dreams of limitless possibilities and implant in her mind an "impossible ideal" that was "all the more compelling and haunting because of its very unobtainability."[28] She associates similar ideals with her father, an air force officer who encouraged Kay to pursue her interests in science and literature. However, he was not a wholly affirmative force in her life, particularly as he tended to shuttle between "soaring" moods that filled the house with "warmth and joy" and "grimmer" moods that she remembers as "bleak emotional withdrawal," especially when he loses his post-military job at Rand.[29] Despite this uneven emotional landscape, Kay's first manic-depressive episode as a high school senior happened on her own terms when she experiences an exhilarating high followed by a period of self-torture. These mood swings are not untypical of adolescence, but for Jamison they set a horizon that darkened during her years as a medical student.

By her late 40s, Jamison had discovered a vocabulary that she lacked as a student and young professor when she was desperate to conceal her depressive episodes, her financial recklessness, and the scrambled thinking of her manic phases.[30] Her bleakest times were the seemingly endless periods of depression, which, as Elizabeth Wurtzel reminds us, can often lead to paralysis where it is not possible to "think straight" and when meaningful words prove elusive.[31] Whereas Wurtzel embraces prescription drugs as a feature of her self-absorbed life—even though she realizes they might dam her creativity—Jamison concludes that her resistance to drug therapy proved costly. In addition to dark moods and nightmares, she becomes painfully thin and her intimate relationships begin to show signs of strain. She learns little of personal benefit about mood disorders on professional residency programs: these were dominated by psychoanalytic approaches that she, like many in the profession at the time, were becoming skeptical about. She nevertheless sees psychotherapy as a means for locating a calming "sanctuary," which she describes as a barrier against "the crushing movement of a mental sea" that had enough permeability to "let in fresh sea-water."[32]

When she finally started taking lithium in 1974, Jamison found that she slept better but accomplished less and missed her manic intensity. She experienced some side effects of lithium, such as blurred vision, nausea, a loss of concentration, and "a lack of enthusiasm and bounce," but she had become attached to her exhilarating highs, seeing them as both dangerous and as a doorway to "energy, fire, enthusiasm, and imagination."[33] Lithium was a necessary crutch that made everyday life bearable, protecting her from suicidal impulses and potential institutionalization. It was only when her lithium dose was lowered, though, some years after she started, that she experienced renewed clarity in her thinking and color in her sensory experiences. This was by no means the end of her mood swings or her life dilemmas (such as the painful decision not to have children because of her family's history of depression), and she looked to genetics and neuroscience for answers that medicine, psychiatry, and psychopharmacology could not provide.

In essence, Jamison neither ultimately rejects drug treatment nor sees it as a panacea. Lithium was the preferred treatment for manic depression until the appearance of Prozac, and it had relatively few of the side effects of anti-depressants. *Prozac Nation* takes this a step further by documenting the combination of drugs that Elizabeth Wurtzel took from 1990 onward after being given both lithium and Prozac following an overdose of the antidepressant Desyrel.[34] Even though it takes time for Jamison to respond to Prozac and she is initially skeptical about its effects, she recognizes its potential for lifting the fog that clouds her thoughts and for others whose daily lives are "clouded by constant despair."[35] Despite such admissions, Wurtzel and Jamison each contributed to the popular trend of romanticizing euphoric moods that made a smart drug like Prozac cosmetically desirable rather than necessary for functioning.[36]

This romantic strain is encapsulated in the 1995 teen-pic *Mad Love*, starring former child protégé Drew Barrymore as the out-of-control and recently hospitalized college student Casey Roberts. The film plays off Barrymore's real-life story of addiction and rehabilitation, as explored in her 1990 autobiography *Little Girl Lost*. It focuses on an illicit road trip Casey and her boyfriend Matt Leland (Chris O'Donnell) take from Seattle to the Mexican border, before Casey's mood swings thwart their attempt to escape her concerned but controlling parents. Although *Mad Love* addresses the topic of overmedicated children, it seems to conclude that care and love cannot replace medical intervention when mood swings need to be recalibrated. Despite this, the film celebrates Casey's elemental wellspring of energy. This contrasts with the disengaged slacker culture of Wurtzel's generation, captured in the opening of the film by grunge band Nirvana's debut single, a repetitive yet discordant cover version of the 1969 psychedelic rock track "Love Buzz."[37]

Borderline States

The accounts discussed above associate mood fluctuations with the kind of fundamental questions about identity that prompted Patty Duke to reflect that her "life seems to have happened to someone else."[38] This expression of dissociation is characteristic of a range of conditions, but whereas mood disorders involve shifting states of mind, *DSM-III* describes a personality disorder as "an enduring pattern of inner experience and behavior that deviates markedly from the expectations of the individual's culture."[39] These "pervasive" traits cluster individuals into one of three groups: "odd or eccentric" (classified alternately as paranoid, schizoid, and schizotypal); "dramatic, emotional, or erratic" (including borderline, histrionic, and narcissistic types); or "anxious or fearful" (encompassing avoidant, dependent, and obsessive-compulsive disorders).[40] Because of the ingrained nature of these character traits, personality disorders are more difficult to treat with drugs than mood disorders and often require a therapist to understand the "underlying intrapsychic dynamics" that might break a destructive cycle or can help the patient find new significance in a world where there is sometimes either too little or too much meaning.[41] The expanded section dealing with personality disorders in *DSM-IV* uses a more refined multiaxial system than *DSM-III*, yet it notes that patients display traits that blur the lines between the three groups, leaving room for a "mixed personality," of which depressive personality disorder is given as a key example.[42] This suggests that disorders of mood and personality are not as distinct as they first seem and that phases of depression and mania are common to both.

In this and the next sections I focus on two personality disorders of the "dramatic, emotional, or erratic" type that struck a chord with broader patterns in American culture in the 1980s and 1990s and that problematize the unsubstantiated claim of the *DSM* authors that these conditions "deviate from the expectations of the individual's culture." Borderline and narcissistic personality disorders were by no means new, but they reflected the volatility and self-obsession that Tom Wolfe and others associated with the 1970s and that grew in intensity in the following decades. Whereas previous chapters looked at deceptive voices in addiction and anorexia narratives, the personality disorders of this chapter profoundly question the notion of a unitary and cohesive voice. By focusing on these two disorders, we can analyze liminal states in which the self and voice are open to risk through distortion, exaggeration or diminishment.

DSM-IV characterizes borderline personality disorder as having a "pervasive pattern of instability of interpersonal relationships, self-image, and affects" and a particular fear of abandonment that is often imaginary yet can at times lead to intense anger.[43] Although "borderline" suggests a "not-quite" disorder—and can overlap with a diagnosis of mood disorder—the experiencer can often feel deeply immersed and unable to control passionately felt emotions or suicidal impulses. There is sometimes an intense moral charge to these feelings, but individuals have reported that at other times they feel empty or "have feelings that they do not exist at all," particularly when they are alone or lack support.[44] The disorder can, at times, be traced to child abuse or parental loss at an early age which is then repeated through subsequent transitory relationships. This can lead to an intense need for attachment mixed with bouts of anxiety or rage.

There was some disagreement about whether the *DSM* description accurately captured the essence and variation of borderline experiences, an issue the *DSM-III* advisory group tried to tackle in the mid-1970s when they met to consider the ways personality disorders often seep into, or emerge from, everyday life.[45] Not only is the symptomology of borderline disorder sometimes misread variously as dependency, paranoia, food obsession, or substance addiction, but, as Theodore Millon, the founding editor of the *Journal of Personality Disorders*, noted in 1992, it is both "overdiagnosed and elusive," especially when it refers to more general behavioral patterns of the "impulsive, unpredictable, and often explosive" kind.[46] Borderline individuals tend to experience separation anxiety and long for affirmation yet sometimes reject support when it is offered. Millon discerns that this impulse stems from a "lack of inner harmony" and an "immature, nebulous, or wavering sense of identity," but he also takes external pressures into account.[47] While Robert Jay Lifton finds much to celebrate in the dynamism and potential of the "protean self," Millon sees the "fluid and inconsistent" practices of late capitalism seeping into consciousness and eroding ego stability, leaving vulnerable individuals "groping and bewildered."[48] In fact, an authentic voice and a resilient ego are most at risk, with overwhelming impulses often leading to violent outbreaks.[49]

We can identify this symptomology in a number of 1970s cultural texts, for example in the behavior of the unstable and manipulative Evelyn Draper (Jessica Walter) who becomes obsessed with the California DJ Dave Garber (Clint Eastwood) in the 1971 psychological thriller *Play Misty for Me* and the erratic behavior of the Los Angeles working-class housewife Mabel in John Cassavetes' 1974 film *A Woman under the Influence*. Both films focus on psychological struggles, but the increasingly violent behavior of the female leads has an obsessive intensity that exceeds everyday behavior. The most sustained cycle of films in which unstable characters could be imputed to have borderline personality disorder were produced in the early 1990s, although these conditions are rarely diagnosed as such and the films focus on violence rather than on treatment or care. This is most obviously linked to identity confusion in *Single White Female* (1992), in which a bond that develops between New Yorker Allie Jones (Bridget Fonda) and her new roommate Hedra Carlson (Jennifer Jason Leigh) becomes an unhealthy process of identification that leads to the murder of Allie's husband and undermines the stability of both women.[50] The film developed the stalker theme from the 1987 revenge thriller *Fatal Attraction*, itself a derivation of *Play Misty for Me*. For its depiction of psychopathic violence, feminist critics read *Fatal Attraction* as a backlash against the rise of the independent career women in favor of Reaganite family values: Alex Forrest (Glenn Close) turns into an unstable, almost monstrous, character as she seeks vengeance on the family of Dan Gallagher (Michael Douglas) when their brief affair ends.[51] The film deals with borderline disorder only loosely, though, as did another domestic horror film, *The Hand that Rocks the Cradle* (1992), and two mid-1990s releases, *Malicious* and *Thin Line between Love and Hate*, which also depict young women who feel betrayed by male suitors and whose overwhelming feelings tip over into vengeance.[52]

Feminist critic Susan Faludi cites evidence that mental health problems were more often associated with single women than married women, a view that correlates with filmic portrayals that link borderline diagnoses with young women's anxieties about identity.[53] We see this at play when Susanna Kaysen dwells on her diagnosis in the closing pages of *Girl, Interrupted*. The label of "borderline" gives her more cause for concern than the vague clinical description that was made when she was first hospitalized in April 1967: "psychoneurotic depressive reaction" and "personality pattern disturbance, mixed type. R/O Undifferentiated schizophrenia." The case reports Kaysen quotes illuminate her mood patterns, including one "episode of depersonalization" that lasted six hours when "she felt that she wasn't a real person, nothing but skin" and felt an urge to harm herself. Kaysen was told she had a "character disorder" when she was discharged from McLean Hospital in September 1968, but her final diagnosis of "paranoid type (borderline)" pushes her to consult *DSM-III*.[54] Frustrated with the new classification of borderline personality disorder, she tries to make sense of it in her own words: "a way station between neurosis and psychosis: a fractured but not disassembled psyche," a borderline between "common unhappiness" and behavior that teeters on the dangerous.[55]

Kaysen believes that while the diagnosis is fairly accurate for her teenage self, it is not a profound classification that defines her being. Although she continues to face uncertainty, she thinks the symptoms (some of which she associates only with adolescence) have lost their intensity, leaving her feeling generally unhappy rather than on the threshold of psychosis. This section of Kaysen's text is written with wry irony shot through with defiance as she gives voice to an experience that cannot easily be captured in abstract language. She concludes, too, that the classification hides a gender bias, imputing moral categories of promiscuity and "self-damaging activities" that have no male equivalents.[56]

The poetic ending to the book muses on the idea of an interrupted life to consider how the clinical record of her two years of institutionalization creates an indelible text. She does not totally dismiss the insights she gained during her stay in hospital, yet she longs for a different kind of light by which she could observe herself afresh. The final pages of *Girl, Interrupted* evoke a moment of stillness, inspired by the seventeenth-century Vermeer painting that lends an abbreviated version of its name to the text. This mood is in direct contrast to the violent, unstable characters that populate the psychological thrillers of the early 1990s, and it played out in the 1999 film adaptation through the contrast between Winona Ryder's portrayal of Susanna, who longs for stillness and calm, and Angelina Jolie's Lisa Cody, who is an appealing but disruptive force that Susanna must learn to reject before she can recover. In this way, the screenplay turns Kaysen's subtle reflections into a hospital melodrama where the borderline is played out through the dyadic relationship between Susanna and Lisa—or, figuratively, between everyday adolescent neurosis and dangerous psychosis.[57]

The fact that "borderline" has mythic implications or can better be explained in poetic terms (Laura Slater calls it "the line of the horizon, a flat world, a ship tipping over into the star-filled night") makes it an even more elusive.[58] Although there were some realistic accounts of this often-confusing diagnostic category—such as the 1989 documentary *Borderline Syndrome: A Personality Disorder of Our*

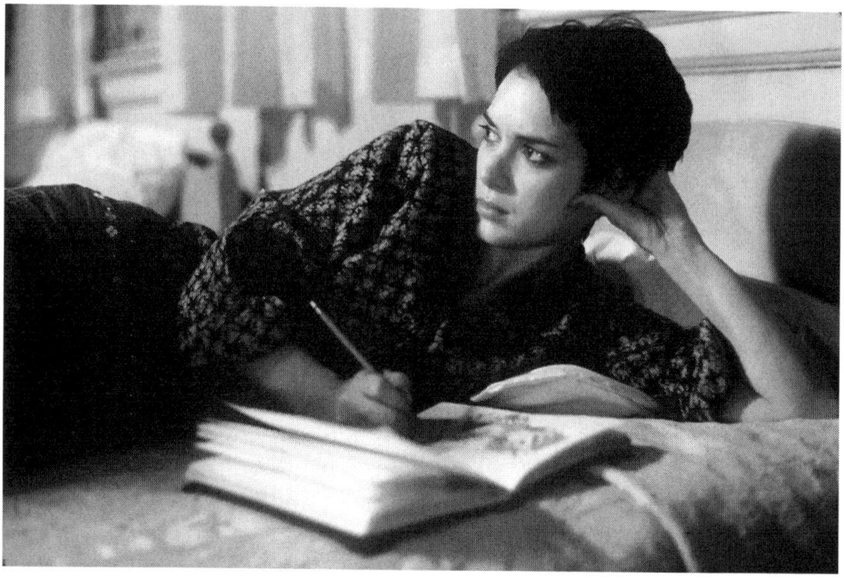

Figure 7.1 A contemplative Susanna Kaysen (Winona Ryder) in *Girl, Interrupted* (dir. James Mangold, 1999) during her eighteen-month stay at McLean Hospital. Columbia Tristar/The Kobal Collection/Suzanne Tenner.

Time, which links personal stories to clinical overviews based on the *DSM-III* classification—it is the enigmatic dimension that is often amplified in cultural accounts through amorphous characters or other characters who are splintered versions of each other.[59] The film of *Girl, Interrupted* can be read through this lens, as can another resonant late-nineties text, Chuck Palahniuk's novel *Fight Club*, through the double image of the shadowy narrator and the mercurial Tyler Durden. The expanded *DSM-IV* classification of borderline personality disorder resonated with broader cultural trends too, such as the highly publicized suicide of Nirvana singer Kurt Cobain, who, just days before his death, had escaped from the Exodus Recovery Center in Los Angeles, where he was being treated for heroin addiction.[60] Cobain was never diagnosed with a psychiatric disorder, yet there is evidence in his art, lyrics, and interviews to suggest that he was struggling with an identity disorder that involved a family history of suicides and unstable parental relationships, sustained drug use, digestive problems, and bouts of depression and that tilted him toward violence and emptiness.

Narcissistic Selves

The *DSM* classification places both narcissistic and borderline personality disorders within the "dramatic, emotional, or erratic" cluster. Research into the likelihood that narcissistic and borderline types would be attracted to each other was being conducted in the early 1990s, but it was the narcissistic type that took a stronger hold of the public imagination, mixing psychoanalytic ideas with the belief that American cultural values had taken a wrong turn after the 1960s.[61] The clinical etiology of narcissism reaches back to Freud's attempt in his 1914 essay "On Narcissism" to explain it in psychoanalytic terms as an ego ideal that emerges in early sexual development. A half-century later, two Austrian émigré analysts, Heinz Kohut and Otto Kernberg, were key to developing this basic framework. Kohut's 1971 book *The Analysis of the Self* molds Freud's tenets into his theory of "self psychology" in which narcissism is a fight to locate an authentic voice that could combat feelings of low self-esteem, whereas Kernberg's *Borderline Conditions and Pathological Narcissism* (1975) focuses on early ego development but distinguishes between different types of narcissism, not all of which are pathological. The fault lines between Kernberg and Kohut are important because they show both how narcissism remained a vexed clinical issue and how conflicting psychiatric, psychoanalytic, and cultural uses stretched it across a broad spectrum that blurred with other conditions.[62]

This broader expression was captured in Christopher Lasch's *The Culture of Narcissism* and shaped what *DSM-IV* described as "a pervasive pattern of grandiosity, need for admiration, and lack of empathy." The *DSM* classification was constructed at a significant historical juncture (appearing soon after President Clinton's health insurance bill had failed), when both purposeful individualism and cohesive communities appeared to be under strain.[63] Jimmy Carter had stressed the need to renew civic values fifteen years earlier, in part to address the potential pathological impasse of self-absorption and self-gratification that Lasch had identified. This narcissistic trend appeared only to worsen in the 1980s, though, at a time when heightened competition and a more aggressive marketing industry normalized self-importance and extreme careerism as ways of advancing in business.

However, not all theorists agreed that narcissism is invariably pathological. For example, in one of his most popular books of the 1950s, *The Art of Loving*, neo-Freudian Erich Fromm promoted "self-love" as the productive foundation for loving others based on the theory "that love is an attitude which is the same toward all objects, including myself." Fromm believed that only in extreme forms did self-love become an incapacity or a disorder.[64] Fromm's humanist conception of self-love seemed to have little purchase a quarter of century later, though, when selfishness seemed to be becoming the kind of "bottomless pit" that Fromm believed could never be satiated.[65] Although this theory of narcissism can be read as an attempt to overcompensate for a "basic lack of love," Fromm's description of a swelling up of the self in reaction to feelings of self-depletion was not far from Lasch's use of the term, particularly the self-interested "survival mentality" that Lasch explored in his 1984 book *The Minimal Self*.[66]

Swiss psychologist Alice Miller was another influential thinker who explored narcissism from a psychoanalytic perspective. In her 1979 study *The Drama of the Gifted Child*, first translated in 1981, she rescued the term from its derogatory association with selfishness to make it at least possible to experience healthy narcissism, which she describes as the "ideal case of a person who is genuinely alive with free access to the true self and his authentic feelings," in contrast to narcissistic disorders which take root "within the prison of the false self."[67] Retaining a model of depth psychology, Miller realized that a degree of self-love is vital to preventing ego disintegration or a state that leaves the individual vulnerable to false thoughts or abuse.[68] This middle ground between exaggerated forms of narcissism and the "solitary confinement" of depression is a strong theme of *The Drama of the Gifted Child*, which draws upon Miller's own experience of child abuse, as she discusses in a preface to the 1986 edition.

Miller's thoughts are aligned with Kohut's theory that narcissism is an inner battle between feelings of inferiority and over-estimation of self-worth. Depression and mania are thus encoded within narcissism, together with a fear of rejection and failure that sometimes shades into diagnoses of borderline personality disorder. Written while Kohut was lecturing in psychiatry at the University of Chicago, *The Analysis of the Self* focuses on the role of objects "either used in the service of the self and of the maintenance of its instinctual investment, or objects which are themselves experienced as part of the self."[69] His argument is that the narcissistic self is intimately bound up with "objects which are not experienced as separate and independent from the self," meaning that these individuals "remain fixated on archaic grandiose self configurations" in which they experience a "compelling need for merger with [a] powerful object."[70] While he noted that the narcissistic self is often impoverished because of the narrowing of the individual's lifeworld, Kohut believed that narcissists usually retain a "cohesive self," certainly much more often than do those with borderline conditions.[71] This does not mean there are no pathological elements of narcissism or that the narcissistic self is necessarily resilient. Kohut contrasts the "formation of a nuclear cohesive self" at a young age with a "hollow," "brittle," and "fragile" self that is grafted on top in adulthood.[72] Moreover, narcissism can shift rapidly between relative normalcy (positive self-esteem and admiration for others) and psychosis ("delusional reconstitution of the grandiose self" and overinvestment in omnipotent objects), depending on circumstances or relationship patterns.[73]

An instructive literary example of this battle between pathological and healthy narcissism is Don DeLillo's debut novel *Americana* (1971), which depicts the sharp transition of television executive David Bell from corporate life in Manhattan to a self-defining journey westward. DeLillo clearly wants us to see David Bell as an arch-narcissist. At the "end of another dull and lurid year" living and working in Manhattan, Bell proclaims that he has the "same kind of relationship with my mirror that many of my contemporaries [have] with their analysts."[74] While the mirror offers Bell some comfort, it is also a reflected image that can disappear in the blur of the image industry in which he works. Kohut notes that the mirror might be a symbol of vanity or "unbridled ambitions," but individuals who constantly check themselves in the mirror can harbor feelings of failure and emptiness.[75] Bell soon realizes that he is covering up existential fears with empty behavioral patterns: "when I began to wonder who I was, I took the simple step of lathering my face and shaving."[76]

Seduced initially by the power of the image, which he believes feeds into "the circuitry of my dreams," he comes to recognize that because of his amoral lifestyle, he is "living in the third person."[77] Bell's memories of his mother offer a clue to his anomie (she also experienced depression) and push him into a cycle of short-lived sexual relationships that may stem, it is implied, from an unresolved oedipal relationship.[78] To combat the narcissistic dead end in which he finds himself, Bell decides to head west on a journey to discover a new identity in the hope that he can "match the shadows of my image and my self."[79] Bell's quest can be interpreted as an extreme form of self-indulgence, but it has both therapeutic and expressive possibilities, especially because he plans to make "a long unmanageable movie full of fragments of everything that's part of my life."[80] This search for an authentic voice links DeLillo's novel to Kohut's clinical experiences: some of Kohut's patients dream about losing their voice and he hears other patients speaking with odd intonations and in different pitches. The film Bell makes in *Americana* (in which he plays an alter ego) is perhaps his saving grace. But Bell's literary descendants cannot evade their condition as easily, such as the serial killer Patrick Bateman in Bret Easton Ellis's *American Psycho* and the split protagonist in Chuck Palahniuk's *Fight Club*, both of whom try to escape an imprisoning world through gratuitous acts of violence.

In the 2000 film adaptation of *American Psycho*, we see an updated version of David Bell's relationship with his mirror when Patrick Bateman applies a face mask after his morning shower. The novel's description focuses on the cleansing routine and other consumerist rituals involving popular music and breakfast items, whereas the filmed scene pauses with the peeling off of the semi-transparent mask, giving the visual illusion that this is Bateman's split-off face, simultaneously a replica and a negation of himself. The novel also contains numerous scenes involving mirrors in which Bateman obsessively checks his hair and skin tone. He believes he has supreme agency in choosing high-quality cleansing products and designer clothes, but he is actually in danger of losing himself within a world of fetishistic objects: what Georgina Colby perceptively reads as a "merging of the subject with the economic apparatus."[81] When he peels off the face mask early in the film, his composite face symbolizes this liminal state between self-affirmation and self-erasure.

While David Bell seeks an antidote for an unforgiving culture that pushes him inward, Patrick Bateman is seemingly beyond help, although it is not always clear where the lines between fantasy and reality meet or where his ironic detachment from Reaganite values becomes pathological indulgence, such as his overuse of Nancy Reagan's anti-drug catchphrase Just Say No. While Bell is confident that his western travel movie will reveal a deeper truth than corporate life in Manhattan does, Bateman continually empties out meaning, for example when he claims that he wants to understand two call girls by "filming their deaths," only to comically distract himself with the technical specifications of his movie camera.[82] Neither text has a clearly defined healer figure who could play the role of a therapist or help the characters reestablish a stable reality. If, as Heniz Kohut and Alice Miller surmise, narcissism is a result of a lack of empathy at an early age then the absence of parents—together with hints of an unhealthy maternal relationship—seem to be the key to both narcissism and the repetitive cycle that Bell goes some way to breaking and in which Bateman is imprisoned. Although both Kernberg and Kohut emphasize the relationship between self and objects, Kernberg differs from Kohut in examining forms of regression that can be traced to primitive emotions and that account for "the intense oral-aggressive quality" of narcissistic fixations.[83] Not only do narcissists tend to distrust others and see the world outside themselves as insubstantial, they can be drawn toward paranoid thinking in which "shadowy external objects sometimes suddenly seem to be invested with high and dangerous powers."[84]

The primitive world that Bell manages to sublimate through his quest envelops Bateman and makes it impossible for him to evaluate his behavior. Instead, he is drawn toward fetishistic cleansing and clothing rituals as a sublimation of his viscerality. As literary critic James Annesley detects, Bateman becomes "screened off from reality" and inhabits a place where "his violent acts become, in his imagination, indistinguishable from the unreal images he sees around him," leading to what Colby calls the "liquidation of subjectivity."[85] This ontological state of derealization correlates with what Kernberg calls the "hungry, enraged, empty self, full of impotent anger at being frustrated, and fearful of a world which seems as hateful and revengeful as the patient himself."[86] When *American Psycho* ends with the taut phrase "no exit," it prompts the reader to question whether Bateman is a villain or a victim, despite his history of bloodshed and abuse.[87] It is the violence of this world, which Kernberg describes as "rage reactions" precipitated by feelings of isolation and futility, to which I turn next.[88]

Violent Eruptions

Peter Kramer appends a short essay on violence to his largely affirmative account *Listening to Prozac*. Based on a case study of a suicidal patient who was taking Prozac, Kramer concludes that the health risks of the drug are low, even though he notes with concern that the media tends to inflame stories about the side effects of Prozac "because they are meshed with science-fiction images of chemicals that turn Jekyll into Hyde."[89] Evoking the image of a split self, Kramer touches on how private and public stories involving certain psychiatric disorders entwine, particularly when violent behavior makes an otherwise internal condition public. While depression might be experienced inwardly, mania, erratic states of being, and aggression are the more obvious social faces of mental illness. In the final two sections of this chapter, I turn to these twin images—violent selves and split selves—to understand better how unstable and multiple voices complicate the faith that many therapists and health groups have in the patient's authentic voice.

Jamison's and Wurtzel's memoirs both contain violent episodes—sometimes they are taking prescription drugs and sometimes not—that seem to be symptomatic of how violence increasingly encroached on everyday life during and beyond the 1970s. We saw earlier how *Taxi Driver* became a keynote for the sense of disillusionment and social instability that took hold in the wake of the Vietnam War and how the mass media caught onto stories of armed veterans running amok.

Despite the caricature of the rampaging veteran that Tim O'Brien evoked in his 1979 *Esquire* article (as discussed in chapter 2), there is some truth in these stories, particularly as the number of homicides at the hands of veterans diagnosed with schizophrenia (such as the murder of an elderly Sacramento woman by traumatized veteran Manuel Babbitt in 1980) increased. The assassination attempts on Presidents Ford and Reagan in 1975 and 1981, respectively, added to concerns about social instability.[90] While Travis Bickle of *Taxi Driver* cannot be seen as a narcissist, despite his periods of lonely contemplation and the "you talkin' to me?" sequence when he faces himself in his bedroom mirror during his transition from quiet taxi driver to punk assassin, the film became notorious for prompting a young man who was later diagnosed with narcissistic personality disorder, John Hinckley Jr., to start collecting firearms and reading about Lee Harvey Oswald, the former marine who assassinated President Kennedy.[91]

Yet even in the cases of Hinckley and Oswald, the loose label of psychopathology is tricky to pin down in clinical terms. The staff psychiatrist at the juvenile home Oswald lived in during his teenage years claimed that he combined "traits of dangerousness"; "explosive aggressive, assaultive acting out"; a "cold, detached outer attitude"; and "intense anxiety."[92] DeLillo's 1987 novel *Libra* tries to inhabit Oswald's psychological world, portraying him as a boy who veers toward "emotional instability" and "erratic behavior" but who grows into an intelligently quiet man who struggles with dyslexia, a condition that makes it difficult for him to read situations clearly.[93] Similarly, Norman Mailer's semi-factual book *Oswald's Tale: An American Mystery* (1995) explores Oswald's childhood in more depth, drawing on interviews with his school teachers that suggest, contrary to early psychiatric reports, that Oswald was not experiencing any exaggerated disturbances or disorders, despite his distance from the other boys and his feelings of "being able to do anything he wanted."[94]

Hinckley has not received such sensitive literary treatment, but he found himself caught in a web of identities and texts that connected the literary source of *Taxi Driver*—Arthur Bremer's diaries, published in 1973, in which Bremer plots to assassinate President Nixon before shifting his focus to Governor George Wallace—to Hinckley's infatuation with actress Jodi Foster, whose character Iris symbolizes *Taxi Driver*'s themes of precarious innocence and clouded vision.[95] At his trial in the spring of 1982, the prosecution claimed that Hinckley had only borderline tendencies despite evidence that he was maladjusted, that he identified closely with Travis Bickle (after seeing the film fifteen times), that he had stalked Foster, and that he had collected firearms. The trial nevertheless concluded with an insanity defense that led to Hinckley's incarceration in St. Elizabeth's Hospital rather than a prison sentence.[96] Certainly he was depressed, thought of himself as marginalized, and became caught up in the fantasy world of *Taxi Driver*. Yet the trial showed that he was also capable of executing complex plans and had an IQ that put him on the bright side of normal.[97] Despite the verdict, Hinckley's case revealed a complex personality that was masked by psychiatric labels and the media furor around his attempt to assassinate President Reagan.[98]

This culture of violence, which is often linked to drug crime, was an ongoing concern for the Reagan and Bush administrations, but in terms of personality disorders it was frequently linked to a concern that late-capitalist culture exacerbated conditions rather than ameliorating them. We can see the most obvious and notorious examples of this in *American Psycho* and *Fight Club*, which both portray scheming yet unstable protagonists who are drawn toward violence and often find it hard to separate reality from fantasy. It is significant that both texts are told in the first person, partly to prevent the reader from establishing a stable frame of external reference and partly to allow the reader to explore a world in which banality and extravagance are entwined, as symptomatic of what Robert Jay Lifton calls "collective patterns of dissociation" in the late twentieth century.[99] Both characters inhabit seemingly privileged worlds—Bateman is an executive in a Wall Street firm and the white-collar narrator of *Fight Club* spends his working life traveling between airports—yet the two characters are manifestations of environments in which hidden violence is encoded in everyday activities. My commentary here primarily focuses on the two literary texts, but the beginning of David Fincher's and Mary Harron's film adaptations of the novels (released in 1999 and 2000, respectively) visualize how these external and internal worlds collide. The opening sequence of *Fight Club* takes us on an immersive inner journey through close-ups of brain neurons and synapses, while *American Psycho* begins with the blood-letting that dominates the film subtly on display in the delicate servings of haute cuisine that are a feature of Bateman's yuppified Manhattan world.

Bateman displays narcissistic and sociopathic tendencies early on in Ellis's novel. He constantly checks his looks and is able to explain in detail the features of all his consumer products. But his seemingly ironic detachment from the world is shown to be a façade and his empty recitation of politically correct attitudes about equality, tolerance, and rights leads historian David Eldridge to describe his language as "pure media-speak, delivering a string of soundbites with no sense of consistent political philosophy."[100] Bateman is symptomatic of a world in which social privilege is built upon a knowledge vacuum, which Bret Easton Ellis describes in an interview as "a consumerist kind of void."[101] This culture of dissembling is exemplified by the grossly misinformed view of Bateman's friend Timothy Price, who extends his belief that AIDS can be caught through unprotected sex to a whole range of other conditions, including Alzheimer's, anorexia, cancer, and cerebral palsy—a parody of the public misinformation about the HIV virus that artist Mary Fisher tackled in her impassioned "A Whisper of AIDS" speech at the Republican National Convention the following year.[102]

Simulated reality is a major theme of both *Americana* and *American Psycho*, as if naming psychiatric conditions or consumer brands or restaurant names is Bateman's attempt to mask the "nameless dread" and "existentialism chasm" that he habitually faces and that often leads him to take Xanax or go shopping.[103] Within this simulacrum, violence becomes Bateman's raison d'être and a technique of self-affirmation in which he exerts control over his victims—although there is a danger that even his most violent acts are meaningless and his adoption of alternative names and assumed identities pushes identity evasion to pathological extremes. The first-person voice of the novel only reveals glimpses of character development as Bateman descends into psychological mayhem and is increasingly unable to assert the cleansing rituals that dominate early sequences.

Fight Club also eschews straightforward narrative development in favor of immersing the reader in a twilight world in which the protagonist repeatedly wakens at major urban airports with little recognition of what has occurred in between. The unreality of the novel is appreciated only after the first reading, when it becomes easier to identify subtle clues that Tyler Durden is the unnamed narrator's alter ego, such as the almost disembodied line "Tyler had been around a long time before we met."[104] It is hard to determine whether the narrator has a mood disorder or whether there is an underlying personality disorder that would explain his violent eruptions. The fact that Tyler burns the shape of his lips onto the narrator's hand with lye might suggest a narcissistic condition, as does his early obsession with designer labels, even though he learns to reject the fetishistic side of consumerism. But the narrator reveals borderline tendencies too, particularly regarding the triangular love-hate relationship between Tyler, him, and the neurotic and elusive Marla, who he first encounters in group therapy and who initially speaks of herself in the third person.

When the narrator's condominium is mysteriously blown up, he moves into Tyler's deserted warehouse of a home, where Tyler establishes a fight club as a means of asserting a primitive selfhood that cuts beneath the banality of the narrator's white-collar job. It is difficult to ascertain if the fights are sadistic or masochistic, depending on whether we see the characters as distinct or as two faces of a split self. However, images of the narrator's battered body—the "big O of my mouth with blood all around it" and "the hole punched through my cheek doesn't ever heal"—suggests both extreme forms of violence and a void at the core of his identity.[105] The fight club, at least at first before it takes on cult status for its followers, is seen to be more therapeutic than a talking cure, but a rage continues to burn inside the narrator—"I am Joe's Raging Bile Duct . . . I am Joe's Enraged, Inflamed Sense of Rejection . . . I am Joe's Boiling Point"—that cannot easily be allayed.[106] When his boss stumbles across a paper that describes the rules of fight club, the narrator caricatures the kind of person who would indulge in such behavior as "a dangerous psychotic killer" who "could probably go over the edge at any moment and stalk from office to office with an Armalite AR-180 carbine gas-operated automatic."[107] While physical fighting gives him an outlet for his rage, the narrative progression is toward random violent acts of terrorism on a macro scale. Out of this violence the anarchistic collective Project Mayhem emerges with a life force of its own that ushers in a paranoid world in which motives and identities blur and only secretly planned acts of violence against corporate culture bring meaning to the narrator's "psychogenic fugue state."[108] The final chapter suggests that he is in fact institutionalized, for how long it isn't clear, yet even this may be another form of paranoid unreality.

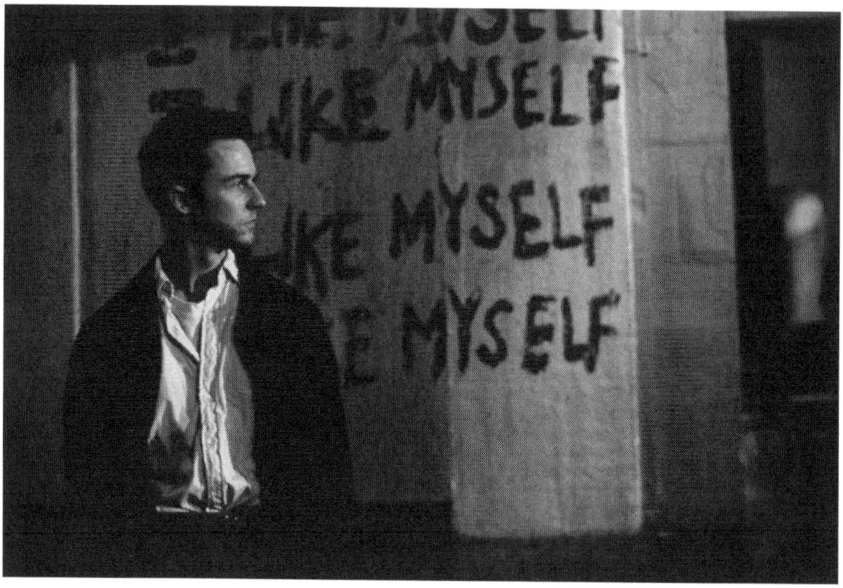

Figure 7.2 Edward Norton plays the unnamed white-collar protagonist of *Fight Club* (dir. David Fincher, 1999), filmed against a wall of therapeutic graffiti. 20th Century Fox/The Kobal Collection.

American Psycho and *Fight Club* blur reality and fantasy from an overtly masculine perspective. The obsession with violence and death in the two films reflects the increase in gun crime, but it can also be traced to hints about the protagonists' childhoods and their destabilizing relationships with their parents. The violence of Jamison's *An Unquiet Mind* is no less disturbing, even if it is more domesticated. She notes that outbursts among young women are "not something spoken about with ease," giving credence to the reading of vengeful psychotic female characters in early 1990s films as a male backlash against (supposedly) inappropriate female emotions.[109] The power of Jamison's description is that she retains the double perspective of observer and agent, acknowledging the failure of vocabulary to give voice to the experience without losing its visceral nature: "Being wildly out of control—physically assaultive, screaming insanely at the top of one's lungs, running frenetically with no purpose or limit, or impulsively trying to leap from cars—is frightening to others and unspeakably terrifying to oneself. . . . I have in psychotic, seizurelike attacks—my black, agitated manias—destroyed things I cherish, pushed to the utter edge people I love, and survived to think I could never recover from the shame."[110] Such experiences are painful for all concerned, but the fact that Jamison feels ashamed of her actions indicates that her ego remains intact despite her mania and that she retains a regard for others, putting her in a different category than the narcissist who is either oblivious to the other person's pain or relishes inflicting violence.

The extreme violence of Patrick Bateman and Tyler Durden can be read as attempts of the authors to rework in the context of late capitalism what the popular CBS television show *The Incredible Hulk* did for the socially unstable 1970s.

Whereas the etiology of Bateman's and Durden's instability is only hinted at, in the case of the physician and laboratory scientist David Banner (played by Bill Bixby) we know that the transformation that he undergoes when testosterone builds in his system is the result of gamma radiation, following a miscalibrated experiment in his quest to understand how the body can sometimes draw on hidden strengths when faced with danger. Suffering from depression in the wake of an accident in which he failed to muster the strength to help his wife escape from a car crash, in the two pilot episodes of November 1977 Banner uses himself as a test case to see if increased gamma activity can be channeled to make the body more resilient in stressful situations.

Mental health problems are only hinted at prior to the gamma radiation experiment, but afterward Banner periodically dissociates into a seven-foot bulky green monster, particularly when he feels trapped or when another person faces danger, often a young woman who resembles his wife. The primary trauma of his wife's death is exacerbated by the death of his scientist friend, Eleana Marks, in a fire at the radiation test center. In order to escape discovery by a self-seeking reporter (who carelessly started the fire), we see Banner drifting across the country. His underlying melancholia and isolation are emphasized by the closing credits in which he walks alone while "The Lonely Man" theme song plays.

The choice of bodybuilder Lou Ferrigno to play the oversize alter ego created a figure whose body contrasted starkly with the fine features and small physique of Bill Bixby. The title sequence presents a visual of the split personality (Bixby on the left, Ferrigno on the right), while the metamorphosis (which typically happens two or three times per episode) focuses on facial transformation, accompanied by dramatic music, the ripping of clothes, and the widening and clouding of his pupils during moments of stress and anger. That Bixby makes no efforts to bulk up to improve his chances of fighting his way out of dangerous situations himself suggests that he is not suffering from muscle dysmorphia. However, at a time when the bodybuilding craze (epitomized by the 1977 film *Pumping Iron*, starring Lou Ferrigno and Arnold Schwarzenegger) was leading to the recreational use of anabolic steroids and emerging cases of "reverse anorexia," the roots of Banner's condition are more complex than they first seem, making *The Incredible Hulk* a show that is both populist in its exaggeration of and seriously engaged in its exploration of personality disorders. The key issue for many of these texts is that the coherence of identity and voice is undermined by experiences of dissociation that makes individuals oblivious to (or quick to forget) their violent outbursts.

Dissociated Lives

David Banner is certainly not a narcissist, and *The Incredible Hulk* series (which ran for five seasons, from 1978 to 1982) only occasionally uses split or fractured facial reflections to emphasize Banner's occluded view of himself. In fact, the Hulk is only ever violent toward those involved in criminal or abusive activities, and his strength is guided by a primitive moral drive to rescue those in peril. The second season deals with mental illness more directly, even though Banner is often the voice of reason in the face of disoriented characters, despite undergoing a phase when his rage becomes more unstable as he starts to intuit his hidden life. The show was suspicious of authority figures, but it included some good healers such as the kind yet ailing psychologist Carolyn Fields early in the second season and the blind Chinese philosopher Li Sung, whose philosophy is being misused by a former pupil. The psychological theme is less obvious in later seasons, except for the opening episodes of season four, which show the protagonist suspended halfway between his dual identities of David Banner and The Hulk, and thus more vulnerable to agents of power.

While narcissistic personalities are frequently associated with violent protagonists, as is the case of *American Psycho* and *Fight Club*, the genesis of *The Incredible Hulk* points to another form of violence that is perpetrated on the individual. Whereas the television series uses the deaths of Banner's wife and his scientist friend Eleana as the primary and secondary traumas that emotionally explain his dissociating states, in the original Marvel comic, The Hulk's split personality is given an infantile etiology: as a boy, Banner experiences his father physically abusing both him and his mother. Feelings of inadequacy and powerlessness underpin the storylines of both versions, but the split-personality narrative is taken much further in late-1990s issues of the Marvel strip, in which four distinct personalities emerge that make The Hulk even more unstable and threatening. This is an example of the narrative of abuse and childhood trauma that was often closely linked to the splitting of personalities, particularly when cases of multiple personality disorder (as it was called before 1994) started to emerge in clinical literature in the late 1960s and 1970s.

Multiple personality disorder was just one of five dissociative disorders outlined in *DSM-III*, but it is the one that has received most cultural attention. The most famous published account is the biography *Sybil* (1973) written by the journalist Flora Rheta Schreiber, in collaboration with the patient and her therapist. *Sybil* recounts the case of a Minnesota patient who began experiencing multiple personalities during a lengthy period of therapy with Michigan psychiatrist Cornelia Wilbur, who had been trained in treating cases of hysteria in the early 1940s. Wilbur and Sylvia collaborated closely for over a decade, and Schreiber also worked closely with the pair in the latter stages to record the encounter. The case was remarkable because Sybil displayed sixteen distinct personalities during her lengthy course of therapy, including the first recorded case of two cross-gender personae. Wilbur believed that the split personalities—some of whom were aware of each other, others of whom were not—stemmed from an extended period of severe child abuse by Sybil's mother that had led to periods of amnesia, fugue states, and other forms of dissociation.[111]

Sybil was published at a time when cases of child abuse (usually involving fathers) were coming to public attention, leading Alice Miller to contemplate the relationship between abuse and silence, which she believed often led to "self-destruction on a gigantic atomic scale."[112] *Sybil* functions as a keynote for the 1970s as an "age of fracture," to recall Daniel Rodgers's phase—particularly the popular made-for-TV film *Sybil* (1976), starring Sally Field and Joanne Woodward.[113] Child abuse could lead to uncontrollable "feelings of terror, of despair and rebellion, of mistrust," psychic splitting, and, sometimes, biological symptoms—such as diabetes and color-blindness—that are apparent only when a particular personality is dominant.[114] However, this symptomology did not prevent psychoanalysts from being generally skeptical about Wilbur's methods and her diagnosis of so many alters, particularly as a good proportion of cases where multiple personality disorder was diagnosed were under her care. It also returns us to the issue of selective recall, in which the patient becomes their own storyteller or fabulist. Socio-cognitive thinker Nicholas Spanos describes this mode of self-presentation as an "indecipherable mix of fantasy and reality" that seems to preclude any stable reality or therapeutic cure.[115] This comment seems to propel us into a realm of absolute relativism. But despite the epistemological and ontological fissures Sybil's case poses, in the book, Wilbur helps Sybil reconstitute reality, fusing and reconciling her different selves by solving the mystery of her repressed childhood abuse.

While multiple personality disorder suggests a specific condition, its nosology remained unstable and the term did not make it into *DSM-IV* in 1994, when it was reclassified as dissociative identity disorder.[116] However, it featured in popular films, particularly through the image of the split self or the double, which in the cases of *Doppelganger* (1995), another Drew Barrymore film, and cult director David Lynch's *Mulholland Drive* (2001) are linked to supernatural occurrences (and in the former to a pattern of long-term sexual abuse). These popular accounts—plus others such as Brian De Palma's 1992 horror film *Raising Cain*, which portrays a child psychologist with multiple personality disorder—exploit (more than they elucidate) mind-body questions that are difficult to resolve through therapy. In fact, philosopher Ian Hacking remains skeptical about the scientific veracity of such disorders.[117] So although we might link such cases to the fractured decade of the 1970s, only 300 cases had appeared in medical literature by 1983 and it was not until after the work of NIMH psychiatrist Frank Putnam Jr. in the early 1980s on the vocal range and brain waves of individuals who were suspected to have multiple selves that the condition came to the fore, both as a more frequent clinical diagnosis and as a distinctive form of testimony.[118]

The most publicized of these texts was upstate New Yorker Truddi Chase's 1987 autobiography *When Rabbit Howls*, which recounts the sexual abuse she experienced as a child and teenager in the 1940s at the hands of her stepfather and of the dissociated adult life that followed. Chase, who appeared on *The Oprah Winfrey Show* in May 1990, helped raise public awareness of a condition that often remains hidden behind a host of mood disorders and the psychological aftershocks of deep-seated abuse, including versions of PTSD that could be likened to post-combat experiences.[119] A six-year course of intensive treatment with sexual abuse specialist Robert Phillips Jr. helped Chase shift from a state of periodic amnesia to a functioning awareness of her condition, but neither therapist nor patient favored a therapeutic model that could assimilate her ninety-two separate identities (which she labels "The Troops") into a single whole.[120] In order to depict this sense of multiplicity, *When Rabbit Howls* shifts fluidly between pronouns and explores what it means to write as a group of multiple selves, only some of whom acknowledge each other.

With this in mind, I now turn to two self-reflexive accounts of dissociative states published in the 1990s to conclude this chapter. Both raise searching questions about voice and identity. The first of these, *The Flock*, follows *Sybil* in exploring the transference dynamic between a dissociating teacher and a healing therapist who is pictured as the good maternal figure in contrast to the patient's abusive mother. The second text, *Prozac Diary*, returns us full circle to thinking about the place of medication (specifically Prozac) in balancing a combination of mood and identity disturbances.[121]

Published in 1991, a time that the Bush administration was promoting the Show You Care program to prevent child abuse, *The Flock* deals with dissociative states that are eventually traced back to parental maltreatment. Dissociation begins to occur when the author Joan Frances Casey starts consulting with clinical social worker Lynn Wilson. She first sees Wilson in Chicago in the spring of 1981, a time when she was harboring suicidal thoughts in the wake of a marital breakdown. Casey thinks that she will soon feel better, but this marks the beginning of a six-year course of therapy during which she reveals twenty-four distinct personalities that cluster around a history of sexual abuse as a child perpetrated by her father and emotional abuse by her mother. Joan's story is interrupted with extracts from her case files, which form a hybrid text that shuttles between subject positions as both women attempt to understand a story that is punctuated by Joan's memory lapses. Wilson suspects multiple personality disorder three weeks into analysis, especially as the patient responds to alternative names that correlate with her different faces. Joan herself is aware of at least four different identities, but the therapist tries to persuade her that these are "a lot more than a voice," especially when other identities emerge that are only dimly aware of each other.[122]

The Flock does not have a compelling narrative, though one of its most interesting aspects is the search for a symbolic language that can speak to the multiplicity of selves that have their own temperaments and life histories but that are intricately connected. The image of the photograph album, for example, suggests snapshots of a past that cannot be linked together as a cohesive whole.[123] Only when a second (male) analyst joins the sessions does the therapeutic narrative shift gears. The metaphor of "the flock" proves to be an enabling one for Casey as she comes to recognize that birds instinctively create a "perfect formation" within what seems like "whirling confusion."[124] This imagery also converges with the maternal theme when Casey decides that she needs a symbolic object that speaks both to Wilson's nurturing role and her desire to integrate her personalities. Casey finds this symbol in a toy, "a translucent plastic egg, constructed of many intricate pieces, all fitting snugly together."[125] She sees this egg as a homology of her "whole being coming together in a new, coherent way," and by running glue over the cracks she ensures that its parts cannot again separate. The toy egg has a catalyzing effect, enabling Casey to accept her given name (Joan) and to think singular thoughts for what seems the first time. She expresses this new realization and inner flow in romanticized language: "I was the thought, the voice of all who were, of all that I could be. Evolving, growing. A person."

In contrast, Lauren Slater's *Prozac Diary* deals with dissociative identity disorder in a more diffuse way, perhaps because she was not undergoing therapy during the writing of the text but also because cases of multiple personality disorder were on the wane after the shift in diagnostic language in *DSM-IV* and a series of legal cases against a Minnesota therapist who misdiagnosed the disorder and linked it to a satanic cult.[126] Whereas *When Rabbit Howls* and *The Flock* view dissociation as a survival mechanism, Slater sees her creative voices as a way of expressing herself as a multiplicity. When she begins a course of Prozac in 1988, she is immediately exhilarated by fresh possibilities and a newfound confidence, yet she is also worried because Prozac jeopardizes the strength of those voices. While the etiology in *Prozac Diary* is vaguer than either *The Flock* or *When Rabbit Howls* and questions might be asked about the veracity of the account, Slater follows Kaysen in printing her psychiatric record. This reveals a number of related conditions, including obsessive-compulsive disorder, anorexia, self-mutilation, suicidal tendencies, and depression, the latter of which she traces to her parents and manifested itself in an unhappy marriage. The first of these brief reports reveals that she was diagnosed with borderline personality disorder in 1982 (at age 19) and was hospitalized five times in the period 1977 to 1985. Although she segues into a lyrical reflection of her childhood (which she remembers mostly as a source of joy), Slater's experience of illness had been so lengthy that she finds the notion of a cure disorienting, a "new, strange planet, pressing in."[127] A sense of wellness makes her feel more confident and gives her renewed appetite for adventure, but it is also a quieter state of being and mutes the voices she had lived with so long. There are echoes of *Wasted* and *An Unquiet Mind* here, especially in Slater's desire to hold onto an ontological state that brings her suffering and comfort in equal measure.

The text also raises the question of whether the voice during drug therapy is any more authentic than the inner voices that she had listened to from an early age. Like Joan in *The Flock*, Slater moves into a realm of alters that have creative lives of their own, but unlike Joan or Sybil, she seems to be able to summon these voices at will. She mentions eight alters, but "blue baby" has the "most interesting things to say," sending her into a semi-trance in which she seems to channel alternative voices.[128] There are hints of mysticism and ventriloquism in her claim to be able to write poetry automatically in a different voice, plus an aesthetic sensibility that ebbs as soon as Prozac starts improving her sense of well-being. Although Prozac gives her space to move, glimpses of her past soon recede and she feels that words are "dull, dead" because they separate her functional self from her inner being.[129] Instead of listening to Lauren's concerns or to the nuance of her language, her doctor prescribes a higher dose, and the longer she stays on it the more she orients herself to a more monochrome reality, largely unaware of the long-term risks of the drug.[130]

In truth, Slater's alternative identities play a minor role in her narrative, partly because the text begins when she starts taking Prozac and she only sporadically returns to her childhood, a time in her life she explores further in later books after she left her job as director of Boston's AfterCare services to become a professional writer.[131] The fact that five of her eight alters in *Prozac Diary* are children and that Slater's psychiatric troubles began at a young age provides a clue to the fact that she only reluctantly grows up, and there are hints that she is still intricately bound to her mother, especially when she describes her psychological dependency on Prozac as "suckling my pills."[132] While Prozac gives her the stimulus to move on from the past, she worries that it lends her an inauthentic self and buries other selves under chemical layers. At times, Slater thinks that the drug might be fusing different facets of herself, but she also muses that it might furnish her with alternative (possibly false) memories of the past to support her transformed condition. This recalls Nicholas Spanos's idea of "an indecipherable mix of reality and fantasy" and what could be called "pastmaking" in which the personal history is reorganized and rewritten.[133] Thus, the book is a form of personal testimony that appears, in places, to operate on the level of fiction as a willful breaking down of diagnostic "border policing."[134]

Despite claims that Slater's account is more fiction than fact, her worry about how authentic her life is now that she is reliant on Prozac is a central theme that runs through accounts of mood and personality disorders. *Prozac Diary* steers away from the child abuse theme that links *Sybil* and *The Flock* to later accounts such as the abusive psychiatrist in Todd Solondz's 1998 ironically titled film *Happiness* and Cameron West's *First Person Plural: My Life as a Multiple* (1999), but it leaves us with two profound questions that are in fundamental tension with each other. First, to what extent do mood stabilizers offer a functional lifeline for individuals whose impulses are otherwise too extreme to bear? And second, to what extent is the drug an enforced compromise that turns an expressive person who struggles with everyday life into an acceptably productive one? Although she is critical of Peter Kramer for being too utopian, Slater is caught between these two questions, and ultimately resists deciding if this "capitalist pill" is friend or foe.

8 *Mental Health at the Millennium*

In July 1992, President Bush acknowledged that a quarter of the nation would "suffer from a mental health disorder" over the course of their lives.[1] Bush had announced a program for comprehensive health reform six months earlier, but he tended to be evasive on health matters. Notably, he went quiet on the subject of HIV/AIDS after his term as Reagan's vice-president, then passionately defended his own AIDS policy in the first presidential debate of October 1992, not long after Los Angeles Lakers basketball star Magic Johnson had resigned from the National Commission on AIDS on the grounds that the Bush administration had "dropped the ball."[2] While the criticism that Reagan saw AIDS primarily as a budgetary and public relations problem cannot easily be leveled at his successor, it was in the sphere of employment rights and public access for the disabled that Bush most obviously displayed the "moral leadership" that Magic Johnson was demanding.[3] The progressive aim of empowering disabled citizens so that they might "blend fully and equally into the rich mosaic of the American mainstream" was embodied in the Americans with Disabilities Act of July 1990, which President Bush thought was as critical as the fall of the Berlin Wall for safeguarding freedoms.[4] Although the ADA embraced health coverage for citizens with a diagnosable mental illness, this did not prevent ambiguous language and funding restrictions from at times eroding the very patients' rights the act was intended to protect.[5]

Indeed, although the Department of Health and Human Services made mental health a priority in its 1990 report *Healthy People 2000*, the speed of reform was slow. Bush mentioned mental health only twice in his public speeches during his four years as president, and the only specific pieces of legislation on the topic he signed were the District of Columbia Mental Health Program Assistance Act (1991) and the Alcohol, Drug Abuse, and Mental Health Administration Reorganization Act (1992). The latter act was intended to increase federal resources for three medical areas that had been aligned during the Nixon administration, although much of the additional financial investment was targeted at substance abuse disorders. Nonetheless, in announcing the act, Bush spoke favorably about cross-fertilizing ideas and said that he looked forward to the "sharing of expertise in neuroscience and behavioral research within the biomedical research community," primarily through the National Institutes of Health, which Bush viewed as an exemplary model of scientific commitment and compassion, especially on AIDS research.[6] This statement was in keeping with the president's proclamation that the 1990s would be the "Decade of the Brain," a phrase that symbolized a paradigm shift from a psychoanalytical-psychiatric to a biological-neurological explanatory framework, a defining feature of what has more recently been called the "brain revolution."[7]

Bush's "Decade of the Brain" pronouncement might have been shaped by his position as chair of the board of pharmaceutical giant Eli Lilly in the late 1970s, but it also chimed with an interest among philosophers and scientists to better understand the neurological underpinning of consciousness. There were ethical issues to consider as well. Inconclusive discussions about whether the individual, state authorities, or the federal government was ultimately responsible for personal health marked the early decade as a troubled period for health advocates.[8] There were some encouraging signs, though. In 1989, the president pledged an increase of $3 billion for Medicaid, and he appointed Louis Wade Sullivan as his secretary of health and human services. Wade was an African American physician from Georgia with a strong record of profiling the medical and nutritional needs of minority and rural groups. At Sullivan's swearing-in ceremony, Bush voiced his concerns about the risks to environmental health of hazardous waste, his aspiration for a "kinder and gentler nation," and the crucial need for the Department of Health and Human Services to focus on AIDS and drug addiction.[9] In 1990, Sullivan was tasked with reviewing the "quality, accessibility, and cost of our national health-care system," but it took three years for a health plan to emerge as part of Bush preparation for his reelection campaign. But the focus of the health plan on tax credits did not shift substantially from Reagan's market-competition approach.[10] So, when Bill Clinton entered the White House, he faced a paradox: twelve years of relative federal neglect of healthcare reform sat uncomfortably with the cultural obsession with "healthism" that made it difficult to know how much health is healthy.

The story of federal neglect is much more straightforward than this knotty paradox. Arthur Barsky tried to capture it in a 1988 essay that explored the tension between general improvements in health and declining satisfaction with healthcare services. Barsky encouraged a longer historical view as a way of understanding how the impasse had come about, noting that the paradox was particularly acute for mental health issues.[11] The trouble was that although University of Pennsylvania psychiatrist Aaron Beck had been highlighting the complex cognitive and affective processes involved in major depressive episodes for twenty years, depression was often seen either in symptomatic terms or as a single-effect illness that could be simply treated by chemical means.[12] The publication of *DSM-IV* in 1994 marked a moment of diagnostic advances: for example, the pharmaceutical company Pfizer designed a self-reporting Patient Health Questionnaire (PHQ-9) that was more specific and sensitive than earlier tools to the symptoms, duration, and severity of depression.[13]

However, there were still deficiencies in a panoramic understanding of depression as a common but complex experience. As earlier chapters have discussed, this was the legacy, at least in part, of the dismantling of Carter's Mental Health Systems Act in 1981 and its replacement with the Omnibus Budget Reconciliation Act, which ceded responsibility to the states while cutting funding for mental healthcare by 26 percent. Even though it is unlikely that Carter's legislation would have resolved the health paradox, its aim was to protect the needs of minority groups, the poor, and the underserved and to achieve parity of provision. The Carters were devastated by the fact that the President's Commission did not have a direct effect on policy and funding, but Rosalynn Carter continued to campaign, most visibly through the Carter Center that opened in Atlanta in 1982 and as the chair of the center's Mental Health Task Force, which formed in September 1991. In fact, I would argue that this legacy of the Carter administration was vital in refocusing President Clinton's health priorities in the mid-1990s. Following the defeat of the Health Security Act of 1994, federal attention shifted to children's illnesses (a pressing issue for the first lady) and mental health through the vice-president's wife, Tipper Gore, whom Clinton had appointed as his mental health policy advisor a year earlier.[14]

Sustained advocacy for healthcare for the mentally ill in the second half of the decade culminated in the first White House Conference on Mental Health, which was held at Howard University in June 1999. The conference took its stimulus from grassroots efforts, the testimony of public figures, and new scientific developments. Nine years earlier, the report *Healthy People 2000* had noted encouraging signs, claiming that suicide rates among the elderly were falling and that more Americans with emotional problems were seeking support. In terms of depression, though, there had been little change. Only an estimated 35 percent of those experiencing depression were seeking treatment in the 1990s, a far cry from the aspiration that 54 percent would be receiving effective treatment by 2000.[15] This correlated to the estimate of the National Comorbidity Survey, conducted between 1990 and 1992, which revealed that less than 40 percent of those with psychiatric disorders (as defined by the revised version of *DSM-III*) were seeking help.[16]

This is the point where the story of neglect intersects with the story of a national obsession with health. When smart drugs such as Prozac were released to the market, the desire to effectively treat moderate and severe depression was bound up with a pharmaceutical cure that arguably raised more problems than it solved. Tipper Gore was suspicious of seeing medication as a panacea but was also convinced that mental and physical illnesses are just variations of one another. This was the view of the Mental Health Parity Act of September 1996, which required that annual lifetime dollar benefits for mental healthcare be equal to those for surgery. However, Mrs. Gore realized that it was more than a matter of reforming medical insurance. Calling mental illness the "last great stigma of the twentieth century," she sought to challenge "the myths and the disillusionments and the misperceptions" that bring shame to those experiencing depression, as she claimed had been recently the case for those suffering from cancer and AIDS.[17]

While AIDS was the most visible health crisis of the 1980s, I would argue that a spectrum of depressive experiences was equally critical for the 1990s, including AIDS-related depression and postpartum depression. The rise of recorded cases of these two forms of depression in that decade tallied with the claim of the World Health Organization that unipolar depression was one of the great "disease burdens" of developed nations, second only to coronary heart disease and over three times more prevalent than bipolar disorder.[18] Given these emerging statistics, not everyone was so sure about Tipper Gore's message of hope, particularly Republicans and some psychiatrists who still felt that complex conditions were being simplified to create bureaucratic solutions.

In order to contextualize 1999 as a pivotal year in the history of mental health, the following sections address three topics: first, advances in and impediments to healthcare reform during the Clinton administration; second, new writing on depression, including powerful expressions by William Styron, David Foster Wallace, and Andrew Solomon that spanned generations and sexualities; and, third, a fresh wave of women's health activism that often focused on motherhood and aging. These are linked to a more generalized set of anxieties that I illustrate through a reading of Todd Haynes's 1995 film *Safe*, about a debilitating physical and psychological condition that is triggered by late twentieth-century life. Although these examples gave new credibility to experiences of depression in the 1990s, they all raise a theoretical tension that places the personal and existential experience of depression (which often eludes language and causal explanation) in a strained relationship with the medical belief that as a form of brain disorder, depression is both diagnosable and treatable. While I acknowledge the historic importance of the 1999 White House Conference and the first Surgeon General's Report on Mental Health published later that year, instead of celebrating the late 1990s as a high point in public health culture, I conclude this chapter by thinking beyond the health paradox to consider ongoing shortfalls in mental health provision, particularly for minority groups and the homeless.

Clinton's Healthcare Reforms

At a lunchtime press conference on 21 September 1993, in the Old Family Dining Room of the White House, President Clinton, just eight months into his presidency, began by making a joke about one of his most ferocious critics, the right-wing talk radio host Rush Limbaugh, who had turned the recent suicide of the depressed Deputy White House Counsel Vince Foster (one of Clinton's boyhood friends) into an unsubstantiated conspiracy theory. The president took the opportunity to poke fun at Limbaugh, but his real topic was the healthcare reform bill that was to be announced the following day. Clinton had been consistent on the topic from early in his election campaign, favoring a "managed competition" approach that he felt would provide choice while guaranteeing equity, spurred on by the fact that healthcare was the most frequent topic that the electorate raised with him on the campaign trail.[19] These concerns stimulated the "new covenant" that Clinton outlined in his nomination speech in July 1992, in which he echoed Presidents Ford and Carter by claiming it was "time to heal" the country after "falling behind" on social commitments during the Reagan-Bush years.[20]

The belief that health insurance would become a hot campaign issue also motivated President Bush to belatedly outline his healthcare plans that year. Whereas Bush's strategy was to push for efficiencies in the private system with an emphasis on consumer choice, Clinton took lessons from the health policy workshop that he had convened at the Democratic Party mid-term conference in the winter of 1978.[21]

Even though his role models were both liberals, Clinton believed that the fusion of Senator Kennedy's idealistic commitment to comprehensive coverage and President Carter's pragmatic approach provided him with the tools he needed "to cross party lines and put the interests of the American people first," as he described it, on the issue of health insurance.[22] Bush continued to stereotype the Democratic line as tax-and-spend politics, but Clinton resisted simplifying the human dimension of health to a fiscal equation, even if his primary focus was insurance.[23] Indeed, four years later he regretted the fact that the Health Insurance Portability and Accountability Act (which was designed to simplify healthcare coverage, extend long-term care, and make it tougher for employers to shirk responsibilities) did not contain "the provision to eliminate that differential treatment of mental health coverage" that the Mental Health Systems Act had sought.[24]

Clinton was determined that his attempt at healthcare reform would make a historic mark, achieving what Truman had failed to do in the late 1940s. The time was ripe, because what Clinton described as "the escalating costs and the escalating dysfunctions" in the health system had become a liability. Herb Block cleverly illustrated these systemic dysfunctions in his May 1991 *Washington Post* cartoon "Health Coverage." As illustrated overleaf, one patient is crushed by "multi-billion-dollar paperwork costs" in his hospital bed while his fellow patient, who is uninsured, lies shivering on the adjacent bed with no covers.[25] Clinton and Bush agreed that it was necessary to contain the federal portion of the Medicare and Medicaid budgets, but they divided along party lines about whether healthcare should be a right or a privilege. At the 21 September 1993 press conference, Clinton returned to his twin beliefs that the nation's health was the cornerstone of daily life and that urgent reform was necessary. He saw this as a pivotal phase in the long history of health reform. The first lady, who regularly faced the press as chair of the President's Health Task Force, echoed the belief that the nation was at a historic juncture the following month: "History is on our side now because—today—Americans from all walks of life are making their voices heard."[26]

The second year of the Clinton administration was an important moment for defining the healthcare horizon of the millennium. Following Mrs. Clinton's vigorous public relations campaign (which included a persuasive address to the American Medical Association) and a month-long bus tour of the nation in which the president's supporters promoted the benefits of the Health Insurance Portability and Accountability Act (known unofficially as the Health Security Act), President Clinton outlined his plans for Congress. In October 1993, the *New York Times* triumphantly proclaimed that the Clinton proposal was "Alive on Arrival," but less than a year later plans were floundering in the face of strong Republican opposition and a downturn in approval ratings.[27] This was not helped by the series of "Harry and Louise" television commercials made by the Coalition for Health Insurance Choices (CHIC), in which a middle-class white couple aired their concerns about federal meddling in their right to choose healthcare insurance plans. Like most Republicans, Richard Nixon was opposed to Clinton's plan, describing it as "a blueprint for the takeover by the federal government of one seventh of the

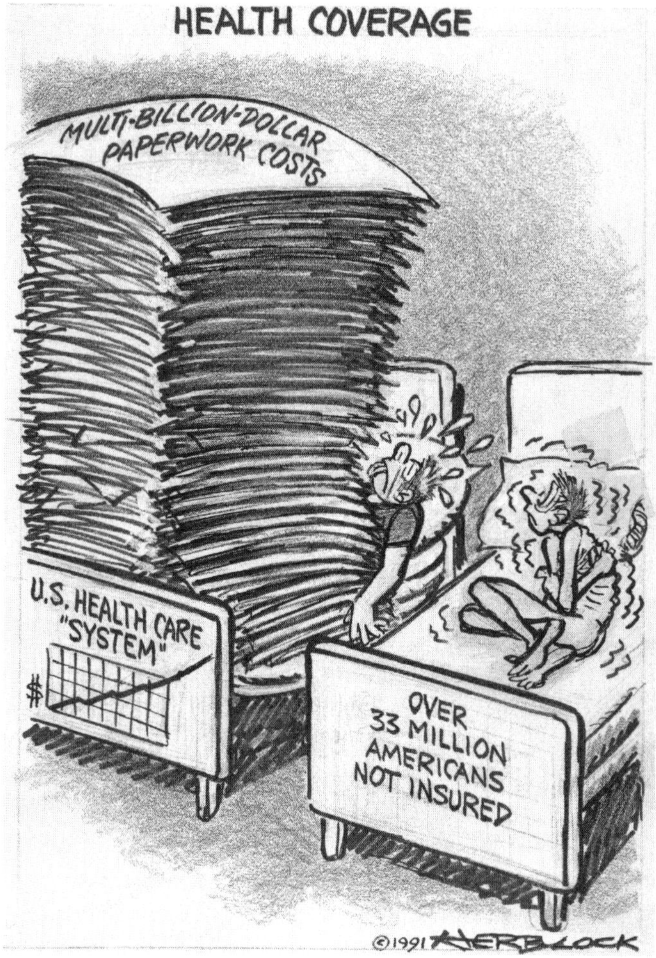

Figure 8.1 Herb Block, "Health Coverage," *Washington Post*, 3 May 1991. Courtesy of the Library of Congress Prints and Photographs Division, Herbert L. Block Collection.

nation's economy" that would "represent the ultimate revenge of the 1960s generation" against business-friendly Republican policies.[28] Buying into the culture wars of the mid-1990s, Nixon described Clinton's proposal as "mass produced, compulsory universal conscription," although he did not go as far as Limbaugh (who was working with CHIC), who claimed that if Clinton's healthcare policy became law, the president would be directly managing a fifth of the economy. Nixon's comments on health insurance were unsurprising. He endorsed a free market approach that he claimed was more cost effective than Medicaid and Medicare and he bemoaned the rise of healthcare costs and the rising numbers of administrators at a time when patient numbers were falling.[29]

The Health Security Express bus tour and a number of forceful public appearances by the first lady did not prevent a sense of confusion about what the plan meant to the general public. It did not save the plan from defeat at the hands of

Republicans the following year, when the bill did not even reach the voting stage in Congress. In his bleak book *Dead on Arrival* (2003), historian Colin Gordon sees the turnabout in support for the reform of the health insurance industry of 1993–94 as "an appropriate postscript to nearly a century of frustrated reform."[30] The collapse of Clinton's plans pivoted on the vexed question of financing and the fact that he tried to balance contradictory interests, especially between the expectations of employees and overall cost control. As political scientist Alex Waddan points out, although elements of Clinton's health plans were rescuable—notably portable insurance for workers and the Children's Health Insurance Program of 1997—they were marginal wins in the face of his initial ambitions. The fact that a conservative majority took control of Congress in 1995 meant that there was little room for maneuver in his second term in the face of aggressive attacks on Medicare and Medicaid.[31] However, while Gordon reads "the Clinton debacle" as a moment when "health politics collapsed into a pattern of piecemeal reform and persistent anxiety," I would argue that, at the very least, it offered the opportunity for the second-term Clinton administration to focus on more localized issues linked to children's health and mental health.[32]

Tipper Gore, who was at a slight remove from the political fray, took every opportunity to point out that mental health was due closer attention as a major public health issue affecting more than 20 percent of Americans.[33] While Mrs. Gore was the most visible face of advocacy for mental health and the prevention of substance abuse, the national conversation was much broader than this and included former First Ladies Rosalynn Carter and Betty Ford, who both testified in Congress in March 1994 about the importance of including mental health in healthcare reform.[34] Clinton's secretary of health and human services, Donna Shalala, and Ira Magaziner, one of his senior policy advisors, also played important roles in the conversation on health insurance. Shalala, who had served as secretary of housing and urban development in the Carter administration, helped tackle urban health needs and articulate the president's philosophy of managed competition.[35] Magaziner ran the White House Health Care Working Group, spoke frequently with senators, and took time to address questions relating to the administration of healthcare at the state level. For example, at a Tufts University conference in April 1993 (at which Magaziner appeared by satellite link), Senator Ted Kennedy praised Magaziner for being receptive to regional issues. However, Kennedy also stressed at this conference that mental health was one of the categories for which debates about insurance were insufficient, pointing out that three out of seven mental hospitals in Massachusetts were being closed because they were deemed unfit for purpose.[36]

Tipper Gore echoed the emphasis of this 1993 conference on close collaboration between different kinds of health officials, but to her mind the key to the reform was to see mental health as organically grounded and empirically observable. In line with the research shift toward neurobiology (as highlighted in a June 1998 *Scientific American* article on the biological determinants of depression), Mrs. Gore argued that treating a problem of the brain was little different from treating liver problems and that stigma would be reversed only if the public saw all illnesses on the same spectrum.[37] Not everyone was convinced that such a breakthrough in treatment for and attitudes toward mental illness could be achieved. New Jersey psychiatrist Yale Kramer, for example, argued that her messages were just "upbeat abstractions" that were blind to the multiple causes of mental illness and ignored the real cost of healthcare.[38]

As the debate repeatedly returned to these kinds of economic considerations, Tipper Gore was a key figure in keeping human stories front and center. Her psychology degree and the humanist impulse of her photography shaped this perspective, whereas others, including Hillary Clinton, were worried that extending universal health coverage to all forms of mental illness risked spiraling costs. The second lady was convinced that her proposal to extend health coverage only to diagnosable disorders as codified in *DSM* would not be a financial strain. Nevertheless, there were real concerns about needing to limit the cost of psychotherapy and rehabilitation and disagreements between some states and the federal government about who would pay for what.[39] In some ways, then, mental healthcare reform was linked to the fate of the Clintons' general healthcare plan. However, as I discuss here, it also had a strong afterlife, culminating in the 1996 Mental Health Parity Act and profile-raising advocacy in which issues of language, voice, and personal experience came to the fore. This, in part at least, realized the hopes of Rosalynn Carter of two decades earlier.

Depression beyond Expression

Against the backdrop of the 1992 election and Clinton's promises to fix the healthcare system, the early 1990s was a breakthrough moment for testimonies about depression. The specter of the Thomas Eagleton case twenty years earlier and the stigma attached to psychiatric treatment for those in the public eye lingered, despite the increasing number of published first-person accounts of depression that gave others the confidence to speak out with fewer fears that their careers would suffer as a consequence. The risks to public life were clear when the press and Republicans latched onto speculations about the mental health of Democratic presidential candidate Michael Dukakis in the run-up to the 1988 election, linked to the suicidal breakdown of his brother earlier in life. His wife, Kitty Dukakis, also came to attention for the treatment she had received in 1982 for amphetamine addiction.[40] Such rumors lost their traction as the 1990s advanced, and the speculation that Michael Dukakis had mental health issues was shown to be false when he made his medical record public (Kitty's addictions worsened after her husband lost the 1988 election race to George Bush).[41] With these speculations in mind, and before returning to the topic of depression and gender, I want look at three accounts published in high-profile national magazines—*Vanity Fair*, *Harper's*, and the *New Yorker*—that pose searching questions about the experience and language of depression that were often masked in public statements. These three pieces focus on unipolar depression—an experience that clinical psychologist Martha Manning also addressed in *Undercurrents: A Life Beneath the Surface* (1994) and southern journalist Tracy Thompson explored in *The Beast: A Journey through Depression* (1995).[42]

The first of the three was written by Virginia author William Styron, who published a condensed account of his depression in the December 1989 issue of *Vanity Fair*. Styron had first broached the subject at a symposium on affective disorders in Baltimore that May, and he revisited the subject the following year in his book *Darkness Visible*. Styron focused on the depressive feelings that descended on him while living in Paris in 1985, although such feelings had nagged at him since he was a young man in the early 1950s.[43] The packaging of Styron's two published accounts are worth noting: the issue of *Vanity Fair* that included Styron's article had an exuberant Michael Jackson on the cover and a feature on "The 1989 Hall of Fame: The Media Decade," whereas the Random House publication had a plain cover that presented the author's name, title, and subtitle "A Memoir of Madness" in a stately, classical font. Otherwise the two versions are very similar, focusing on the fluctuations in Styron's life between being totally consumed by the experience of depression and his periodic ability to abstract himself enough from his condition to adopt the role of "a wraithlike observer who . . . is able to watch with dispassionate curiosity as his companion struggles against the oncoming disaster."[44] The fact that he does not address contemporary cultural pressures and that his experience of psychic doubling is largely internalized lends *Darkness Visible* an existential tone that jars with the glossy format of *Vanity Fair*.

Styron thought that one cause of his depression might be bound up with his decision to stop drinking at age 60, but an equally significant cause was his unresolved childhood emotions (his mother died when he was 13) and the sense of powerlessness that often accompanies the onset of old age.[45] He found touchstones, but little comfort, in the experiences of writers and public figures, especially because a number of these—Ernest Hemingway, Sylvia Plath, Randall Jarrell, Jean Seberg, Abbie Hoffman—ended in suicide when their anguish became too much to bear. (The *Vanity Fair* version begins with a reflection on Hoffman's recent suicide from an overdose of prescription drugs mixed with alcohol.) These suicides struck a chord with Styron's own mood. He found that his earlier capacity for hope had diminished and that previously harmless household objects had metamorphosed into potential tools of self-destruction. Acknowledging that there was no quick remedy for these impulses, Styron offered a subtle critique of his prescription drugs (Halcion, Ativan, Ludiomil, and Nardil), which seemed to intensify suicidal impulses.[46] However, the aim of *Darkness Visible* was not to critique psychoactive drugs or electroconvulsive treatment (Styron is actually more critical of the group therapy and art therapy he was expected to participate in when he finally checked himself into a hospital in December 1985). Rather, his focus was on the shift from hope to hopelessness as he grappled with an experience that turned a productive life into one of utter stasis.[47]

Although in the previous year, 1988, Philip Roth had disclosed the "emotional and mental dissolution" that prompted him to start his autobiographical account *The Facts* (although Roth did not "delve into particulars"), there were few literary precedents for Styron to draw upon that steered between a medical understanding of depression and the inner life of the individual.[48] This was one reason perhaps that Styron felt utterly isolated, with no guide or touchstone, and also why he questioned the clinical language of depression that he believed lacked the poetry of "melancholia" and the creative energy of "brainstorming." He found the "bland tonality" of the word depression especially inadequate for conveying the "anarchic disconnections" in his mind and the "gathering murk" of his dark moods that typically descended in the afternoon and intensified in the evening.[49] Early in the text, he stated that as a mood disorder, depression is "so mysteriously painful and elusive in the way it becomes known to the self . . . as to verge close to being beyond description," and he later repeated his belief that it was "beyond expression."[50] Foreshadowing Lauren Slater's description in *Prozac Diary* of depression as the "language of emptiness," Styron asserted that the pain was indescribable and that there was no physical correlative. Enclosed in "interior gloom," he felt that his voice was diminishing and that even occasional words seemed meaningless and drawn out, leaving him with only a "hoarse murmur," the voice of an aged man, "faint, wheezy and spasmodic."[51]

Given this emphasis on voice, it is important that the moment that Styron resolved to commit suicide was when he dispensed with the notebook in which he had jotted thoughts and feelings over a long period. Throwing the wrapped notebook in the garbage can was in effect an abandoning of his second self (the self that observes) for a complete immersion in a condition that appeared to be veering toward self-annihilation. It was only when a Brahms rhapsody pierced through his all-enveloping gloom that he realized he might sidestep death by admitting himself for a three-month stay in a hospital which, despite his skeptical attitude toward some of the therapeutic practices there, helped him "return from the abyss."[52]

Styron's motivation for publishing *Darkness Visible* was not primarily to raise the profile of depressive disorders, although he did appear on an August 1990 ABC *Prime Time* show to discuss the subject.[53] And although he managed to cling to a sense of authentic voice and believed that this "vile and detestable illness" was "conquerable," *Darkness Visible* did not represent closure for him.[54] He continued to face depression, especially in the summer of 2000, when he could barely write a letter, and in early 2002, when he believed that antidepressants had transformed his "mental disorder" into a "physical breakdown."[55] Styron's personal account is often cited for the ways it gave voice to a voiceless condition, but it was another writer, nearly four decades younger, whose literary emergence in the mid-1990s brought the issues of depression and addiction to the public eye.

Although David Foster Wallace had been on the literary scene since 1987, it was his sprawling postmodern novel *Infinite Jest* of 1996 that led to his acclaim as one of the leading voices of his generation, equally adept at writing incisive cultural criticism and self-reflexive fiction.[56] The series of health excursions in Wallace's near 1,100-page novel includes a meditation on clinical depression, which the book distinguishes from "anhedonia" (or "numb emptiness") because the latter suggests a feeling rather than a void. The character associated with this theme is the young suicidal Kate Gompert, who cannot find words for her "nausea of cells and soul" except for the elusive yet clinging term "It," which reveals "a level of psychic pain wholly incompatible with human life . . . in which any/all of the alternatives we associate with human agency . . . are not just unpleasant but literally horrible."[57]

While *Infinite Jest* explored the relationship between language and mental health on both experiential and philosophical levels, it was Wallace's January 1998 *Harper's* story "The Depressed Person" that more effectively tackled the language and symptomology of depression. *Harper's*, for which Wallace had been an associate editor since 1996, allowed him a degree of literary freedom that would have been difficult in a glossy such as *Vanity Fair*, and the tale took its place in the magazine among other cultural and social critiques, including a "Notebook" piece on omens related to the coming millennium in the same January issue and an article that was critical of managed healthcare (titled "The Doctor is Not In") two months later.[58]

Wallace's tale reads as a fable written at a high level of abstraction. It avoids Styron's first-person voice and instead moves between perspectives, often imperceptibly, through a technique of free indirect discourse. The central female character is never named or given physical characteristics (although it is arguably based on Elizabeth Wurtzel, with whom Wallace had an uneasy relationship).[59] The depressed person finds that she can neither share nor articulate her psychic pain, and although she reflects on her parents' divorce when she was a child, those feelings of "neglect or abandonment or even outright abuse" do not explain the "bottomless, chronic adult despair she suffered every day and felt hopelessly trapped in."[60] She has a network of friends that she calls on for a reality check, but she appears to feel guilty and ashamed that she is leaning on them and boring them with a condition that varies very little. She shares this persistent feeling that she is a "joyless burden" with her therapist, who encourages her to go on a weekend retreat focusing on inner-child therapy. The retreat only leaves her feeling emotionally exhausted, though, and when the therapist dies suddenly (from a "toxic combination of caffeine and homeopathic appetite suppressant") she sees this as another form of abandonment that puts even greater strain on her support network.[61]

Her dependency on the therapeutic relationship is conveyed in a very long footnote, which might be a version of one of the entries in her "Feelings Journal" we are told about in another footnote. Wallace's use of footnotes lends the story a multi-voiced aspect despite the suffocating experience of the central character (the fourth footnote virtually fills the sixth page of the *Harper's* story and spills onto the following page), but he also subverts the expectation that the notes will clarify or explain things.[62] This subversion of expectations is taken further in a long final passage where the self-absorption of the depressed person becomes all consuming after the death of the therapist (who, she realizes—or imagines—might have been suffering from similar pain herself). She begins to yearn for a journey that could lead her out of the "bottomless emotional vacuum" in which she finds herself after the therapist's death, but there is a hint that this journey might equally be a therapeutic cliché that offers little meaningful direction for either her or the reader.[63]

"The Depressed Person" does not present any direct solutions, especially as it is written in a tone that wavers between sincerity and irony. It probes the relationship between the psychological world in which the protagonist is consumed and a social reality that she both yearns for and fears. When she asks her friends to share candid opinions about her condition, it is not clear if she desires to know the truth independently of herself or if this is another layer of manipulation intended to draw her friends further into her world of dependency. Wallace pushes this ontological instability further in his *Brief Interviews with Hideous Men* collection, in which "The Depressed Person" was published the following year. Here, the equally fable-like "Suicide as a Sort of Present" depicts an emotionally fraught mother who experiences "self-loathing, terror, and despair" from a young age and carries "very heavy psychic shit" around with her.[64] To compensate for this, she places "impossibly high" expectations on both herself and her son. She nurtures her child and absorbs his growing pains, but it is not clear where her consciousness ends and his begins—he is sometimes referred to as "it" and is described as a facet of the "mother's own reflection in a diminishing and deeply flawed mirror." When he terrorizes the neighbor's pets and steals from classmates she forgives him, but as a consequence her self-loathing only heightens. By the time he enters adulthood, she is in a worse state than she was as a young woman, when her depressive and borderline experiences had sharper definition. The narrator tells us that the mother is unable to speak about any of this and implies that the son's actions are akin to a prosthetic voice that destroys her despite her ideals.

Wallace's two fables and the meditations in *Infinite Jest* can be interpreted autobiographically as a sublimated working through of depressive experiences that would otherwise be too painful to voice. These were linked to depression Wallace had experienced as a child in the early 1970s, experiences of drugs and alcohol during his undergraduate years at Amherst, and a major depressive episode as a graduate student at Harvard. Although he was influenced by Styron's account, Wallace was aware that confessional memoir could be read as a form of indulgence in which the outside world is transformed into a solipsistic mindscape. Literary fiction is not a mask for Wallace but a way of revealing a more complex reality than the clinging first-person "I" can easily render. The notion of an authentic expressive voice is thus left hanging by a slender ontological thread. Although Wallace's ironic dark comedy might be read alternatively as survival or subversion—or as a concerted attempt to get beyond the specifics of the illness—the search for a community that exists beyond the self speaks to his attempts to better understand both the mediated nature of reality in the 1990s and the psychic need for support structures that are sometimes a lifeline and other times a fantasy.[65]

New York writer and activist Andrew Solomon published an autobiographical piece, "Anatomy of Melancholy" in the *New Yorker* the same month that Wallace's "The Depressed Person" appeared. The essay self-consciously echoes Robert Burton's early seventeenth-century medical-philosophical work of virtually the same name and is a first run on ideas that Solomon expanded in his 2001 book *The Noonday Demon: An Anatomy of Depression*, in which he explores depression both as an extreme version of sadness and as an entirely discrete illness category.[66] Solomon's goals in the *New Yorker* piece are to move beyond a singular first-person account and to avoid "sweeping generalizations extracted from haphazard anecdotes" in order to think through the personal experience of depression and to better understand its "temporal and geographical reach."[67] This combination is an antidote to what Wallace calls the incapacity for empathy that sometimes accompanies severe clinical depression and the inability to look outside of the "universal pain that is digesting [the self] cell by cell" that we see in "The Depressed Person."[68] In contrast, Solomon manages to modulate his voice to think through the narrative pattern of depressive episodes: what he calls the experience of "rusting" or "emotional decay" that usually precedes a breakdown and the broader sociocultural factors that shape the likelihood and contours of depression.[69]

Even though he knew that depression can sometimes take on a life of its own and consume the self, Solomon was determined to avoid solipsism; he tried to write "a coherent narrative" that was supplemented by empirical research on the biological and psychological aspects of a wave of late-century depression that, he predicted, would by 2020 "claim more years than war and AIDS put together."[70] The prelude to his depression was a period of boredom following the publication of his debut novel *A Stone Boat*, when he found he was unable to connect to people or things and experienced suicidal ideations. But the psychological triggers had a longer arc, relating to his mother's planned suicide following ovarian cancer, as he had documented in a *New Yorker* essay three years earlier and reflected upon in *A Stone Boat*.[71] Finding his sleep disturbed and his appetite suppressed, in the autumn of 1994 Solomon began to experience panic attacks. During one distressing episode, he found that he had "forgotten how to talk," that words suddenly became complicated, and that he felt a peculiar kind of sensory experience: a "physical need, of impossible urgency and discomfort, from which there was no release—as though I were constantly vomiting but had no mouth."[72]

Solomon was initially prescribed a combination of Zoloft and Xanax (the former a serotonin-inhibitor like Prozac and the second a medication to control anxiety attacks) and he quickly entered a world of "confusing, dream-heavy sleep" policed by pills.[73] He documented a range of other prescriptions, some of which had fewer side effects, but the initial combination helped him only a little during a grueling reading tour when he barely kept his public persona from disintegrating. He supplemented a balanced account of prescription drugs (perhaps because his father was chair of a New York pharmaceutical company) with comments on the personal cost of depression: an estimated $70,000 in the forty months between the first prescription and the time he wrote the article. Interwoven with his personal story are reflections on the Mood Disorders Support Group of New York, established in 1981, which he started attending primarily for research purposes. This group gave him a new perspective on depression, medication, and electroconvulsive treatment that—perhaps surprisingly, given the fact that the media tended to fixate on barbaric depictions such as that of the 1975 film of *One Flew Over the Cuckoo's Nest*—they saw as a positive alternative to prescription drugs that involved only minor memory loss. Solomon experienced distressing withdrawal symptoms when he chose to quit his prescriptions. He entered an agitated state and started taking risks, including having unprotected sex in the hope that he would contract AIDS, feeling that a physical disease, would give his self-destructive impulses more tangible significance. (He does not explicitly discuss his sexuality in this essay, except to say that Xanax suppressed his sexual drives.)

After managing to struggle through this phase, Solomon acknowledged his reliance on antidepressants and, thinking politically, worried that the "rising tide of depression" might be due to "cost-economizing managed-care" that would lead to prescriptions that were blind to an individual's life story. This prompted him to conclude that in a late-capitalist, technologically driven culture, "basic social and psychological needs are not being met." At the same time, this culture was turning "anhedonia and internal emptiness" into "hip and cool" commodities, as Wallace described it.[74] Putting these broader worries aside, Solomon closed the essay with the knowledge that depression would always be just around the corner for him, but accompanied by a new belief that life can be "vital, even when it's sad."[75]

Solomon's essay echoed Styron's personal and Wallace's depersonalized accounts in its attempts to fashion a functional self that could navigate between reality and fantasy and between what psychotherapist Emmy Gut called productive and unproductive depression (the former is a mode of adaptive behavior toward deep-seated troubles that cannot be easily tackled directly).[76] Although Solomon realized that there is "no essential self that lies pure as a vein of gold under the chaos of experience and chemistry," he came to view therapy as the art of rescue.[77] He elaborates on this in *The Noonday Demon*, which credited drug therapy with the capacity to hack "through the vines" of depression. Yet he recognized, too, that this might just be a way of propping up the self, which for full recovery requires "love, insight, work, and, most of all, time."[78]

Gendered Voices of Depression

Of these three accounts, only David Foster Wallace's "The Depressed Person" and "Suicide as a Sort of Present" deal with the ways depression is often bound up with women's life changes. The previous two chapters looked at how particular phases of life bring their own emotional stresses: teenage neuroses for Marya Hornbacher, student anxieties for Kay Jamison, a fear of maturing for Lauren Slater, mid-life worries in *The Flock*. The marketization of Prozac at the turn of the 1990s offered a smart drug that promised to help women navigate these difficult phases, but the shaping factors of depression were still shrouded by myths and very often lacked attention to particularities. While the three voices of the previous section offered individualized responses (albeit at an emotional remove for Wallace), the emergence of a public voice on women's depression in the 1990s linked the singular and the collective and worked to raise awareness of gender issues and lobby for better representation in health research. This was crucial. A 1991 study emphasized the common elision of the loss of self and loss of voice among depressed women that often led to a retreat from interpersonal conflict and complexity into isolation and silence.[79]

When the Boston Women's Health Collective updated their landmark text *Our Bodies, Ourselves* in 1992, its members noted that two-thirds of the prescriptions for psychoactive drugs were for women and that this was often linked to the onset of menopause.[80] The updated edition, *The New Our Bodies, Ourselves*, is generally negative about the cost of healthcare and the ease with which women could obtain prescriptions. Without ignoring the positive effects that exercise, psychotherapy, and acupuncture can have, the more specific passages on depression are linked to childbirth, premenstrual tension, and aging. The authors of *The New Our Bodies, Ourselves* were worried about the damaging myths surrounding menopause (this is one of the reasons the collective had published a companion book, *Ourselves, Growing Older*, in 1987), but they acknowledged that symptoms that last more than a month relating to appetite, sexuality, sleep, and general enjoyment might indicate a depressive disorder. The same is true of postpartum depression, which the book stresses should not be mistaken for the physical, hormonal, and psychological transitions that accompany the shift from pregnancy to motherhood. It gives reassurance that fluctuating mood patterns and feelings of exhaustion (the loss of regular sleep or anemia) are not uncommon and distinguishes between "baby blues," mild to severe depression, and postpartum psychosis, a rare condition stimulated by hormonal changes that requires medical attention.[81] *The New Our Bodies, Ourselves* eschews a drug-based solution to postpartum depression and recommends that women experiencing the condition (an estimated 13 percent of American mothers) should combine exercise with support from parents' groups, women's centers, and formal therapy (although the authors recognize that talk therapy can be expensive and it puts the onus on doctors to offer responsible advice).[82]

The emphasis on knowledge, self-help, and responsibility in *The New Our Bodies, Ourselves* highlighted women's health networks and publications such as *Women Wise*, which began circulation in New Hampshire in 1978 with the intention of sharing knowledge among feminist health centers.[83] It also linked laterally to the work of high-profile feminists such as Betty Friedan and Carol Gilligan and to the ongoing advocacy of Rosalynn Carter, who co-authored two important publications in the 1990s. The first of these, *Helping Yourself Help Others* (co-written with Susan Golant), argued that caregiving requires knowledge, patience, honesty, trust, humility, hope, and courage. Carter and Golant blamed medical bureaucracy for neglecting the crucial role of the voluntary caregiver and highlighted the human cost of a medical system that many in the women's health movement felt was failing them.[84]

Rosalynn Carter published her second volume, *Helping Someone with Mental Illness* in 1998, a year after Tipper Gore presented her with a National Mental Health Association Into the Light award for her "tireless leadership, her vision, and her compassion for people with mental illnesses and their families and caregivers."[85] This book (again written with Golant) offered deeper analysis and advice on a range of mental health issues, including depression. Based on a decade of events at the Carter Center, the book had a three-fold purpose: to tackle stigma, to outline new treatments for pervasive mental health conditions, and to assess caregiving and advocacy. The chapters on depression and bipolar disorder range from a discussion of genetic vulnerability to the triggers of depression, including low self-esteem, divorce, retirement, legal problems, bereavement, and physical illness.[86] Focusing on neurological overreactions to stress and the effects of serotonin on sleep and anxiety, Carter considered the effects of depression on bodily rhythms, sex drive, and sadness.[87] Although she noted the bad press that aggressive treatments such as electroconvulsive therapy had received, she saw the contemporary practice as much safer for "patients with severe depression who have not responded to several medications," even though she admitted that more research was required to establish its effectiveness.[88] The chapter on clinical depression ended with the hopeful message that new treatments could bring relief to individuals and families and that the growth of organizations and websites meant that advice is available on a level that had not been available when Mrs. Carter had chaired the President's Commission on Mental Health twenty years earlier.

Carter's work continued to have a public face. In 1997, she initiated Carter Center fellowships to improve journalism on mental health topics and collaborated with a number of celebrities who had testified about their depressive experiences. This group included actor Rod Steiger, who silently suffered eight years of depression after a heart bypass operation, and Joan Rivers, who became depressed following the suicide of her husband Edgar Rosenberg in 1987.[89] Although Rivers and Rosenberg had recently separated, it was a combination of grief and anger that destabilized Rivers, a version of which the aging Steiger faced when Hollywood stopped offering him leading roles. While Steiger worked with Mrs. Carter as a survivor of suicidal depression, Rivers was her own spokesperson, offering "stand-up therapy" and weaving into her public persona the admission that she was periodically bulimic.[90] Steiger's advocacy work seemed more honest than that of Rivers: he spoke eloquently about his suicidal ideations and fugue states, his career disappointments, and the poor self-image that led him to undergo facial cosmetic surgery, which Rivers also chose to an extreme degree.[91] Steiger distinguished between clinical depression based on chemical imbalance from social depression (he experienced both), but he would not be pressed on his medication because he did not want to endorse a treatment that might play into the hands of pharmaceutical companies or prove damaging to others.

Depression is most frightening when the cause cannot be identified or when it seems that the world is too bewildering to be able to cope. While this is more often the case for the elderly, Todd Haynes gave eloquent expression to this form of depression in his 1995 film *Safe*. The film looks at the declining health of Los Angeles housewife Carol White (played by Julianne Moore), who develops a rare form of chemical intolerance and spirals into a depression. Haynes deliberately evokes the height of the AIDS epidemic by setting the story in 1987 but then complicates the resonance between AIDS and environmental illness by focusing on a repressed suburban wife and mother whose lifestyle is diametrically opposite to those at highest risk from the HIV virus. When Carol starts reacting adversely to upholstery, perming chemicals, and car fumes, it appears that her condition is caused by external factors, reflecting what a 1997 environmental report called the nation's "toxic ignorance" of top-selling chemicals. Yet she also experiences pressures from within that seem to stem from the existential ennui of her lifestyle. Although her regular doctor can find nothing tangibly wrong and advises her to change her diet, she continues to experience headaches, sickness, sleeplessness, and an intense panic attack at a baby shower during which she can neither breathe nor utter words. The viewer is prompted to wonder if Carol's panic attack is caused by the shallowness that surrounds her, a tangible medical condition, toxins in the environment, or a sense of emptiness within, especially because when she closes a mirrored bathroom door at the baby shower both her reflection and her identity seem to be wiped out. Julianne Moore's restrained acting and the lack of meaningful dialogue in the film shrouds this "twentieth-century disease" in mystery and links it to fundamental questions about gender, identity, and voice. Thus, the focus upon Carol's collapsing immune system is an ontological meditation on what anthropologist Emily Martin calls a "death from within" in which boundaries between self and non-self are threatened or actually dissolve.[92]

We begin the story with Carol and her husband returning to their spacious suburban home in the San Fernando Valley, where all the neighboring houses are lit in fluorescent shades of green, yellow, and silver-blue, but she ends the story sealed off from the world in a tiny safe house at Wrenwood recovery center outside Albuquerque that features "white, ceramic-tiled walls, ceiling, and floor" that give "the impression of an antiseptic space capsule."[93] Permanently attached to an

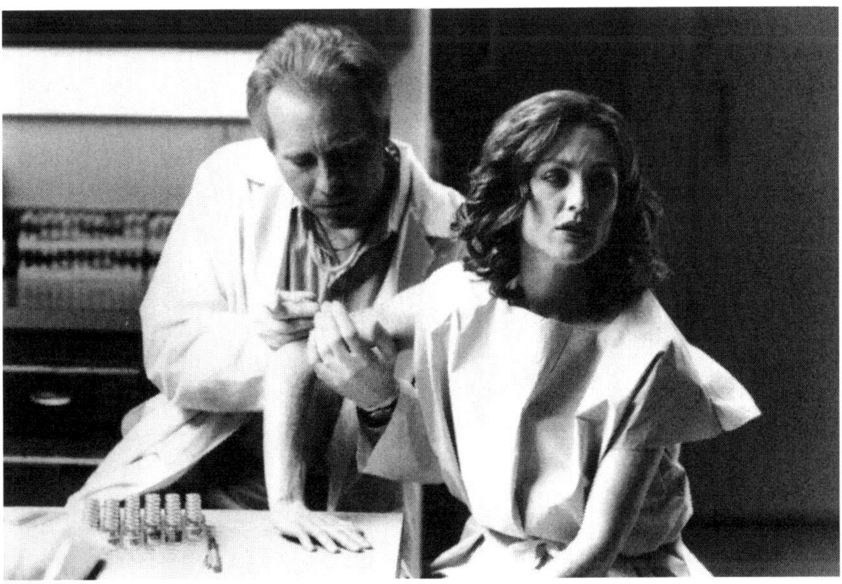

Figure 8.2 Carol White's (Julianne Moore) doctor tests her in an effort to determine the cause of her symptoms. *Safe* (dir. Todd Haynes, 1994). American Playhouse/Channel 4/The Kobal Collection.

oxygen tank in the rural seclusion of Wrenwood, with lank hair, bad skin, and a lesion on her forehead, Carol can barely manage to find her voice. At Wrenwood, she is cocooned by the new age philosophy of its founder, a HIV-positive self-help guru, and his zealous director, who together give Carol a language with which to express herself, even as the viewer realizes this is at best vacuous and at worst a form of false consciousness.[94] Although Carol is always quiet and bewildered (again aligning the depressed self and a loss of voice), by the end of the film she can articulate some words of self-affirmation, although she can barely move her mouth or any muscles in her face. The film ends with an uncomfortable close-up of Carol staring at herself in the mirror, waiting for something to happen.

Even though Carol's journey from a vibrant yet polluted California to a bleached-out New Mexico safe house is presented in a melodramatic mode, the film suggests that many women were enduring depressive conditions in silence, despite the affirmative message of *The New Our Bodies, Ourselves* and other initiatives of the women's health movement. Whereas Robert Jay Lifton saw the "protean self" of the late century as possessing inherent resilience, at the end of *Safe* Carol has no dynamism and no perspective apart from what film historian Rob White calls the "obedient and defeated" "I" by which she addresses herself in the mirror.[95] This feminist reading of *Safe* resonates with influential voices of the women's movement who argued that the patriarchal structures of medicine had changed little from the early 1970s, even though the Women's Health Equity Act of 1990 ensured gender equality for NIH research, particularly on cancer and AIDS. (The act was extended in 1998 to cover cardiovascular diseases and screenings for breast and cervical cancer.) Sandra Morgen discusses this view in her important book on the women's health movement, especially the concerns that the neoliberal language of the "empowered consumer" spoke to affluent women but left minority and poor communities untouched.[96] Although significant strides in women's health advocacy were made in the 1990s, the silences around the causes and experiences of depression—as Carol White faces in *Safe*—also informed the 1999 White House Conference on Mental Health.

The 1999 White House Conference

Tipper Gore did not go public about being treated for clinical depression until 7 May 1999, only a few weeks before the White House Conference. The media was more interested in her disclosure in *USA Today* than in the conference schedule, even though it had been previously documented that Mrs. Gore had been depressed at the turn of the 1990s, after her son Albert was nearly killed in a car accident. In this new interview, she admitted that she had undergone counseling and had been on medication but disclosed no details about the nature of the therapy or drug treatment, commenting that "when someone singles out a particular medication," some readers are likely to try it, whether or not it is the right drug for them.[97] Although Mrs. Gore conducted other interviews prior to the conference, she regularly avoided details about her medical treatment. When she appeared on *The Oprah Winfrey Show* on 2 June, for example, she was guarded about specifics and especially about her mother, whom she revealed in 1996 had battled with depression too.[98] Some journalists were suspicious that Mrs. Gore had gone public for political reasons and to prevent the issue from harming her husband's presidential campaign.[99] Nonetheless, the disclosure offered credence to her social commitment to give a "voice for the voiceless," building on the "Homeless in America" photography exhibit she had curated with the National Mental Health Association, which toured for two years.[100]

Tipper Gore did not point a finger at particular publications or institutions for perpetuating negative stereotypes about depression. Instead, she conjured the rather hackneyed stereotype of Freudian analysis as portrayed in Woody Allen's films. Wanting to demystify "Woody Allen syndrome," as she called it, Gore used the White House Conference to develop a holistic view of mental health that featured an equal focus on parity of provision, coverage for mental and physical health, scientific advances, the importance of community, and enabling personal stories.[101] Instead of gathering writers and intellectuals who may have focused on the ontological and existential themes discussed earlier in the chapter, the conference sought a more practical approach that involved "a broad coalition of consumers, providers, advocacy groups, business leaders, state, local, and national elected officials, and leaders in the mental health research and pharmacology, service delivery and insurance coverage" and, by satellite, "communities across the country."[102] Inspired by initiatives such as the National Alliance on Mental Health's "In Our Own Voice" education program (which initially focused on schizophrenia when it started in 1996), the White House conference emphasized the importance of voice on both the personal and the political level. The central event was chaired by Mrs. Gore and included contributions from the vice-president, the first lady, the president, and guests who offered a range of private and professional experiences.

After her initial remarks and a brief description of her own depression, Mrs. Gore interviewed three guests who had also come out about their experiences: CBS journalist Mike Wallace, who had experienced depression periodically since the mid-1980s and had recently featured in the HBO documentary *Dead Blue: Surviving Depression*; John Wong, a Californian born in Hong Kong who had experienced schizophrenia since the age of 16 and was now receiving support from the Asian Pacific Family Center based in Rosemead, east of Los Angeles (where he was now working); and 19-year-old Jennifer Gates from Scotch Plains, New Jersey, who was recovering from anorexia that, at its most severe, saw her food intake falling as low as twenty calories per day and her weight to 100 pounds (the briefing notes confirmed that Jennifer had experienced bouts of depression, was still receiving treatment, and continued to obsess about her academic grades and weight). Mrs. Gore's interventions focused mainly on family structures and the importance of medication, even though for Wallace and Wong this was a long-term prescription. In line with her own emphasis on "from discovery to recovery" (the title of a 1998 speech), she was very keen to elicit positive stories and looked uncomfortable when Wallace dwelled on his dark moods and Wong on violent outbursts against his father—perhaps because she was trying redress the media tendency to associate mental illness with psychopathology.[103]

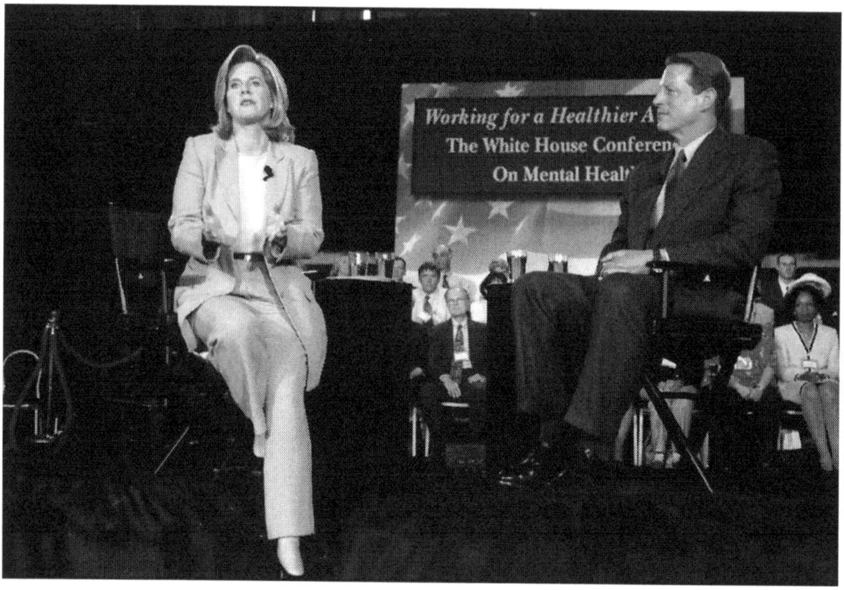

Figure 8.3 Tipper Gore and Al Gore lead the discussion at the White House Conference on Mental Health (7 June 1999). Courtesy of the Presidential Materials Division, National Archives and Records Administration, Washington, DC.

Following these three interviews, Mrs. Gore switched the focus to the need for better pediatric care and support for seniors with clinical depression. The vice-president followed her by emphasizing the importance of family and community and by announcing a hike in block grants for mental healthcare, with a particular focus on the plight of the homeless, unemployment caused by mental illness, and the health needs of crime victims. He mentioned the ripple effects of the Oklahoma City bombing of April 1995, which had led to a number of suicides, including that of police officer Terrance Yeakey, who had struggled for a year with the fact that he had not been able to help more people in the blast zone.[104] The vice-president must also have been thinking of the Columbine High School massacre in Littleton, Colorado, that spring, especially as the Clintons had spoken about the shootings on ABC's *Good Morning America* three days earlier. But Gore did not let these events distract him from two measured interviews with a mother whose son had been diagnosed as bipolar and the vice-president of Bank One Corp, a Chicago-based company that had recently invested a great deal in mental health support for its workers. The focus on the Oklahoma and Colorado tragedies was reinforced by a satellite link to the Carter Center, where Surgeon General David Satcher was holding a discussion with child psychiatrist Betty Pfefferbaum, who had developed a mental health service in Oklahoma City and had investigated the causes and consequences of the U.S. embassy bombings in Nairobi the previous year. Satcher emphasized that mental health in communities is "everybody's business" and reiterated the vice-president's emphasis on integrating community facilities with medical and paramedical care and faith-based services.

The emphasis then switched to scientific developments, including Tipper Gore's interview with Steven Hyman (the National Institute of Mental Health director since 1996 and a key figure in pushing the *DSM* categorizations toward a neurobiological paradigm) and Harold Koplewicz (director of New York University's Child Study Center), who spoke about dismantling stigma, early interventions for children (he felt that the Columbine School shooting was preventable), and the importance of public awareness and testimony. Hyman stressed that despite socioeconomic complexities, a spectrum of mental illnesses could be treated by better understanding the brain through a combination of medication and therapy. Dismissing the refrigerator mother construct in early theories of autism, Hyman and the first lady focused on genetic breakthroughs and the importance of the Human Genome Project, which had been initiated in 1990 during the Bush administration through a series of coordinated biotechnology projects in the United States and Europe (its total cost was over $3 billion). Hyman did not ignore the effects that psychotherapy can have on the brain but maintained that mental illness was fundamentally a brain disease and could be treated like "general medical illnesses."

When Bill Clinton took to the podium he admitted that he had learned about depression by reading Styron's *Darkness Visible*, but he called the experience of listening to personal testimonies "stimulating, moving, humbling . . . something so real, that touches so many of us."[105] While he noted that these shared stories can bring hope, he also felt that new scientific research was needed that could lead to a "unified theory of mind and body." The president emphasized that care should make it possible for sufferers to lead more productive lives in the "mainstream of American life"—a phrase that echoed presidential statements by Kennedy and Carter—and outlined work incentives, employment responsibilities, and insurance programs that might facilitate this.[106] He returned to the 1996 Mental Health Parity Act and admitted that the Department of Labor still had a long way to go before "the rights under the existing law" are observed "because a lot of people don't even know it passed."[107] His emphasis on the "economic burden" of mental illness might suggest that the pendulum was swinging back toward health finance, but a balance between practical measures, advocacy, and community support ran through the president's speech, while statistics about suicide among the young and the recent Columbine shootings gave his words humanity and urgency.

The White House Conference broke ground by emphasizing human stories and the integration of research, professional care, and community services. It succeeded in bringing to life distinct stories about clinical depression, schizophrenia, anorexia, and bipolar disorder and helped launch a broad-based National Mental Health Awareness Campaign. The event felt a little self-congratulatory with so much praise expressed toward Mrs. Gore, especially at the end of the headline session, when she and Mrs. Clinton embraced and guests were invited to join them on camera. It was nevertheless a balanced event in the sense that it took the secular scientific approach that mental illness is a form of brain disease yet did not overlook the importance of faith and hope as key values for ensuring that individuals did not feel isolated from networks of support.

In this respect, the conference went beyond the "science and services" approach of the surgeon general's report of late 1999, even as it shared the 450-page report's renewed optimism.[108] In fact, perhaps the most significant feature was the emphasis on new technologies of different types: for illuminating affected areas of the brain in cases of schizophrenia and depression by means of neuroimaging and tomography, for revealing the ways neural circuits can be stimulated during therapy, and for highlighting communication channels that can enhance public education. Mrs. Gore evoked the power of digital technologies in her opening remarks by mentioning the importance of Internet conversations and the 6,000 downlink sites that were transmitting the conference to states, districts, and communities. President Clinton returned to communication technologies in his closing speech by evoking the tragedy of Columbine and outlining a Learning First Alliance program that would be seen in more than 1,000 school districts through satellite dishes donated by the communications company EchoStar. Although the conference centerpiece had the feel of a chat show, Mrs. Gore's sincerity, the president's mention of suicide among gay teenagers, and the emphasis on new forms of communication as a way of breaking silence about isolated experiences revealed a commitment to mental healthcare reform as a shared responsibility that was rooted in local communities but stimulated by federal action.

Health Challenges at the Millennium

A quarter of a century after Christopher Lasch published *Haven in a Heartless World*, his jeremiad about the decline of the American family, Al and Tipper Gore, in the aftermath of the unsuccessful Gore-Lieberman presidential campaign, offered a rejoinder. The Gores' co-authored 2002 book *Joined at the Heart: The Transformation of the American Family* was an attempt to resuscitate the vitality of American families, not by harking back to the postwar nuclear family but by identifying synergies between flexible structures of family and community. The book was released along with a photographic volume *The Spirit of Family*, which echoed the humanist sentiment of the Museum of Modern Art's famous mid-century exhibition *The Family of Man* by focusing on a spectrum of contemporary families—although in this case they were national rather than global families. The domestic perspective was stimulated by the shocking events of 9/11 and tapped into an annual gathering that the Gores had held since 1991, the Family Re-Union in Nashville, in which families and communities were encouraged to knit together in a rapidly changing world.[109] They saw this "family-centered approach" as especially valuable in the field of health, from caring for sick family members at home to sharing information within communities and educating future generations. Although they focused on positive stories rather than gaps and silences, this emphasis on shared health voices was not intended just for suburban neighborhoods but was also evident in densely populated urban areas such as Cudahy, southeast of Los Angeles, a neighborhood with many Hispanic immigrants and a high crime rate in which a school and a hospital were joining forces to offer free healthcare and health education.[110]

The inflection here was certainly a liberal one. But despite the emphasis on drug therapy and communication technologies at the White House Conference, the Gores did not offer a technocratic solution and they did not see a single replicable model as beneficial for every community. They were particularly idealistic about health education. Evoking the community health model of the Kennedy-Johnson years, they envisaged the future of health education as a linking of hands and hearts to create "vibrant connections" that could shape shared futures and reinforce the right to education, healthcare, and an unspoiled environment. Aside from the fact that they did not address domestic abuse toward family members experiencing mental health challenges, the Gores would not have disagreed with a *Time* article of the summer of 1999 that saw no easy fix to the complex patchwork system that President Carter had criticized over twenty years earlier or the lack of data on minority and rural communities. They nevertheless maintained the hope that a fusion of scientific research, federal investment, and public advocacy could offer flexible and meaningful direction.[111] Flexibility is often seen as having therapeutic potential (as we saw in the quotation from Gregory Bateson in this book's preface), but the danger is that it might equally serve to align human health with the late-capitalist emphasis on adaptability. Thus, while new technologies can offer meaningful advances in communication and delivery of services, they may also give rise to fresh forms of vulnerability in the wake of "psychopharmacological over-enthusiasm" or from immersive experiences with video gaming, for example.[112] These forms of vulnerability were largely unacknowledged in political statements and policy documents of the time and required the kind of deep exploration in the cultural realm that I discussed earlier in this chapter.

Within this context, radical leftist journalists Alexander Cockburn and Jeffrey St. Clair offered a critical response to what they called "the coercive therapeutic liberalism" of the Clinton administration. They evoked the conclusion of *Haven in a Heartless World*, in which Christopher Lasch posited that the state controls both the individual's body and spirit by subtly persuading Americans to adopt technocratic solutions to often intractable social problems.[113] Cockburn and St. Clair believed that this was especially the case with mental health reform; they argued that pharmaceutical companies such as Prozac manufacturer Eli Lilly were in cahoots with White House officials (they might have mistakenly been thinking of George H. W. Bush's boardroom connections) and exaggerating the number of cases of depression that can be effectively treated by drugs (they did not provide evidence for this claim). This is an example of the polarization that was common in the culture wars of the 1990s, although here the attack was from the Left rather than the Right (the latter was epitomized by the frequent charges leveled at Bill Clinton by the likes of Rush Limbaugh). Nevertheless, the critique pushes us to consider whether the positive messages that accompanied late-century federal initiatives were as straightforward as they first seem, especially as questions about personal experience, veracity, and cultural mediation that the literary accounts of Styron and Wallace explored were rarely considered at the policy level.

I will return to these issues in my conclusion, but I want to finish this chapter by reflecting on the problems that the Clinton administration faced in advancing the therapeutic liberalism of the 1999 White House Conference. In the fields of women's and children's health, there were real advances in the 1990s—although, as chapter 5 discusses, it was sometimes difficult to untangle science from pseudoscience in efforts to understand the spike in the cases of autism late in the decade. An emphasis on children's and teenagers' mental health came to the fore after Columbine, including a White House Conference on Teenagers in May 2000 that addressed the topic of "responsible and resourceful youth" after a spate of articles on the uncontrolled rage of young Americans.[114]

A commitment to the health of minority groups also returned to the agenda and there was more inclusivity—such as the contribution to the Health Care Task Force of Raul Yzaguirre, president of the National Council of La Raza, a Hispanic advocacy group—but the mental health needs of other ethnic groups did not receive as much attention.[115] For example, the briefing notes for the 1999 White House Conference reveal that President Clinton's speech was meant to include the announcement of a dedicated initiative for young Native Americans in the face of rising suicide rates, but the notes outline the topic only in general terms. Clinton did not mention health at all in his speech about shared visions and new technologies during a visit to Pine Ridge Indian Reservation in South Dakota the following month.[116] Others, such as Paul Simms, president of the Black Caucus of Health Workers, acknowledged in 1993 that reducing the cost of healthcare and widening access were both vital goals, but he argued that African American and Hispanic American communities often faced a "politics of exclusion" (despite the endeavors of the federal Office of Minority Health to address this) because their doctors remained the most disenfranchised.[117] Prompted by his suspicion that managed care would not deliver to underserved communities, Simms argued for a pluralistic public health culture and promoted regional health councils as a way of aligning policy with community services.

The Clintons were aware that much more attention was needed to assess the health needs of women and minority communities. AIDS research, for example, revealed a significant disparity related to gender and age: black men represented just over a quarter of the male population with AIDS, but the proportion of blacks with AIDS rose to over 50 percent of cases when women and children were included, and this proportion continued to rise during the 1990s.[118] Research into the psychological and neurological effects of the virus on mood, cognition, and onset dementia was only just getting under way at Johns Hopkins University and through the American Academy of Neurology AIDS Task Force; these early studies identified significant levels of depression in high-risk groups and those who were HIV-positive, especially women.[119] Grassroots organizations such as the National Black Women's Health Project sensed the looming crisis for African American women and initiated education and treatment programs to ensure that women were seen as victims and not just vectors of the HIV virus.[120] The president was not unaware of these issues. He launched a grand project in 1997, "One America in the 21st Century," which sought to raise the profile of diverse minority groups and to close the disparity in access to healthcare by 2010.[121] It would be an overstatement, though, to claim that such initiatives were winning the battle against inadequate services or that the healthcare needs of ethnic groups were being fully addressed, especially treatment for alcoholism and suicide prevention.

The inner cities were also a major problem and were full of health scare stories. For example, in his speech at the 1999 White House conference, President Clinton mentioned being "incredibly moved" by a recent *New York Times* story that examined the uncoordinated mental health facilities that led to the release from the hospital of 29-year-old schizophrenic Andrew Goldstein despite his record of violence. Soon afterward, he pushed 32-year-old Kendra Webdale under a Midtown Manhattan subway train.[122] This had been headline news in January, but in this May feature, journalist Michael Winerip gave a more reflective account, detailing Goldstein's medical history (disorganized thought patterns and disconcerting inner voices) and pointing to the lack of investment in community residences by Governor George Pataki.[123] Two years of research at a Long Island group home for the mentally ill had shaped Winerip's view that anti-psychotic medicine offers only quick fixes for patients in need of long-term care or supervision. Noting that there are more than three times more cases of mental illness in jails than in state hospitals, he claimed that individuals with cognitive disabilities were now better represented (through the Americans with Disabilities Act) than those with diagnosable mental illnesses. In Goldstein's case, Winerip blamed the politics of deinstitutionalization and the lack of halfway house community programs.[124]

There were some positive accounts to offset this bleak picture. President Bush established a Task Force on Homelessness and Severe Mental Illness to consider issues of housing, safe havens, and rehabilitation (its 1992 report was titled *Outcasts on Main Street*), while Clinton proposed over $1 billion in 1994 for programs to assist the homeless, including improved urban shelters and mental health facilities.[125] In Massachusetts, in particular, progressive improvements to benefit the homeless took place, but the national statistic that one-third of homeless individuals were veterans (40 to 60 percent of whom had served in Vietnam) pointed to ongoing problems with the VA and a lack of integration in health services.[126] It is debatable whether health facilities in inner cities improved markedly in the 1990s, but the Clintons and Gores nevertheless placed great faith in medical science and genetic research to provide breakthroughs in treatment and contribute to destigmatization. The fact that Ralph Nader, always the champion of social justice, ran as the Green Party candidate in the 2000 presidential campaign against what he called the "the two-party duopoly" was a strong indication that the Left did not feel well represented and that grassroots groups remained disenfranchised.[127] Nader argued that the Clinton administration was a "RepDem hybrid" that accommodated big business and only paid lip service to certain communities. This view undercuts the emphasis of the White House Millennium Project on interconnectedness and the new spirit of "openness and dynamism" in Clinton's New Year's Day 2000 address, a speech that reprised the positive energy that Ford had tried to mobilize at the bicentennial.[128]

Nader's campaign was arguably the primary factor that kept Al Gore from entering the White House as the 43rd president; if he had been elected, Tipper Gore would have had at least four more years to extend the advocacy and policy work that Rosalynn Carter had begun in 1977. Given that Al Gore had promised to make mental health a chief focus of his presidency, with his loss in the election there was a danger that the momentum of the late 1990s would be squandered or that it would repeat the cycle of twenty years earlier when Carter's reforms were overturned almost instantly by the Reagan administration.[129] Nevertheless, there were some positive continuities beyond the millennium. While the health paradox with which I began this chapter was far from being resolved, the George W. Bush administration was keen to affirm the importance of community health. President Bush may well have been motivated by the view that community centers were ultimately cheaper than crowded emergency rooms.[130] However, there were some positive signs too. The New Freedom Commission on Mental Health of 2003 strongly emphasized communities and in 2005 the coalition-based Campaign for Mental Health Reform released an "emergency response" roadmap that sought to tackle the ongoing "mental health crisis," initiatives to which I turn in the conclusion as a coda to thirty turbulent years for American mental healthcare.

Conclusion

NEW VOICES, NEW COMMUNITIES

Walker Percy's apocryphal novel *Love in the Ruins* centers on the efforts of psychiatrist Tom More to devise a new machine he can use to diagnose contemporary soul sickness. Percy's More is a reincarnation of Thomas More, the Renaissance humanist who envisioned a pristine New World free from the social problems of sixteenth-century Europe. However, even though the novel is set in the appealingly named Perfection, Louisiana, More does not live in a modern-day utopia, and he is prone to mental lapses and bouts of drinking as he endeavors to assess the malaise of his fellow Americans.[1] *Love in the Ruins* was published in 1971, the year that a poll revealed that 45 percent of young Americans thought they were living in a "sick society." More complains about a dysfunctional nation run by corrupt leaders: "Is it even possible that from the beginning it never did work? That the thing always had a flaw in it."[2] As a physician-turned-novelist with a Catholic sensibility, Percy's intention in *Love in the Ruins* was to analyze the experience of mental illness and test the spiritual barometer of the nation.

In its portrayal of divisive factions and the disappearance of collective cause, *Love in the Ruins* foreshadowed the alarmist views of a number of social theorists in the 1970s. The antidote, it seemed, required both a massive reform of the system and a moral reorientation to community in line with sociologist Robert Bellah's warning in *The Broken Covenant* that in an "age of fracture" (to recall Daniel Rodgers's phrase), social bonds need to be reforged. We see the convergence of reform and reorientation in President Carter's efforts in the late 1970s to fix the patchwork medical system and his commitment to health as a right rather than a privilege—prompted, in part, by pressure from his Democratic rival, Senator Edward Kennedy. Carter realized that there was no quick fix, but he wedded pragmatic reform (in contrast to Kennedy's call for sweeping reform) to a belief that public advocacy can make a real difference and prevent inertia from setting in. When Indian tuberculosis expert Hafdan Mahler, director general of the World Health Organization, wrote to Carter in August 1978 to stress that the WHO's chief aim was "health for all by the year 2000 as the world social goal for the end of the twentieth century," he chimed with Carter's belief that health was much more than a fiscal consideration and that it could provide "a platform for peace."[3]

As I have discussed in this book, the fact that the legacy of Carter's investment in mental health reform paid off, albeit over a longer arc than he or Rosalynn Carter would have liked, is a testament to his belief in the social covenant. This suggests that healthcare is not just an administrative system but also a moral imperative that is in fierce tension with the persistent sense, particularly (but not exclusively) within the Republican Party, that the health budget is a drain on the life force of the nation. These misgivings have not ebbed in the early years of this century, despite the fact that President Clinton's surgeon general, David Satcher, described the mid-2010s as an "inflection point" in the longer history of healthcare reform in the United States.[4] In this respect, we need to look beyond partisan debates over health insurance and personal responsibility to see how questions of parity, stigma, research, and equitable care—together with the experiences of patients, ex-patients, and caregivers—offer a more nuanced and layered narrative than a tight focus on healthcare economics offers.

There is an instructive historical story to tell here. Bill Clinton's second term was in many ways the culmination of a process that the Carters began (or at least gave shape to) in the late 1970s, leading to the first Surgeon General's Report on Mental Health and the historic White House Conference of June 1999. But given the endemic social and medical problems that Percy's *Love in the Ruins* brings into focus, there is also an equally interesting cultural story in which mental health becomes a barometer of national values. This means that the events of 1999 did not really mark a moment of closure, especially since the WHO claimed in 2007 that the United States had the highest prevalence of mental health disorders in the world and in 2012 that depression had become "a global crisis."[5]

Far from the millennium closing a challenging period for mental health advocacy, then, Carter's concern that he was inheriting a "haphazard, unsound, undirected, inefficient non-system" was reprised in a 2003 report produced by the New Freedom Commission on Mental Health, an initiative of the George W. Bush administration. After fourteen months of research led by Michael F. Hogan, director of the Ohio Department of Mental Health, the commission's report, *Achieving the Promise: Transforming Mental Health Care in America*, described mental health services "as a patchwork relic" and concluded that support is "fragmented, disconnected and often inadequate."[6] The tone was milder than that of earlier reports, though, asserting that "recovery from mental illness is now a real possibility" and that the goal should be "a life in the community for everyone."

The fact that this project was launched early in Bush's first term suggests that the social covenant is not just the province of Democrats. For example, it reflects the prominence of disability rights during George H. W. Bush's term and the shift from "paternalism to productivity" embodied by the Americans with Disabilities Act of 1990.[7] But in other respects—and despite ongoing arguments that healthcare inequalities for minority groups and working-class women are widening, not shrinking—Bush's emphasis on overcoming stigma, improving service delivery, and addressing "unfair treatment limitations placed on mental health in insurance coverage" was not that different from that of the Clinton administration.[8] It also fits within the broad paradigm of "civil religion" that Robert Bellah outlined in the late 1960s and 1970s and that fed through to the rhetoric of renewal and healing in a number of late twentieth-century presidential speeches.[9] In a speech at the University of New Mexico in April 2002, Bush, in fact, sounded like a hybrid of Jimmy Carter and his father: "We must work for a welcoming and compassionate society, a society where no American is dismissed and no American is forgotten. This is the great and hopeful story of our country."[10]

We may be suspicious of the rhetoric here, particularly because Bush's emphasis on community centers in his second term seemed to be primarily a way to contain the costs of emergency treatment rather than an extension of Johnson's Great Society program or an admission that the Republican administrations of the 1970s and 1980s had underestimated the importance of community health services. But the emphasis that Bush's first secretary of health and human services, former Wisconsin governor Tommy Thompson, placed on screening for emergent mental health problems among preschool children and increasing the research budget implied a long-term commitment. This topic was reprised in the Campaign for Mental Health Reform report of July 2005, *Emergency Response: A Roadmap in America's Mental Health Crisis*, in the shape of seven steps and twenty-eight action points.[11] Given its emphasis again on parity and ending discrimination, this report reminded Gerald Grob of earlier iterations in the Carter and Clinton years, suggesting that "roadmaps and action agendas can guide the way" but impetus can be quickly lost through lack of leadership or disinvestment between programs.[12]

Long-term planning was certainly preferable to lurching into panic mode in the face of new health crises. This was most obviously the case in the month after the appearance of the *Emergency Response* report when Hurricane Katrina devastated the Louisiana coastline in August 2005. In the aftermath of the hurricane, low-income families of New Orleans were faced with a range of physical and mental health challenges relating to trauma, disruption, and displacement that recalled the health effects of the massive Buffalo Creek tidal wave that hit West Virginia mining towns in early 1972 and that gave rise to its own psychiatric syndrome.[13] When Bush spoke three years before Katrina, one might have hoped that he would have been focusing more on long-term planning and how community health facilities could better serve minority and low-income groups as part of a responsive infrastructure that could lower the health risks of such environmental disasters. Reform was clearly too slow in coming, and Ralph Nader, among others, argued vociferously that Bush did little to protect the health of the poor. Nevertheless, in a San Jose speech that coincided with a new initiative, the New Freedom Commission on Mental Health, the president at least recognized the diversity of the American people and the need for a compassionate government. In this speech he placed equal emphasis on public education, community self-help, and federal responsibility to support the poor and help seniors with the cost of health insurance.[14]

Bush's primary emphasis on that occasion was on community activity rather than the paternalistic hand of welfare that the George H. W. Bush administration tried to cast off with the Points of Light volunteer initiative of 1989, in which the president lauded organizations from California to Florida that served individuals with cognitive, developmental, and physical disabilities. There were some suspicions that the Points of Light Foundation favored businesses over volunteer initiatives, but the central premise was to encourage "every individual, group, and organization in America to claim society's problems as their own by taking direct and consequential action"—a message that Clinton's surgeon general, David Satcher, also emphasized at the 1999 White House Conference on Mental Health.[15] George W. Bush also echoed this tone of responsibility (in 2008, he signed amendments to the ADA that sought to eliminate discrimination), but linked to the Republican belief that the federal government should not be expected to find solutions to all social problems.

This message of compassion and the need for communities to mobilize grassroots energies nevertheless reveals continuities with the priorities of the Clinton years and Carter's emphasis on "competence and compassion" on the 1976 campaign trail.[16] Such a line of continuity is a reminder that successive administrations do not always follow what Theda Skocpol has called the "boomerang effect," a term she uses to characterize the back-and-forth health politics of the late twentieth century.[17] Incremental mental health reform during the Bush and Obama presidencies is to be welcomed, of course, but continuity is not without its downside, given persistent problems with drug addiction, suicides among veterans, and hidden health problems within the prison system. The neglect of prisoners is especially alarming; the National Institute of Mental Health estimated in 2016 that 50 percent of all U.S. prisoners had mental health problems and that fewer than half of these had received any form of treatment.[18]

Aside from the compassion agenda, one of the key ingredients of a responsive public health culture is a robust and flexible infrastructure that enables meaningful inputs from both above and below. As the 2002 Institute of Medicine report *The Future of the Public's Health in the 21st Century* attests, public health should address both a wide variety of evidence-based factors that link physical and mental health and the broader relationship between "social connectedness, economic inequality, social norms, and public policies."[19] This involves a combination of prevention and access; finely granulated health data; health education free of ideology; public participation in events and meetings at which health priorities can be discussed and debated; and open channels for lobbying for rights and against inequities at local and state level. Putting aside the issue of how to adequately fund such a platform, the danger of a layered and pluralistic system across such a large country—as a plethora of health reformers found, from Julius Richmond in the late 1960s to Michael Hogan in the early 2000s—is that it can result in "a maze of services, treatments, and supports" that is either too bureaucratic on the one hand or too reliant on market forces on the other. A public health culture that can be facilitated nationally but involves multiple channels and modes of participation might seem idealistic, but it is also potentially transformative. Two examples of how this could work at the national and state levels—at least in part—are the Bring Change 2 Mind nonprofit initiative (launched by actress Glenn Close in 2010), which encourages people to share their mental health stories via YouTube, and the 2015–16 "Epidemic Ignored" project, which shares through print and social media the stories of low-income, uninsured Oklahomans facing mental health and addiction challenges while they await services that may never come (this is led by *The Oklahoman* journalist and Carter Center fellow Jaclyn Cosgrove).

The Clinton administration grappled with this "maze of services" in the 1990s, and President Obama returned to the issue in 2009 when he again prioritized healthcare reform in the face of an unresponsive system that he believed failed to emphasize prevention and wellness. The Patient Protection and Affordable Care Act of 2010 brought healthcare to the fore of the national conversation in terms of what David Satcher calls "a reinvigorated infrastructure that expands access" to healthcare "as one of the most essential and basic human rights."[20] The Affordable Care Act was significantly influenced by the advocacy of Ted Kennedy, whose death in August 2009 ironically threw the reform into crisis; when Kennedy's Massachusetts seat was subsequently lost it made it easier for the Republicans in Congress to block Obama's plans. The primary aim of what quickly became known as Obamacare was to increase access to underinsured and uninsured Americans. But from 2014—a year after Obama had hosted the second White House Mental Health Conference—it also sought to align itself with the Mental Health Parity and Addiction Equity Act.[21] Bush signed this piece of legislation in 2008 in an attempt to close loopholes in the original Mental Health Parity Act and to ensure that mental health is seen as an "essential health benefit" of insurance plans. Obama pushed further by seeking to improve mental health facilities for veterans (a policy issue that Hillary Clinton and Donald J. Trump each emphasized during the fiercely contested 2016 presidential campaign) and by signing the Mental Health Reform Act and the 21st Century Cures Act during his final year in office.[22]

Despite Trump's campaign threat to either "repeal and replace" or significantly amend the financial mechanisms of Obamacare, this narrative of incremental reform suggests real advances during the Clinton, Bush, and Obama years rather than a swinging between opposing ideologies and programs. The 2003 report *Achieving the Promise* was an example of this long-term approach. Instead of arguing for a magic-bullet solution, it identified a number of research pathways, including an assessment of healthcare facilities in minority communities, the consequences of long-term medication, the effects of traumatic injury, and a need to develop new information and communication technologies for refining health record databases and enhancing public education.[23] Although *Achieving the Promise* offers a balanced view, it might have said more about how communities can be empowered to help shape their own health facilities instead of simply seeing healthcare in consumerist terms. It is important, also, to remember that the idealistic rhetoric of political speeches and high-level reports can sometimes hide profound shortcomings and inequities in the system. On this point, in March 2016, Kimberlé Crenshaw spoke persuasively about how endemic "intersectional failures" lurk within public systems and mask institutional violence toward those whom these systems fail. Crenshaw highlighted the case of 37-year-old African American Natasha McKenna, who had been diagnosed with schizophrenia and depression earlier in life but died in police custody in February 2015 after being forcibly restrained and tasered. The lid on such intersectional failures is only slowly being lifted.[24]

More broadly, it is the issue of citizenship that has concerned disability studies scholars since the millennium, not only in striving for tighter legislation to ensure voting rights and due process but also to close the gap between "legal signification" and "the lived reality of citizenship."[25] This raises fundamental questions about social status, voice, and narrative that demand sensitivity to the kinds of cultural and environmental factors that are often difficult to square with medical and neuroscientific models.[26] It also focuses attention on, first, how to secure an appropriate amount of care that can preserve agency instead of pushing citizens into the role of passive patients, and second, how to ensure that the "voiceless" have access to mental health facilities that are often out of reach for poor families and new immigrants.[27] Within such discussions of citizens' rights there are usually tensions between the data-driven social categorization that informs healthcare policy and explorations of selfhood and identity that have endured in the arts and humanities despite the seemingly triumphant "brain revolution" of the 1990s.

At its root, mental health lies on the fulcrum of these seemingly incommensurate ways of accounting for human life and prompts the kinds of questions that paleontologist Stephen Jay Gould addressed in his 1981 book *The Mismeasure of Man* about how much is left out when we turn abstract categories into fixed entities and seek deterministic explanations for complex epistemological, ontological, and cultural issues.[28] We could use a similar argument to propose that health economics and the management of healthcare on a macro-level will always be at the expense of the felt, intimate experience of life in which the personal drama of health and illness plays out. But the language of health management does not necessarily erode personal health experiences, which in their textual form—literary, autobiographical, journalistic, cinematic—weave through the chapters of this book.

There are now many more published survivor narratives written by ex-patients than there were in the early 1990s, but the tendency for such stories to be edifying does not mean that personal accounts of mental health are always healing ones. Nor do they inevitably link to the kind of consciousness raising epitomized by law professor Elyn Saks, whose personal and medical experiences—as captured in the bestselling 2007 memoir *The Center Cannot Hold*—led her to found the Saks Institute for Mental Health Law, Policy, and Ethics at the University of Southern California as a forum for addressing the legal intersections that Kimberlé Crenshaw highlights.[29] A powerful example of a health narrative that does not heal is Joyce Carol Oates's 2015 essay "The Lost Sister: An Elegy" about her mute and severely autistic younger sister Lynn Ann, whom she has chosen not to see since their parents institutionalized her in a Buffalo inpatient facility in 1971 as a 15-year-old. That Oates uses written expression to probe a relationship for which she says she has "no access" and no way of speaking "across a deep chasm" again highlights the politics of voice and the need to think carefully about the language and ethics of mental health.[30] And for every Susan Sontag who is suspicious of figurative language that cloaks health and illness in myth there is a critic like Mary Sykes Wylie, editor of the *Family Therapy Networker*, who shows how potentially damaging the diagnostic language of *DSM* is if left unchallenged, particularly as *DSM* categories relate directly to medical insurance claims.[31]

However, we cannot simply flee the world of policy and provision to reclaim a romantic conception of authentic experience that can only be expressed in the first person. Unreliable narration, fragmentary memories, distorted perceptions, the erosion or loss of self, and the inability to articulate are all markers of the health conditions examined in this book that pose far-reaching questions about veracity, authority, and authenticity. It would seem that only a discourse that is flexible and responsive enough to bridge the personal and social conceptions of identity can do justice to the at once persistent and slippery conception of mental health while also attending to the intersections between health, race, gender, sexuality, age, place, and economic status. As a number of late-century theorists grasped, narrative and action language are essential therapeutic tools for linking these identity markers, but so too is a sense of meaningful community, citizenship, and social action in which individuals can root themselves in a network of other lives.

With recent clinical research showing that isolation and loneliness have a corrosive effect on well-being, this book has traced a moral dimension to many writings on mental health that bridges the values of 1970s alternative health cultures and what in 2016 David Satcher called "ethical leadership" as a vital ingredient in the pursuit of health equity.[32] In pursuing these issues, *Voices of Mental Health* has sought to develop the sociological insights of Robert Bellah that led him and his collaborators in their 1991 book *The Good Society* to envision the relationship between individuals, groups, and institutions as a "moral ecology" based on genuine caring.[33] Bellah's Christian perspective may have led him to underestimate the gap between reality and ideal that is always tricky to navigate in the sphere of health provision. Nevertheless, this "moral ecology" helps us understand how the mental health consequences of an isolated voice are always likely to be more deleterious than a voice situated within a shared world of others.

Acknowledgments

I began to think of *Voices of Mental Health* as the second in a trilogy of books in 2012, in the latter stages of writing *Therapeutic Revolutions*. For motivating me to pursue this kind of scale and ambition in my research, I first and foremost want to thank Richard King of the University of Nottingham for his inspirational scholarship in the field of U.S. intellectual history and for his guidance throughout my professional life. I am grateful to a number of great friends who have offered me unerring personal support along the way and talented colleagues who have helped me to improve the direction and detail of the book: Peter Bourne, David Brauner, Jennie Chapman, John Dumbrell, Corinne Fowler, Jo Gill, Michelle Green, Andrew Johnstone, Adam Kelly, Prashant Kidambi, George Lewis, Philip McGowan, Catherine Morley, Andy Mousley, Laraine Porter, Jon Powell, Joel Rasmussen, Mark Rawlinson, David Ryan, Annette Saddik, Theresa Saxon, Emma Staniland, Douglas Tallack, Gemma Turton, Robin Vandome, Alex Waddan, Brian Ward, Mark Whalan, Steve Whitfield, and Alex Zagaria. I would also like to thank Kate Babbitt and Anne Hegeman for seeing the book through to publication and my two editors at Rutgers University Press and Edinburgh University Press, Peter Mickulas and Michelle Houston, for their encouragement and positivity (and to Peter for introducing me to the yeti clause).

Since starting the book in 2012, I have presented a number of related papers. These include a keynote at the International Association of University Professors of English Conference at the University of London in July 2016; a panel at the joint Irish and British Association for American Studies Conference at Queen's University Belfast in April 2016; a keynote at the 2nd Social Science and Natural Science Conference at Tanjungpura University, Indonesia, in May 2015; invited talks at the University of East Anglia, University of Glasgow, and Plymouth University; a keynote at the "*Dire les maux (littérature et maladie)*" conference at L'université Michel de Montaigne-Bordeaux in December 2013; and a talk organized by the History and English departments at Dartmouth College, New Hampshire, in November 2013. Elements of chapter 7 are included in an article, "Les gens comme les autres sont extraordinaires. Des troubles dissociatifs dans la culture américaine des années 70," in the special issue "Les écrans de la déraison" of *CinémAction* 159 (July 2016). I am grateful to Jocelyn Dupont of Université de Perpignon (the editor of this special issue) for translating my article and for his conviviality at European Association for American Studies conferences held in Izmir and The Hague in 2012 and 2014. Ideas relating to this book feature in my response to reviews of *Therapeutic Revolutions* by Sue Currell and Jay Garcia, published as a roundtable in the *Journal of American Studies* 50 (December 2016).

I am indebted to the Eccles Centre at the British Library and the Wellcome Trust for funding that enabled me to conduct archival research on both sides of the Atlantic; to the University of Leicester for granting me study leave in 2013 and 2015; and to the Institute of the Americas, University College London, where I was the John Maynard Keynes Visiting Professor in US Studies, 2013–16. My gratitude goes to the directors of the Institute of the Americas during this time, Maxine Molineux and Jonathan Bell, as well as to Iwan Morgan and Nick Witham, for offering me this fantastic opportunity to participate in their intellectual community. I also pay tribute to my colleagues in the British Association for American Studies and the English Association, who continue to make a huge difference for our subjects.

The research for *Voices of Mental Health* has been helped immeasurably by the assistance of archivists at six branches of the National Archives and Records Administration that inform this study: the Richard Nixon Presidential Library in Yorba Linda, California; the Gerald R. Ford Presidential Library in Ann Arbor, Michigan; the Jimmy Carter Presidential Library in Atlanta, Georgia; the Ronald Reagan Presidential Library in Simi Valley, California; the George Bush Presidential Library in College Station, Texas; and the William J. Clinton Presidential Library in Little Rock, Arkansas. I would also like to thank staff who helped me at the Library of Congress; the National Archives (especially Abigail Myrick); the National Library of Medicine; the D. Samuel Gottesman Library at the Albert Einstein College of Medicine in the Bronx; the Matthews-Fuller Health Sciences Library at the Dartmouth-Hitchcock Medical Center; the Medical Center Library at Duke University; the Francis A. Countway Library of Medicine at Harvard University; the Harvey S. Firestone Library at Princeton University; the Louise M. Darling Biomedical Library at UCLA; the Harvey Cushing/John A. Whitney Medical Library at Yale University; the Vere Harmsworth Library at the University of Oxford; the British Library; and the Wellcome Library, London.

For granting permission to use the images that illustrate this book, my thanks go to the National Archives and Records Administration, the Jimmy Carter Presidential Library, the Ronald Reagan Presidential Library, the Wisconsin Center for Film and Theater Research, the Special Collections Research Center of Temple University, the Autism Treatment Center of America, the Herb Block Foundation, the Picture Desk, and Rex Features.

Finally, I want to thank my family for seeing me through both joyful and tough times, and Mary Donovan and Carl Nelson for offering me such a warm and hospitable base on Capitol Hill over these last fifteen years.

Notes

PREFACE

1. Steven Epstein uses the term "credibility struggles" to describe AIDS activism. See *Impure Science: AIDS, Activism, and the Politics of Knowledge* (Berkeley: University of California Press, 1996), 3–4. On health narratives, see Angela Woods, "The Limits of Narrative: Provocations for the Medical Humanities," *Medical Humanities* 37 (October 2011): 73–78.

2. See Centers for Disease Control and Prevention, "Mental Illness Surveillance among Adults in the United States," *Morbidity and Mortality Weekly Report* 60, no. 3 (2011): 1–32, accessed 6 December 2016, www.cdc.gov/mentalhealthsurveillance.

3. The World Health Organization began using the global burden of disease measure in the 1990s to provide a more accurate picture than one that relied only on mortality statistics. See Christopher J. Murray and Alan D. Lopez, *The Global Burden of Disease* (Cambridge, MA: Harvard University Press, 1996). This report predicted that deaths around the world from noncommunicable diseases would account for 73 percent of total deaths by 2020. See also Steven H. Woof and Laudan Aron, *U.S. Health in International Perspective: Shorter Lives, Poorer Health* (Washington, DC: National Academies Press, 2013).

4. "Remarks to the Columbine High School Community in Littleton," 20 May 1999, 2011-0415-S, First Lady's Remarks and Speeches 5/99–12/99 [Columbine High School], First Lady's Press Office–Lissa Muscatine, Box 10, William Clinton Presidential Library, Little Rock, Arkansas.

5. Barack Obama, "Remarks at a Memorial Service for Victims of the Shootings at the Washington Navy Yard," 22 September 2013, *The American Presidency Project*, accessed 6 December 2016, www.presidency.ucsb.edu/ws/index.php?pid=104272&st=&st1=. The crime was committed by discharged sailor Aaron Alexis, who had a history of gun violence, was taking the antidepressant Trazodone for insomnia, and believed that he was being controlled by low-frequency radio waves: "Navy Yard Shooter Aaron Alexis Driven by Delusions," *Washington Post*, 25 September 2013.

6. Obama, "Remarks at a Memorial Service for Victims of the Shootings in Tucson, Arizona," 12 January 2011, in *Public Papers of the Presidents of the United States: Barack Obama, 2011*, Book 1 (Washington, DC: U.S. Government Printing Office, 2014), 14. In early 2016, Obama pledged $500 million to increase service capacity and background checks.

7. See Martin Halliwell, *Therapeutic Revolutions: Medicine, Psychiatry, and American Culture, 1945–1970* (New Brunswick, NJ: Rutgers University Press, 2013).

8. See Audre Lorde, *The Cancer Journals* (Argyle, NY: Spinsters, 1980) and Paul Monette, *Borrowed Time: An AIDS Memoir* (San Diego: Harcourt Brace Jovanovich, 1988). Three influential studies of medical stories are Arthur Frank, *The Wounded Storyteller: Body, Illness, and Ethics*, 2nd ed. (1995; repr., Chicago: University of Chicago Press, 2013); Julia Epstein, *Altered Conditions: Disease, Medicine, and Storytelling* (New York: Routledge, 1995); and G. Thomas Couser, *Recovering Bodies: Illness, Disability, and Life Writing* (Madison: University of Wisconsin Press, 1997). See also the interdisciplinary Hearing the Voice project (2012–2020), run by Durham University's Centre for Medical Humanities, at http://hearingthevoice.org/about-the-project/.

9. Gregory Bateson, *Steps to an Ecology of Mind: Collected Essays in Anthropology, Psychiatry, Evolution, and Epistemology* (Chicago: University of Chicago Press, 1972), 505.

10. Matthew Quick, *The Silver Linings Playbook* (2008; repr., London: Picador, 2012), 7.

11. These letters are more prominent in Matthew Quick's novel, in which voices are less distinct and letter-writing is more entangled.

12. Bradley Cooper spoke at the White House Conference on Mental Health on 3 June 2013.

INTRODUCTION

1. Daniel T. Rodgers, *Age of Fracture* (Cambridge, MA: Harvard University Press, 2011), 3, 5.

2. Walker Percy, *Love in the Ruins* (New York: Picador, 1971), 381–382.

3. On "incoherent texts" see Robin Wood, *Hollywood from Vietnam to Reagan* (New York: Columbia University Press, 1986), 41–62.

4. Richard M. Nixon, "First Inaugural Address," 20 January 1969, *Public Papers of the President of the United States: Richard M. Nixon, 1969* (Washington, DC: U.S. Government Printing Office, 1971), 3.

5. Fred Anderson, "The Growing Pains of Medical Care (I): Paying, More Getting Less," *The New Republic*, 17 January 1970, 15–18; Fred Anderson, "The Growing Pains of Medical Care (II): We Can Do It Better, Cheaper," *The New Republic*, 24 January 1970, 13–16; Fred Anderson, "The Growing Pains of Medical Care (III): Paying for Health," *The New Republic*, 7 February 1970, 17–19. See also the January 1970 issue of *Fortune* magazine, reprinted as Editors of Fortune, *Our Ailing Medical System: It's Time to Operate* (New York: Harper & Row, 1970).

6. Julius B. Richmond, *Currents in American Medicine: A Developmental View of Medical Care and Education* (Cambridge, MA: Harvard University Press, 1969), 70–74.

7. Ibid., 94.

8. Gerald N. Grob, *From Asylum to Community: Mental Health Policy in Modern America* (Princeton, NJ: Princeton University Press, 1991), 364.

9. Richmond, *Currents in American Medicine*, 99.

10. Franklin D. Chu and Sharland Trotter, *The Madness Establishment: Ralph Nader's Study Group Report on the National Institute of Mental Health* (New York: Grossman, 1974),

69. Jimmy Carter, "Speech at the Student National Medical Association, Washington DC," 16 April 1976, in *The Presidential Campaign 1976*, vol. 1, part 1 (Washington, DC: U.S. Government Printing Office, 1978), 130. Nader met Carter at his home in August 1976, but he was later critical of some of Carter's senior appointments.

11. Richard M. Nixon, "Annual Message to the Congress on the State of the Union," 22 January 1970, in *Public Papers of the Presidents of the United States: Richard M. Nixon, 1970* (Washington, DC: U.S. Government Printing Office, 1971), 15.

12. See Nixon's "Special Message to the Congress Proposing a National Health Strategy," 18 February 1971, in *Public Papers of the Presidents of the United States: Richard M. Nixon, 1971* (Washington, DC: U.S. Government Printing Office, 1972), 170–185. For context, see *Towards a Comprehensive Health Policy for the 1970s* (Washington, DC: U.S. Government Printing Office, 1971); David Blumenthal and James A. Monroe, *The Heart of Power: Health and Politics in the Oval Office* (Berkeley: University of California Press, 2009).

13. "Health Care. President Nixon's Rx: Health Care for Everyone with Government Help—But Without Government Takeover" advertisement (May 1972), Box 2, HE 5/1/72–, White House Central Files, Richard Nixon Presidential Library, Yorba Linda, California; Richard M. Nixon, "Annual Message to Congress on the State of the Union," 22 January 1971, *Public Papers of the Presidents: Richard M. Nixon, 1971*, 51.

14. Richard M. Nixon, "Special Message to the Congress Proposing a Comprehensive Health Insurance Plan," 6 February 1974, in *Public Papers of the Presidents of the United States: Richard M. Nixon, 1974* (Washington, DC: U.S. Government Printing Office, 1975), 132–140.

15. Gerald R. Ford, "Address at a Tulane University Convocation," 23 April 1975, in *Public Papers of the Presidents of the United States: Gerald R. Ford, 1975*, Book 1 (Washington, DC: U.S. Government Printing Office, 1977), 208.

16. Jimmy Carter, "Inaugural Address," 20 January 1977, in *Public Papers of the Presidents of the United States: Jimmy Carter, 1977*, Book 1 (Washington, DC: U.S. Government Printing Office, 1978), 1–2.

17. "The Public: Little Confidence in Ford or Congress," *Time*, 17 March 1975, 16.

18. Carter, "Inaugural Address."

19. Timothy Stanley, *Kennedy vs. Carter: The 1980 Battle for the Democratic Party's Soul* (Lawrence: University Press of Kansas, 2010), 2, 81.

20. President's Science Advisory Committee, *Scientific and Educational Basis for Improving Health: Report* (Washington, DC: U.S. Government Printing Office, 1972), 15.

21. See Paul R. McHugh, "The Perspectives of Psychiatry: The Public Health Approach," in *Public Mental Health*, ed. William Eaton (Oxford: Oxford University Press, 2014), 31–40.

22. See, for example, "$14.1 Million Asked for Mental Health," *Atlanta Constitution*, 12 January 1960.

23. An example of this span of conditions is the 1974 statute of the Mississippi Department of Mental Health: see Mario J. Alzvedo, ed., *The State of Health and Health Care in Mississippi* (Jackson: University Press of Mississippi, 2015), 321–325.

24. Gerald N. Grob, "Public Policy and Mental Illnesses: Jimmy Carter's Presidential Commission on Mental Health," *The Milbank Quarterly* 83, no. 3 (2005): 428.

25. For the quotation, see Christopher J. Smith, "Geographic Patterns of Funding for Community Mental Health Centers," *Hospital and Community Psychiatry* 35, no. 11 (1984): 1140. For the report, see Boisfeuillet Jones, ed., *Health of Americans* (Englewood Cliffs, NJ: Prentice-Hall, 1970).

26. Eliot Freidson, *Profession of Medicine: A Study of the Sociology of Applied Knowledge* (1970; repr., Chicago: University of Chicago Press, 1988), 223. See also Steven S. Sharfstein, "Will Community Mental Health Survive in the 1980s?," *American Journal of Psychiatry* 135, no. 11 (1978): 1363–1365.

27. David E. Smith, David J. Bentel, and Jerome L. Schwartz, eds., *The Free Clinic: A Community Approach to Health Care and Drug Abuse* (Beloit, WI: Stash, 1971), xiv.

28. See "Community Mental Health: Problems and Prospects," special issue, *International Journal of Mental Health* 3, no. 2–3 (1974) and Gregory L. Weiss, *Grassroots Medicine: The Story of America's Free Health Clinics* (Lanham, MD: Rowman and Littlefield, 2006).

29. See David L. Snow and Peter M. Newton, "Task, Social Structure, and Social Process in the Community Mental Health Center Movement," *American Psychologist* 31, no. 8 (1976): 582–594.

30. See Tom Wolfe, "The 'Me' Decade and the Third Great Awakening," *New York Magazine*, 23 August 1976, 26–40.

31. Rodgers, *Age of Fracture*, 3.

32. This 1976 survey was devised to replicate a national survey of modern living conducted in 1957 that involved nearly 2500 subjects. See Joseph Veroff, Richard A. Kulka, and Elizabeth Douvan, *Mental Health in America: Patterns of Help-Seeking from 1957 to 1976* (New York: Basic Books, 1981).

33. Peter Marin, "The New Narcissism," *Harper's*, October 1975, 45–56.

34. Philip Rieff, *Fellow Teachers / Of Culture and Its Second Death* (1972; repr., Chicago: University of Chicago Press, 1985), 53–55.

35. Edwin Schur, *The Awareness Trap: Self-Absorption instead of Social Change* (New York: McGraw Hill), 1976), 2–3. See also Christopher Lasch, *The Culture of Narcissism: American Life in an Age of Diminishing Expectations* (New York: Norton, 1979), 118.

36. Schur, *The Awareness Trap*, 7.

37. On Carter's July 1979 speech "Energy and the Crisis of Confidence," see Daniel Horowitz, ed., *Jimmy Carter and the Energy Crisis of the 1970s* (Boston: Bedford / St. Martin's, 2005). An important intellectual resource for Carter was Bellah's *The Broken Covenant: American Civil Religion in Time of Trial* (New York: Seabury, 1975). Bellah was invited to a Camp David summit to discuss domestic affairs on 10 July 1979. See "What the President Reads," *Los Angeles Times*, 8 December 1979.

38. Ted Kennedy called Carter's speech "the most destructive address of the administration": Edward M. Kennedy, *True Compass: A Memoir* (New York: Twelve, 2009), 366.

39. Schur, *The Awareness Trap*, 11.

40. Lasch, *The Culture of Narcissism*, 218.

41. Robert Pirsig, *Zen and the Art of Motorcycle Maintenance: An Inquiry into Values* (1974; repr., London: Vintage, 1991), 16, 77.

42. Ibid., 362.

43. For the 1971 National Health Crusade, see Robert J. Bazell, "Health Radicals: Crusade to Shift Medical Power to the People," *Science*, 173, no. 3996 (1971): 506–509. For the development of the Medical Committee for Human Rights from the mid-1960s, see John Dittmer, *The Good Doctors: The Medical Committee for Human Rights and the Struggle for Social Justice in Health Care* (New York: Bloomsbury, 2009).

44. The Boston Women's Health Book Collective, *Our Bodies, Ourselves* (New York: Simon and Schuster, 1973); Kathy Davis, *The Making of Our Bodies, Ourselves: How Feminism Travels across Borders* (Durham, NC: Duke University Press, 2007).

45. For mental health and minorities, see *Mental and Physical Health Problems of Black Women* (Washington, DC: Black Women's Community Development Foundation, 1975); William David Smith, *Minority Issues in Mental Health* (Reading, MA: Addison-Wesley, 1978); Manuel R. Miranda and Harry H. L. Kitano, eds., *Mental Health Research and Practice in Minority Communities* (Rockville, MD: U.S. Department of Health and Human Services, 1986).

46. Carol Gilligan, *In a Different Voice: Psychological Theory and Women's Development* (Cambridge, MA: Harvard University Press, 1982), 173.

47. Carter, "Cubans Seek Asylum in the United States," U.S. Department of State, Bureau of Public Affairs, Washington DC (14 May 1980), Box 20, Folder 3, Records of the Cuban-Haitian Task Force, Jimmy Carter Presidential Library, Atlanta, Georgia.

48. "Report to the President's Commission on Mental Health from the Special Populations Sub-Panel on Mental Health of Hispanic Americans," 16 January 1978, Box 15, Folder 7, First Lady's Office: Kathy Cade–Mental Health Project, Jimmy Carter Presidential Library.

49. Ibid., 2–3. On the role of cultural psychiatry, see Amado M. Padilla, ed., *Hispanic Psychology: Critical Issues in Theory and Research* (London: Sage, 1995), 107–130.

50. Flora Davis, *Moving the Mountain: The Women's Movement of America since 1960* (1991; repr., Urbana: University of Illinois Press, 1999), 245–248.

51. Robert Jay Lifton, *The Protean Self: Human Resilience in the Age of Fragmentation* (New York: HarperCollins, 1993), 232.

52. Jean Baudrillard, *Simulations*, trans. Paul Foss, Paul Patton, and Philip Beitchman (New York: Semiotext(e), 1983), 54.

53. Philip Cushman, *Constructing the Self, Constructing America: A Cultural History of Psychotherapy* (Cambridge, MA: Da Capo, 1995), 246–247; Gail Sheehy, *Hillary's Choice* (New York: Random House, 1999), 301.

54. Paul Starr, *The Social Transformation of American Medicine* (New York: Basic Books, 1982), x. See also Paul Starr, "Transformation in Defeat: The Changing Objectives of

National Health Insurance 1915–1980," *American Journal of Public Health* 72, no. 1 (1982): 78–88.

55. Starr, *The Social Transformation of American Medicine*, 9; John Harley Warner, "Grand Narrative and Its Discontents: Medical History and the Social Transformation of American Medicine," *Journal of Health Politics, Policy and Law* 29, nos. 4–5 (2004): 765, 769. A more critical account of health policy is Paul Starr, *Remedy and Reaction: The Peculiar American Struggle over Health Care Reform* (New Haven, CT: Yale University Press, 2011).

56. Jonathan Engel, *American Therapy: The Rise of Psychotherapy in the United States* (New York: Penguin, 2008), 194.

57. Ibid., xiv, 167.

58. Robert Crawford, "Healthism and the Medicalization of Everyday Life," *International Journal of Health Services* 10, no. 3 (1980): 368, 385.

59. Editor's Column, *Literature and Medicine* 1 (1982): ix.

60. Enid Rhodes Peschel, ed., *Medicine and Literature* (New York: Neale Watson, 1982), xi.

61. Larry R. Churchill and Sandra W. Churchill, "Storytelling in Medical Arenas: The Art of Self-Determination," *Literature and Medicine* 1 (1982): 75. For a synoptic essay, see Brian Hurwitz and Victoria Bates, "The Roots and Ramifications of Narrative in Modern Medicine," in *The Edinburgh Companion to the Critical Medical Humanities*, ed. Anne Whitehead and Angela Woods (Edinburgh: Edinburgh University Press, 2016), 559–576.

62. Jonathan Cott, "Susan Sontag: The Rolling Stone Interview," *Rolling Stone*, 4 October 1979, 49.

63. Susan Sontag, *Illness as Metaphor and AIDS and Its Metaphors* (1988; repr., London: Penguin, 1991), 73, 41, 36.

64. See Barbara Clow, "Who's Afraid of Susan Sontag? Or, the Myths and Metaphors of Cancer Reconsidered," *Social History of Medicine* 14, no. 2 (2001): 293–312.

65. Roy Schafer, *Language and Insight* (New Haven, CT: Yale University Press, 1978), 7.

66. Jacques Derrida and Paule Thévenin, *The Secret Art of Antonin Artaud*, trans. Mary Ann Caws (Cambridge, MA: MIT Press, 1998), 63.

67. See John Wiltshire, "Biography, Pathography, and the Recovery of Meaning," *The Cambridge Quarterly* 29, no. 4 (2000): 409–422.

68. Melvin Sabshin, "Turning Points in Twentieth-Century American Psychiatry," *American Journal of Psychiatry* 147, no. 10 (1990): 1267–1274.

69. Daniel Dennett, *Consciousness Explained* (1991; London: Penguin, 1993), 67.

70. Erving Goffman, *The Presentation of Self in Everyday Life* (1956; repr., New York: Anchor, 1959); Carl Elliott, *Better than Well: American Medicine Meets the American Dream* (New York: Norton, 2003).

71. See, for example, Jason Tougaw, "Testimony and the Subjects of AIDS Memoirs," *a/b: Auto/Biography Studies* 13, no. 2 (1998): 235–256.

72. Robert N. Bellah, "Civil Religion in America," *Daedalus* 96, no. 1 (1967): 1–21.

73. Robert N. Bellah, Richard Madsen, William M. Sullivan, Ann Swidler, and Steven M. Tipton, *Habits of the Heart: Individualism and Commitment in American Life* (Berkeley: University of California Press, 1985), 8.

74. Ibid., 307.

75. Ibid., 133.

76. See Philip Rieff, *The Triumph of the Therapeutic: Uses of Faith after Freud* (Chicago: University of Chicago Press, 1966).

77. Bellah et al., *Habits of the Heart*, 138.

78. See Peter Levine, *In an Unspoken Voice: How the Body Releases Trauma and Restores Goodness* (Berkeley, CA: North Atlantic Books, 2010).

79. See James Morrison, *When Psychological Problems Mask Medical Disorders: A Guide for Psychotherapists* (New York: Guilford Press, 1997).

80. Catherine Prendergast, "On the Rhetorics of Mental Instability," in *Embodied Rhetorics: Disability in Language and Culture*, ed. James C. Wilson and Cynthia Lewiecki-Wilson (Carbondale: Southern Illinois University Press, 2001), 46.

81. See Kimberlé Crenshaw, *On Intersectionality: The Essential Writings* (New York: Free Press, 2017) and Marcia C. Inhorn and Emily A. Wentzell, eds., *Medical Anthropology at the Intersections: Histories, Activisms, and Futures* (Durham, NC: Duke University Press, 2015).

82. See Jonathan B. Imber, *Trusting Doctors: The Decline of Moral Authority in American Medicine* (Princeton, NJ: Princeton University Press, 2008). On federal authority and intergovernmental relationships, see Gerald N. Grob and Howard H. Goldman, *The Dilemma of Federal Mental Health Policy: Radical Reform or Incremental Change?* (New Brunswick, NJ: Rutgers University Press, 2006).

83. For mental health and AIDS, see Michael B. King, *HIV, AIDS, and Mental Health* (Cambridge: Cambridge University Press, 1993) and Michael Shernoff, ed., *AIDS and Mental Health Practice: Clinical and Policy Issues* (New York: Haworth, 1999).

84. On *DSM-IV* and the media, see Richard G. Frank and Sherry A. Glied, *Better but Not Well: Mental Health Policy in the United States since 1950* (Baltimore, MD: Johns Hopkins University Press, 2006), 134; Jo C. Phelan, Bruce G. Link, Ann Stueve, and Bernice A. Pescosolido, "Public Conceptions of Mental Illness in 1950 and 1996: What Is Mental Illness and Is It to Be Feared?," *Journal of Health and Social Behavior* 41, no. 2 (2000): 188–207.

85. Bruce G. Link and Jo C. Phelan, "Public Conceptions of Mental Illness: Labels, Causes, Dangerousness, and Social Distance," *American Journal of Public Health* 89, no. 9 (1999): 1328.

86. See Ramin Mojtabai, William W. Eaton, and Pallab K. Maulik, "Pathways to Care: Need, Attitudes, Barriers," in *Public Mental Health*, ed. William W. Eaton (Oxford: Oxford University Press, 2012), 415–439.

CHAPTER 1 — HEALTH DEBATES AT THE BICENTENNIAL

1. "The Glorious Anniversary," *Washington Post*, 3 July 1976.

2. American Revolution Bicentennial Administration, *The Bicentennial of the United States of America: A Final Report to the People*, vol. 1 (Washington, DC: American Revolution Bicentennial Administration, 1977).

3. Gerald R. Ford, "Remarks in Philadelphia, Pennsylvania," 4 July 1976, in *Public Papers of the Presidents of the United States: Gerald R. Ford, 1976–77*, Book 2 (Washington, DC: U.S. Government Printing Office, 1979), 1969.

4. Ibid., 1970.

5. Robert N. Bellah, "Civil Religion in America," *Daedalus* 96 (Winter 1967): 19–20; Robert N. Bellah, *The Broken Covenant: American Civil Religion in Time of Trial* (New York: Seabury Press, 1975). See also Robert N. Bellah, "Civil Religion and the American Future," *Religious Education* 71 (May–June 1976): 235–243.

6. For ethnic tensions surrounding the bicentennial celebrations, see Christopher Capozzola, "'It Makes You Want to Believe in the Country': Celebrating the Bicentennial in an Age of Limits," in *American in the 70s*, ed. Beth Bailey and David Farber (Lawrence: University Press of Kansas, 2004), 38–39.

7. Stephen Stills quoted in Johnny Rogan, *Neil Young: Sixty to Zero* (London: Calidore, 2000), 350.

8. Gerald R. Ford, *A Time to Heal: The Autobiography of Gerald R. Ford* (New York: Harper & Row, 1979), 179.

9. For Ford's use of the rhetoric of healing, see Patrick Hagopian, *The Vietnam War in American Memory: Veterans, Memorials, and the Politics of Healing* (Amherst: University of Massachusetts Press, 2009), 32–33. For a broader focus on healing and trauma, see Barbara Keys, Jack Davies, and Elliott Bannan, "The Post-Traumatic Decade: New Histories of the 1970s," *Australasian Journal of American Studies* 33 (July 2014): 1–17.

10. For the transformation of right-wing politics, see Laura Kalman, *Right Star Rising: A New Politics, 1974–1980* (New York: Norton, 2010). For distrust of the government and the military linked to the Vietnam War, see Jerald G. Bachman and M. Kent Jennings, "The Impact of Vietnam on Trust in Government," *Journal of Social Issues* 31 (Fall 1975): 141–155.

11. Ron Kovic's speech is included in *The Official Proceedings of the Democratic National Convention, New York City, July 1976* (Washington, DC: Democratic National Committee, 1976), 379–380. In his acceptance speech as the Republican presidential candidate on 19 August 1976, Ford mentioned Medicare only once: *The Presidential Campaign 1976*, vol. 2, part 2 (Washington, DC: U.S. Government Printing Office, 1979). Carter stressed the need for "a nationwide comprehensive health program" in his own acceptance speech on 15 July 1976, but also said little that was substantive about health: *The Presidential Campaign 1976*, vol. 1, part 1 (Washington, DC: U.S. Government Printing Office, 1978), 350.

12. *Presidency 1976* (Washington, DC: Congressional Quarterly, 1977), 31. See also Richard E. Neustadt and Harvey V. Fineberg, *The Swine Flu Affair: Decision-Making on a Slippery Disease* (Washington, DC: Department of Health, Education, and Welfare, 1978).

13. For the topic of health in the third presidential debate, see "Presidential Campaign Debate," 22 October 1976; and "Vice Presidential Debate in Houston, Texas," 15 October 1976, both in *The Presidential Campaign 1976*, vol. 3 (Washington, DC: U.S. Government Printing Office, 1978), 151, 163.

14. *Joseph A, Califano Jr., to Be Secretary of Health, Education, and Welfare—Additional Consideration, 95th Congress, First Session, 13 January 1977* (Washington, DC: U.S. Government Printing Office, 1977), 19.

15. Congress defeated Nixon's health insurance plan as it was set out in early 1974. For his plan, see "Special Message to the Congress Proposing a Comprehensive Health Insurance Program," 6 February 1974, in *Public Papers of the Presidents of the United States: Richard M. Nixon, 1974* (Washington, DC: U.S. Government Printing Office, 1975), 132–140.

16. Jimmy Carter, *Why Not the Best?* (Nashville, TN: Broadman Press, 1975), 91.

17. Arthur Schlesinger Jr. wrote that "vision" in the first debate "was buried under statistics . . . one got little sense of direction in which either wanted to take the country": "What Happened to Civil Rights?," *Wall Street Journal*, 28 September 1976.

18. Jimmy Carter, "Speech at the Student National Medical Association, Washington DC," 16 April 1976, in *The Presidential Campaign 1976*, vol. 1, part 1, 129.

19. Jimmy Carter, "Address to the American Public Health Association, Miami Beach," 19 October 1976, in *The Presidential Campaign 1976*, vol. 1, part 2, 1057.

20. "Black Voter Concerns," in *The Presidential Campaign 1976*, vol. 1, part 1, 135. For hospital costs, see Peter G. Bourne, "Memorandum for Governor Carter: Priority Administration Decisions on Health," Records of Peter Bourne, Box 4, Health Issues 12/20/76–1/31/77, Jimmy Carter Presidential Library, Atlanta, Georgia.

21. "The Election," *Washington Post*, November 4, 1976.

22. *Playboy* interview with Jimmy Carter (November 1976), reprinted in *The Presidential Campaign 1976*, vol. 1, part 2, 944, 964.

23. Irving M. Levine, "Ethnicity and Mental Health: A Socially Conservation Approach," White House Meeting on Ethnicity and Mental Health, 14 June 1976, Box 35, Folder 3, Jimmy Carter Papers, Pre-Presidential Campaign Issues Office, Jimmy Carter Presidential Library.

24. The meeting was organized by the Office of Public Liaison and the Institute on Pluralism and Group Identity. See "Ethnicity and Mental Health Meeting, June 14, 1976 (2)," Box 10, Myron Kuropas Papers, Gerald R. Ford Presidential Library, Ann Arbor, Michigan. For its influence on Carter's commission, see "Mental Health Care and Euro-Ethnics," Box 37, Folder 14, Jimmy Carter Papers, Office of Public Liaison: Costanza, Jimmy Carter Presidential Library.

25. President's Committee on Mental Retardation, *Mental Retardation: Century of Decision* (Washington, DC: President's Committee on Mental Retardation, 1976), v, iii.

26. For Forrest David Matthews's commitment to citizen participation, see the HEW News Press Release, 25 July 1976, Box 6, Health, Education and Welfare, Dept of. (2), Spencer C. Johnson Files, Gerald R. Ford Presidential Library.

27. President's Committee on Mental Retardation, *Mental Retardation*, v.

28. Ibid., 19.

29. Ibid., 27.

30. Gerald Ford, "Remarks Announcing Plans for a White House Conference on Handicapped Individuals," 22 November 1975, in *Public Papers of the Presidents of the United States: Gerald R. Ford, 1975* (Washington, DC: U.S. Government Printing Office, 1977), 690.

31. Joanne Findlay, "A National Health System for America," Box 35, Folder 3, 1976 Presidential Campaign Issues Office–Sam Bleicher, Jimmy Carter Presidential Library.

32. *Health: United States 1975* (Washington, DC: Department of Health, Education, and Welfare, 1975), 1, https://www.cdc.gov/nchs/data/hus/hus75acc.pdf.

33. Harold H. Goldman and Gerald N. Grob, "Defining 'Mental Illness' in Mental Health Policy," *Health Affairs* 25 (May 2006): 740–741.

34. Gerald N. Grob, "Public Policy and Mental Illnesses: Jimmy Carter's Presidential Commission on Mental Health," *Milbank Quarterly* 83, no. 3 (2005): 427. Grob took these statistics from Paul J. Fink and S. P. Weinstein, "Whatever Happened to Psychiatry? The Deprofessionalization of Community Mental Health Centers," *American Journal of Psychiatry* 136 (April 1979): 406–409. See also Murray Levine, *The History and Politics of Community Mental Health* (New York: Oxford University Press, 1981).

35. John Z. Bowers and Elizabeth F. Purcell, eds., *Advances in American Medicine: Essays at the Bicentennial* (New York: Josiah Macy, Jr. Foundation, 1976), 438–439. See also *Health: United States, 1976–1977* (Washington, DC: Department of Health, Education, and Welfare, 1976), www.cdc.gov/nchs/data/hus/hus7677.pdf.

36. Thomas H. Watkins to Theodore Cooper, February 3, 1976, Box 4, Mental Health and Treatment, 2/3/76–12/14/76, Records of Peter Bourne, Jimmy Carter Presidential Library.

37. "Notes on Improving Federal Programs on Behalf of the Mentally Handicapped," Box 35, Folder 2, 1976 Presidential Campaign Issues Office–Sam Bleicher, Jimmy Carter Presidential Library.

38. Rosemary Stevens, *American Medicine and the Public Interest* (New Haven, CT: Yale University Press, 1971), 528.

39. Frank M. Ochberg, "Community Mental Health Centre Legislation: Flight of the Phoenix," *American Journal of Psychiatry* 133 (January 1976): 61.

40. Allen Ginsberg describes the New York State Psychiatric Institute as a "concrete void" in "Howl": Ginsberg, *Howl and Other Poems* (San Francisco: City Lights, 1956), 15.

41. Lithium had been used medicinally as early as the 1810s, but interest was renewed in the 1950s and 1960s in lithium carbonate as a potential mood stabilizer. See Samuel Gershon and Baron Shopsin, eds., *Lithium: Its Role in Psychiatric Research and Treatment* (New York: Plenum Press, 1973); Joanna Moncrieff, *The Myth of the Chemical Cure: A Critique of Psychiatric Drug Treatment* (London: Palgrave, 2008), 174–203.

42. Michael Douglas quoted in "Lag in Filming Lunacy Symbolism," *Variety*, November 26, 1975, 21.

43. *Inside the Cuckoo's Nest*, dir. Rick Butler, PBS, 1975. Edward Shorter argues that the depiction of electroconvulsive treatment in the film was anachronistic. See Edward Shorter and David Healy, *Shock Therapy: A History of Electroconvulsive Treatment in Mental Illness* (New Brunswick, NJ: Rutgers University Press, 2007), 152–153. See also Irving Schneider, "The Theory and Practice of Movie Psychiatry," *American Journal of Psychiatry* 144 (August 1987): 996–1002.

44. Ronald R. Fieve, *Moodswing*, rev. ed. (New York: Bantam, 1997), 16.

45. Fieve made it clear that lithium can only alleviate bipolar conditions, not schizophrenia and chronic anxiety: ibid., 246. Fieve's use of lithium was covered in "Drugs for the Mind: Psychiatry's Newest Weapons," special issue, *Newsweek*, 12 November 1979.

46. Nathan Hale Jr., *The Rise and Crisis of Psychoanalysis in the United States: Freud and the Americans, 1917–1985* (New York: Oxford University Press, 1995), 322–344.

47. For the Massachusetts trials, see Lester Grinspoon, *Schizophrenia: Pharmacotherapy and Psychotherapy* (Baltimore, MD: Williams & Wilkins, 1972). On the Camarillo and Boston experiments, see David Healy, *Creation of Psychopharmacology* (Cambridge, MA: Harvard University Press, 2002), 144–146.

48. Hale, *The Rise and Crisis of Psychoanalysis*, 328–329.

49. Ivan Illich, *Medical Nemesis: The Expropriation of Health* (1975), republished as *The Limits of Medicine* (New York: Marion Boyars, 1976), 257.

50. Ibid., 63–76.

51. Ibid., 4. For criticism of *Medical Nemesis*, see David F. Horrobin, *Medical Hubris: A Reply to Ivan Illich* (Montreal: Eden Press, 1978). See also Erving Goffman, *Asylums: Essays on the Social Situation of Mental Patients and Other Inmates* (New York: Anchor, 1961).

52. See Erving Goffman, "The Insanity of Place," *Psychiatry: Journal for the Study of Interpersonal Processes* 32 (November 1969): 451–463.

53. See Isadore Rosenfield, *Hospitals—Integrated Design*, 2nd rev. ed. (New York: Reinhold, 1951), 234–258. Rosenfield's work on therapeutic architectural environments continued in her 1971 book *Hospital Architecture: Integrated Components*.

54. See Louis E. Kopolow, "A Review of Major Implications of the *O'Connor v. Donaldson* Decision," *American Journal of Psychiatry* 133 (April 1976): 379–383. For broader considerations, see Robert G. Meyer and Christopher M. Weaver, *Law and Mental Health: A Case-Based Approach* (New York: Guilford, 2006), 131–140; Elyn R. Saks, *Refusing Care: Forced Treatment and the Rights of the Mentally Ill* (Chicago: University of Chicago Press, 2002).

55. See Michael J. Remington, "Lessard v. Schmidt and Its Implications for Involuntary Civil Commitment in Wisconsin," *Marquette Law Review* 57 (January 1973): 68.

56. Robert T. Roth, Melvyn K. Daley, and Judith Lerner, "Into the Abyss: Psychiatric Reliability and Emergency Commitment Statutes," *Santa Clara Law Review* 13 (Spring 1973): 402–403.

57. "Ford's Brush with Death," *Newsweek*, 19 September 1975, 16.

58. Ibid., 22. A *Time* piece grasped for words to describe the incident (a "mad act," a "sprinkling of warped souls") but included an extract from an autobiographical piece by

Fromme that she had hoped to publish. See "The Girl That Almost Killed Ford," *Time*, 15 September 1975, 8, 12. For a more perceptive account, see "The Significance of Squeaky Fromme," *New York Times*, 30 September 1975.

59. "Protecting the President," *Time*, 6 October 1975, 8; Roth et al., "Into the Abyss," 445.

60. Philip Zimbardo, *The Lucifer Effect: Understanding How Good People Turn Evil* (New York: Random House, 2008), viii.

61. Philip G. Zimbardo, "Pathology of Imprisonment," *Society* 9 (April 1971): 4–8; Erich Fromm, *The Anatomy of Human Destructiveness* (1973; repr., New York: Penguin, 1977), 96.

62. See, for example, Robert I. Watson Jr., "Investigation into Deindividuation Using a Cross-Cultural Survey Technique," *Journal of Personality and Social Psychology* 25 (March 1973): 342–345.

63. David L. Rosenhan, "On Being Sane in Insane Places," *Science* 179, no. 4070 (1973): 253.

64. Ibid., 257. Psychologist Lauren Slater replayed Rosenhan's experiment thirty years later by feigning auditory hallucinations in nine psychiatric clinics, each of which diagnosed her as having psychotic depression: Lauren Slater, "On Being Sane in Insane Places: Retracing David Rosenhan's Journey," *Psychotherapy Networker* 28 (March/April 2004): 54–60.

65. For his Pulitzer Prize–winning reports on the "snake pit" conditions of Milledgeville Central State Hospital see Jack Nelson, *Scoop: The Evolution of a Southern Reporter*, ed. Barbara Matusow (Jackson: University of Mississippi Press, 2013), 61–68.

66. A record of this 20 May 1971 phone conversation with an Athens resident is available in the Rosalynn Carter's Special Projects and Events File, Box 131, Mental Health–Central State Hospital, Milledgeville, Carter Family Papers, Jimmy Carter Presidential Library. Peter Bourne's May 1971 speech to the Metropolitan Atlanta Mental Health Association, "Mental Health in Georgia—Where Are We Today?" is helpful for tracing institutional developments in Carter's home state. See Box 131, Mental Health–Articles [1], Jimmy Carter Presidential Library.

67. See Judi Chamberlin, "The Ex-Patients' Movement: Where We've Been and Where We're Going," *Journal of Mind and Behavior* 11 (Summer 1990): 323–336. See also Judi Chamberlain, *On Our Own: Patient Controlled Alternatives to the Mental Health System* (New York: Hawthorn, 1978). For the fate of *Madness Network News* in the 1980s, see Rael Jean Isaac and Virginia C. Armat, *Madness in the Streets: How Psychiatry and the Law Abandoned the Mentally Ill* (New York: Free Press, 1990), 222–224.

68. For a polemical account of the battle over psychiatric truth in the 1970s, see Robert Whitaker, *Mad in America: Bad Science, Bad Medicine, and the Enduring Mistreatment of the Mentally Ill* (Cambridge, MA: Perseus, 2002), 211–226.

69. Jerome Agel, ed., *Rough Times* (New York: Ballantine Books, 1973), xi.

70. Ibid., x.

71. Rick Kunnes, "Detherapizing Society," *Rough Times* 2 (March 1972), reprinted in Agel, *Rough Times*, 88, 92.

72. For an anthology of the Berkeley articles, see Hogie Wyckoff, ed., *Love, Therapy and Politics: Issues in Radical Therapy, The First Year* (New York: Grove, 1976).

73. On "Kill Your Sons" and anti-psychiatry, see Nicola Spelman, *Popular Music and the Myths of Madness* (Burlington, VT: Ashgate, 2012), 39–54.

74. See John Friedberg, *Shock Treatment Is Not Good for Your Brain* (San Francisco: Glide, 1976); J. Friedberg, "Shock Treatment, Brain Damage, and Memory Loss: A Neurological Perspective," *American Journal of Psychiatry* 134 (September 1977): 1010–1014. See also Elliot Valenstein, *Brain Control: A Critical Examination of Brain Stimulation and Psychosurgery* (New York: Wiley, 1973).

75. See Bruce J. Ennis, *Prisoners of Psychiatry: Mental Patients, Psychiatry, and the Law* (New York: Harcourt Brace Jovanovich, 1972). For patients' rights, see Fritz Redlich and Richard F. Mollica, "Overview: Ethical Issues in Contemporary Psychiatry," *American Journal of Psychiatry* 133 (February 1976): 125–136; Bernard L. Bloom and Shirley J. Asher, eds., *Psychiatric Patient Rights and Patient Advocacy: Issues and Evidence* (New York: Human Sciences Press, 1982), 59–82.

76. "Removing the Mental-Illness Stigma," *New York Times*, 18 November 1977, 26.

77. Rosalynn Carter, "We Have to Stop Running Away," *McCall's*, June 1978, 121.

78. "The Campaign: McGovern's First Crisis: The Eagleton Affair" and "The Most Common Mental Disorder," *Time*, 7 August 1972, 11–17. The Montana Association for Mental Health wrote to President Nixon to highlight the unfortunate knee-jerk reaction to Eagleton's "courageous disclosure" and called for a national commitment to mental health. See Mrs. Roy Hellander to President Nixon, 10 August 1972, [GEN] HE 1–5 Mental Disorders 1/1/71–, White House Central Files, Richard Nixon Presidential Library, Yorba Linda, California.

79. See George McGovern, *Terry: My Daughter's Life and Death Struggle with Alcoholism* (New York: Villard, 1996).

80. Fieve, *Moodswing*, 12–13. For an account of the Eagleton case, see Joshua M. Glasser, *The Eighteen-Day Running Mate: McGovern, Eagleton, and a Campaign in Crisis* (New Haven, CT: Yale University Press, 2012).

81. "The Most Common Mental Disorder," *Time*, 7 August 1972, 14, 17; Fieve, *Moodswing*, 160–161. See also Joshua Wolf Shenk, *Lincoln's Melancholy: How Depression Challenged a President and Fueled his Greatness* (New York: Houghton Mifflin, 2005).

82. For the broader context, see Jack Drescher and Joseph P. Merlino, eds., *American Psychiatry and Homosexuality: An Oral History* (New York: Routledge, 2012); Peter Conrad and Joseph Schneider, *Deviance and Medicalization: From Badness to Sickness* (1980; repr., Philadelphia: Temple University Press, 1992), 204–209.

83. "Remarks by Rosalynn Carter, Alexandria, Virginia Rally," 23 October 1976, Box 1, Records of the First Lady's Office: Mary Hoyt's Press Releases and Speeches Files, Jimmy

Carter Presidential Library. For the statistic, see "Carter Proposes $15 Million to Fight 10 Major Killers," *Atlanta Daily World*, 9 October 1973.

84. For context, see Peter G. Bourne, *Jimmy Carter: A Comprehensive Biography from Plains to Postpresidency* (New York: Scribner, 1997), 208. I am grateful for very helpful e-mail correspondence with Peter Bourne in 2013 and 2016.

85. Patrick Anderson, *Electing Jimmy Carter: The Campaign of 1976* (Baton Rouge: Louisiana State University Press, 1994), 123–124. This sensibility was shaped by Carter's Baptist upbringing and his mother's job as a nurse in Plains, Georgia. See Carter, *Why Not the Best?* 134–135.

86. Grob, "Public Policy and Mental Illnesses," 429. Grob discusses the shift in emphasis from "mental illness" to "mental health" in the commission's title.

87. "Rosalynn's Agenda in the White House," *New York Times*, 20 March 1977.

88. Memo from Peter Bourne to Stuart Eizenstat, 27 January 1975, Box 19, Health Care, 4/70–2/75, 1976 Presidential Campaign Issues Office–Stuart Eizenstat, Jimmy Carter Presidential Library. See also Memo from Bourne to Mrs. Carter, December 6, 1976, Box 28, Carter, Rosalynn, 12/6/76–7/11/78, Records of Peter Bourne, Jimmy Carter Presidential Library.

89. Jimmy Carter, "Health Care Legislation Message to the Congress," 25 April, 1977, in *Public Papers of the Presidents of the United States: Jimmy Carter, 1977*, Book 1 (Washington, DC: U.S. Government Printing Office, 1978), 718.

90. Jimmy Carter, "President's Commission on Mental Health," in *Public Papers of the Presidents: Jimmy Carter, 1977*, Book 1, 185.

91. See "Mr. Carter's Class Struggle," *Washington Post*, 7 May 1978.

92. "President's Commission on Mental Health," 186.

93. Rosalynn Carter quoted in Myra G. Gutin, "Rosalyn Carter in the White House," in *The Presidency and Domestic Policies of Jimmy Carter*, ed. Herbert D. Rosenbaum and Alexej Ugrinsky (Westport, CT: Greenwood Press, 1994), 519.

94. "Removing the Mental-Illness Stigma."

95. "President's Commission on Mental Health," 188.

96. Rosalynn Carter, *First Lady from Plains* (Boston: Houghton Mifflin, 1984), 272–277. For the commission's many challenges, see Grob, "Public Policy and Mental Illnesses."

97. Thomas E. Bryant, "The Senate Report on Marijuana," *Washington Post*, 18 October 1974.

98. Memo from Thomas Bryant to Bob Haverly, 3 September 1976, Box 39, Pre-Presidential Campaign, Issues Office, Jimmy Carter Presidential Library.

99. Thomas E. Bryant, introduction to Richard C. Schroeder, *The Politics of Drugs: Marijuana to Mainlining* (Washington, DC: Congressional Quarterly, 1975), vii.

100. Thomas E. Bryant, "Fragmenting the Care System for the Mentally Ill," *New York Times*, 19 June 1981. For comparative hospital costs of fourteen countries, see Table 9 in Government Research Corporation, "Policy Outline on National Health Reform," 4th

draft, 19 January 1989, OA/IO 04810, Health (File I)–National Health Reform [2], Bush Presidential Records, Domestic Policy Council Files, George Bush Presidential Library, College Station, Texas.

101. Carter, "We Have to Stop Running Away," 198. "Health for All" was the slogan of the World Health Organization's Alma Ata Declaration of September 1978. See *Alma-Alta 1978: Primary Health Care* (Geneva: World Health Organization, 1978).

102. "Carter Mental Health Group under Attack," *Washington Post*, 10 August 1977. Bryant wrote a memo to Bourne on 10 February 1977 that stated that he preferred a "qualified citizen" committee membership rather than purely "representational" membership: Box 28, Folder 10, Records of Peter Bourne, Jimmy Carter Presidential Library. For the quotation, see Thomas E. Bryant to Ford H. Kuramoto, 8 March 1978, Box 37, Folder 12, Records of the Office of the Assistant for Public Liaison–Ed Smith's Subject Files, Jimmy Carter Presidential Library.

103. "Mental Health Systems Legislation," 15 May 1979, in *Public Papers of the Presidents: Jimmy Carter, 1979*, Book 1, 859–862.

104. *President Carter 1978* (Washington, DC: Congressional Quarterly, 1979), 47.

105. "Text of the Final Debate between President Ford and Mr. Carter," in *The Presidential Campaign 1976*, vol. 3, 151.

106. Kennedy's speech to the United Auto Workers, Los Angeles Convention Center is often cited as a key moment in the health debates of the 1970s: see "Kennedy Chides Carter on Lack of Health Reform," *Los Angeles Times*, 17 May 1977. For Kennedy's challenge to the Nixon administration, see "Thunder in the AMA," *Newsweek*, 5 July 1971. For Kennedy's single-payer tax-based insurance plan, see Burton Hersh, *The Shadow President: Ted Kennedy in Opposition* (South Royalton, VT: Steerforth Press, 1997), 24–27; Peter S. Callinos, ed., *The Last Lion: The Fall and Rise of Ted Kennedy* (New York: Simon & Schuster, 2009), 198–200.

107. *President Carter 1978*, 47. Kennedy pushed Califano on Carter's health insurance plans in Congress in January 1977: see "Joseph A, Califano Jr., to be Secretary of Health, Education, and Welfare," 18–22. For Kennedy's attack on Carter at the Democratic convention, see Timothy Stanley, *Kennedy vs. Carter: The 1980 Battle for the Democratic Party's Soul* (Lawrence: University Press of Kansas, 2010), 85–87. For the fiscal problems Carter faced, see Philip J. Funigiello, *Chronic Politics: Health Care Security from FDR to George W. Bush* (Lawrence: University Press of Kansas, 2005), 187–193. For the tensions between these incremental and sweeping views of health reform, see Alan Derickson, *Health Security for All: Dreams of Universal Health Care in America* (Baltimore, MD: Johns Hopkins University Press, 2005), 142–143, 150–151.

108. "McGovern Charges Carter Has Broken Economic and Welfare Pledges," *New York Times*, 8 May 1977, 14.

109. "Rosalynn's One Refrain," *Boston Globe*, 27 July 1979, 2. For Rosalynn Carter's view of Califano, see *First Lady from Plains*, 164, 278.

110. "Carter Backs a $500 Million Plan to Improve Mental Health Care," *New York Times*, 28 April 1978.

111. Some reporters thought that Carter's health insurance proposal, which would have been funded by a combination of private and public finances, was not dissimilar to a proposal by Elliot Richardson, Nixon's secretary of health, education, and welfare. See "Califano Gives More Details on Carter Health Plan," *New York Times*, 28 March 1979.

112. See Ruth Daniloff, "Working Out: Behind the Green Door," *Washington Post*, 25 March 1979.

113. Bourne's resignation letter was published in the *New York Times* on 21 July 1978.

114. Garland A. Haas, *Jimmy Carter and the Politics of Frustration* (Jefferson, NC: McFarland & Co, 1992), 63; Carter, *First Lady from Plains*, 277–278.

115. Jimmy Carter, "Mental Health Systems Act: Remarks on Signing S. 1177 into Law," 7 October 1980, *Public Papers of the Presidents, Jimmy Carter, 1980–81*, Book 3 (Washington, DC: U.S. Government Printing Office, 1981), 2098–2104.

116. Rosalynn Carter with Susan K. Golant, *Helping Someone with Mental Illness: A Compassionate Guide for Family, Friends, and Caregivers* (New York: Times Books, 1998), 273.

117. For a view of the "passionless presidency," see John Dumbrell, *The Carter Presidency: A Re-Evaluation* (Manchester: Manchester University Press, 1995), 10, 33.

118. See Grace Robinson, "The End of the Beginning," *The Abolitionist* 9 (September 1979): 1–4. On Szasz's idea of the "therapeutic state," see Jeffrey A. Schaler, *Szasz under Fire: The Psychiatric Abolitionist Faces His Critics* (Chicago: Open Court, 2004), 139–178.

119. Robert N. Bellah, "Human Conditions for a Good Society," *St. Louis Post-Dispatch*, 25 March 1979, 8–11, reprinted in Daniel Horowitz, ed., *Jimmy Carter and the Energy Crisis of the 1970s*, 73–80. For discussion of Bellah and Carter, see Horowitz, *The Anxieties of Affluence: Critiques of American Consumer Culture, 1939–1979* (Amherst: University of Massachusetts Press, 2004), 218–224.

120. On the *National Plan for the Chronically Mentally Ill* (Washington, DC: Department of Health and Human Services, 1980) and its "quiet success" in the 1980s, see Gerald N. Grob and Howard H. Goldman, *The Dilemma of Federal Mental Health Policy: Radical Reform or Incremental Change?* (New Brunswick, NJ: Rutgers University Press, 2006), 115–147.

121. "Removing the Mental-Illness Stigma," *New York Times*, 20 March 1977 and "Rosalynn's Agenda in the White House," *New York Times*, 20 March 1977.

122. *NIMH-Funded Research Concerning Homeless Mentally Ill Persons: Implications for Policy and Practice* (Washington, DC: Department of Health and Human Services 1986), 15. Vice-President Bush lumped together mental illness, homelessness, and drug abuse in the Republican presidential candidates' debate held in Atlanta on 28 February 1988. See also Isaac and Armat, *Madness in the Streets*, 4–5; Christopher Jencks, *The Homeless* (Cambridge, MA: Harvard University Press, 1994), 22–24.

123. See David L. Ginsberg, "Health Care Policy in the Reagan Administration: Rhetoric and Reality," *Public Administration Quarterly* 11 (Spring 1987): 59–70.

124. Margaret M. Heckler, *Report of the Secretary's Task Force on Black and Minority Health* (Washington, DC: Department of Health and Human Services, 1985).

125. Joseph A. Califano Jr., *America's Health Care Revolution* (New York: Random House, 1986), 10. In January 1983, the *American Journal of Public Health* questioned if Reagan could be indicted for betraying the priorities of Carter's Surgeon General Julius Richmond.

126. Ronald Reagan, "Inaugural Address," 20 January 1981, in *Public Papers of the Presidents of the United States: Ronald Reagan, 1981*, Book 1 (Washington, DC: U.S. Government Printing Office, 1982), 2.

127. Reported cases of rape and child abuse were also on the rise; see "Rape and Other Forms of Violence," *American Journal of Psychiatry* 133 (April 1976): 405–437.

128. Albert R. Jonsen and Jeff Stryker, eds., *The Social Impact of AIDS in the United States* (Washington, DC: National Academy Press, 1993), 12.

CHAPTER 2 — WOUNDS AND MEMORIES OF WAR

1. "Ex-Hostages May Suffer Same Effects as POWs, Psychiatrists Say," *Los Angeles Times*, 23 January 1981; "After 'Argo,' a New Spotlight on a Hostage Crisis," *New York Times*, 27 November 2012.

2. Jimmy Carter used the phrase "get the Vietnamese war over with" on the campaign trail through 1976. Three months into Carter's presidency the *Washington Post* noted that he was making "a major effort to make good" on his campaign pledge to "get the Vietnamese war over with": "Those Who Served (Cont.)," *Washington Post*, 11 April 1977.

3. Ronald Reagan, "Restoring the Margin of Safety," Veterans of Foreign Wars Convention, Chicago, 18 August 1980, accessed 8 December 2016, www.reagan.utexas.edu/archives/reference/8.18.80.html.

4. Jimmy Carter, "Vietnam Era Veterans," 10 October 1978, in *Public Papers of the Presidents of the United States: Jimmy Carter, 1978*, Book 2 (Washington, DC: U.S. Government Printing Office, 1979), 1741.

5. Robert N. Bellah, "Civil Religion in America," "Religion in America," special issue, *Daedalus* 96 (Summer 1988): 1–21.

6. "President Awards Medal, Says Troops Weren't Permitted to Win in Vietnam," *Washington Post*, 25 February 1981.

7. See Peter J. Wallison, *Ronald Reagan: The Power of Conviction and the Success of His Presidency* (Boulder, CO: Westview Press, 2004).

8. Vet Centers had counseled over 52,000 Vietnam veterans by the summer of 1981; "Vietnam Veterans Are Wondering Whether They Have a Friend in the VA," *National Journal*, 18 July 1981, 1291–1295. See also "Pulling the Rug from under Vietnam Vets Again," *Washington Post*, 15 March 1981.

9. See, for example, "The Forgotten Warriors," *Time*, 13 July 1981, 18–25.

10. Ronald Reagan, *An American Life* (New York: Simon and Schuster, 1990), 451.

11. *Dog Day Afternoon* is based on the case of Vietnam veteran John Wojtowicz, who tried to rob a bank in 1972 to pay for the sex change of his partner.

12. Tim O'Brien, "The Violent Vet," *Esquire*, December 1979, 96. For the rise of violent crime, see Dane Archer and Rosemary Gartner, "Violent Acts and Violent Times:

A Comparative Approach to Postwar Homicide Rates," *American Sociological Review* 41 (December 1976): 937–963.

13. See Christian G. Appy, *The Working-Class War: American Combat Soldiers and Vietnam* (Chapel Hill: University of North Carolina Press, 1993).

14. See Fred Turner *Echoes of Combat: Trauma, Memory, and the Vietnam War* (1996; repr., Minneapolis: University of Minnesota Press, 2001), 54.

15. Paul Schrader, *Taxi Driver* (1976; repr., London: Faber and Faber, 1990), 1.

16. See Susan Jeffords, *Hard Bodies: Hollywood Masculinity in the Reagan Era* (New Brunswick, NJ: Rutgers University Press, 1994), 17.

17. Keith Beattie, *The Scar That Binds: American Culture and the Vietnam War* (New York: New York University Press, 1998), 5, 7. Beattie notes that Reagan used the language of unity at the National Vietnam Veterans Memorial dedication ceremony (54).

18. Eric T. Dean Jr., *Shook over Hell: Post-Traumatic Stress, Vietnam, and the Civil War* (Cambridge, MA: Harvard University Press, 1997), 10–12. See also Jeremy Kuzmarov, *The Myth of the Addicted Army: Vietnam and the Modern War on Drugs* (Amherst: University of Massachusetts Press, 2009).

19. "Ford says Vietnam Veterans Won't Be Forgotten," *Boston Globe*, 29 October 1974; "Ford Pledges 70,000 Jobs for Veterans," *Washington Post*, 29 October 1974. For criticism of Nixon and Ford, see "The Forgotten Veterans," *New York Times*, 2 June 1974.

20. "Foreword by Peter G. Bourne, M.D.," in *Stress Disorders among Vietnam Veterans: Theory, Research, and Treatment*, ed. Charles R. Figley (New York: Bruner/Mazel, 1978), vii–ix. For the claim about World War II, see Mardi J. Horowitz and George F. Solomon, "A Prediction of Delayed Stress Response Syndromes in Vietnam Veterans," *Journal of Social Issues* 31 (Fall 1975): 67–80 (republished in Figley's volume).

21. Jimmy Carter, "Rural Health," in *The Presidential Campaign 1976*, vol. 1, part 1 (Washington, DC: U.S. Government Printing Office, 1978), 606, 599.

22. Jimmy Carter, "Vietnam Veterans Week, 1979 Remarks at a White House Reception," 30 May 1979, *Public Papers of the Presidents, Jimmy Carter, 1979*, Book 1 (Washington, DC: U.S. Government Printing Office, 1981), 445.

23. See "Carter, and U.S., Forget Vietnam Vets," *Washington Post*, 29 May 1978.

24. "Angry Vietnam Veterans Charging Federal Policies Ignore Their Needs," *New York Times*, 5 February 1979.

25. "Aid Urged for Vietnam Veterans," *New York Times*, 28 January 1979.

26. "For Vietnam Veterans Week: Veterans, Stand Up and Be Counted," *The Veteran* 9 (Spring 1979): 1.

27. See, for example, Peter Sills, *Toxic War: The Story of Agent Orange* (Nashville, TN: Vanderbilt University Press, 2014).

28. Eric Dean notes that estimates of those experiencing PTSD range from 500,000 to 800,000, even though by 1978 only 94,630 veterans had been diagnosed by VA psychiatrists as having neuropsychiatric conditions: Dean, *Shook over Hell*, 15. A mid-1990s survey

identified significantly higher rates of PTSD among African American and Hispanic American veterans. See *Matsunaga Vietnam Veterans Project: Final Report* (Washington, DC: National Center for Post-Traumatic Stress Disorder, 1996). For an earlier discussion of cultural variables, see Erwin Randolph Parson, "Ethnicity and Traumatic Stress: The Intersecting Point in Psychotherapy," in *Trauma and Its Wake: The Study and Treatment of Posttraumatic Stress Disorder*, ed. Charles R. Figley (New York: Brunner/Mazel, 1985), 314–337.

29. For Vietnam as a metaphor, see Michael Anderegg, ed., *Inventing Vietnam: The War in Film and Television* (Philadelphia: Temple University Press, 1991) and Brian Balogh, "From Metaphor to Quagmire: The Domestic Legacy of the Vietnam War," in *After Vietnam: Legacies of a Lost War*, ed. Charles E. Neu (Baltimore, MD: Johns Hopkins University Press, 2000), 24–55.

30. Ron Kovic, *Born on the Fourth of July* (1976; repr., New York: Akashic Books, 2005), 30.

31. For Kovic's speech, see *The Official Proceedings of the Democratic National Convention* (Washington, DC: Library of Congress, 1976), 380. For the case of Erwin Pawelski (who died soon after this incident), see "Helpless Patient 'Lost' for 27 Hours," *Los Angeles Times*, 22 May 1975.

32. The critical Nader Report on the VA was published as Paul Starr, *The Discarded Army: Veterans after Vietnam: The Nader Report on Vietnam Veterans and the Veterans Administration* (New York: Charterhouse, 1973).

33. Jon Nordheimer, "Postwar Shock Besets Ex-GIs," *New York Times*, 21 August 1972. For the Miami Beach demonstration, see Jerry Lembcke, *The Spitting Image: Myth, Memory, and the Legacy of Vietnam* (1998; repr., New York: New York University Press, 2000), 101–105.

34. For a critique of *Coming Home*, see Appy, *Working-Class War*, 310–314.

35. Seth Cagin, "Coming Home," press release, Stills File, Wisconsin Center for Film and Theater Research, University of Wisconsin-Madison; Christopher Lasch, *The Minimal Self: Psychic Survival in Troubled Times* (New York: Norton, 1984), 76.

36. For Kovic's working-class background, see Appy, *Working-Class War*, 13–14, 61–62.

37. See Regula Fuchs, *Remembering Viet Nam: Gustav Hasford, Ron Kovic, Tim O'Brien and the Fabrication of American Memory* (Bern: Peter Lang, 2010), 79.

38. Judith Herman, *Trauma and Recovery* (New York: Basic Books, 1992), 2.

39. See Arthur S. Blank Jr., "The Wounds That Would Not Heal," *Vietnam Veterans Review*, 1 July 1981, 5, 14.

40. For the reception of *Platoon*, see Toby Glenn Bates, *The Reagan Rhetoric: History and Memory in 1980s America* (De Kalb: Northern Illinois University Press, 2011), 81–86.

41. Michael Herr, *Dispatches* (1977; repr., New York: Vintage, 1991), 209.

42. Marita Sturken, *Tangled Memories: The Vietnam War, the AIDS Epidemic, and the Politics of Remembering* (Berkeley: University of California Press, 1997), 2.

43. For these patterns, see Milton J. Bates, *The Wars We Took to Vietnam: Cultural Conflict and Storytelling* (Berkeley: University of California Press, 1996), 137.

44. Robert Jay Lifton, *Home from the War: Vietnam Veterans, Neither Victim nor Executioner* (New York: Simon and Schuster, 1973), 38.

45. Ibid., 65.

46. Ibid., 67.

47. Ibid. For medical neutrality and the goals of the Medical Civic Action Program, see Michael L. Gross, *Bioethics and Armed Conflict: Moral Dilemmas of Medicine and War* (Cambridge, MA: MIT Press, 2006), 175–210.

48. Lifton, *Home from the War*, 37.

49. Beattie, *The Scar That Binds*, 63, 58. On "grunts," see Tim O'Brien, *The Things They Carried* (New York: HarperCollins, 1990), 5, 18.

50. Philip J. Caputo, *A Rumor of War* (1977; repr., London: Pimlico, 1996), xv.

51. Ibid., xix. For narrative memory, see Cathy Caruth, *Unclaimed Experience: Trauma, Narrative, and History* (Baltimore, MD: Johns Hopkins University Press, 1996), 153.

52. See Mardi Horowitz, *Stress Response Syndromes* (New York: Aronson, 1976); Sarah A. Haley, "Treatment Implications of Post-Combat Stress Response Syndromes for Mental Health Professionals," in *Stress Disorders among Vietnam Veterans: Theory, Research, and Treatment*, ed. Charles R. Figley (New York: Bruner/Mazel, 1978), 254–267.

53. Kovic, *Born on the Fourth of July*, 16.

54. Patricia Walsh, *Forever Sad the Hearts* (New York: Avon, 1982).

55. Kathryn Marshall, *In the Combat Zone: An Oral History of American Women in Vietnam, 1966–1975* (Boston: Little Brown, 1987), 14. The prevalence of PTSD among women veterans was not widely recognized until the 1990s; see David H. Price and Jo Knox, "Women Vietnam Veterans with Posttraumatic Stress Disorder: Implications for Practice," *Affilia* 11 (Spring 1996): 61–75.

56. Hagopian, *The Vietnam War in American Memory*, 408.

57. "Honoring Vietnam Veterans—At Last," *Newsweek*, 22 November 1982, 80–86.

58. This line of reasoning follows that of Marita Sturken in *Tangled Memories*, 12–13.

59. "Vets the Victims of Clumsy VA Giant," *Chicago Tribune*, 18 January 1976.

60. "Vietnam Era Veterans Update: Background Report by Office of Media Liaison," 14 October 1978, Box 39, Folder 3, Office of Counsel to the President, Jimmy Carter Presidential Library, Atlanta, Georgia.

61. Penny Coleman, *Flashback: Posttraumatic Stress Disorder, Suicide, and the Lessons of War* (Boston: Beacon Press, 2006), 11.

62. Caputo, *A Rumor of War*, 352.

63. Ibid., 352.

64. See Edward M. Colbach and Matthew D. Parrish, "Army Mental Health Activities in Vietnam: 1965–1970," in *The Vietnam Veteran in Contemporary Society* (Washington, DC: Department of Medicine and Surgery, 1972), III-36.

65. Peter G. Bourne, *Men, Stress, and Vietnam* (Boston: Little, Brown, 1970), 3; Peter G. Bourne, "Some Observations on the Psychosocial Phenomena Seen in Basic

Training," *Psychiatry* 30 (May 1967): 187–197; Peter G. Bourne, "Military Adjustment," in *Human Behavior in a Changing Society*, ed. James F. Adams (Boston: Holbrook Press, 1973), 144–145.

66. On basic training, see R. Wayne Eisenhart, "You Can't Hack It Little Girl: A Discussion of the Covert Psychological Agenda of Modern Combat Training," *Journal of Social Issues* 31, no. 4 (Fall 1975): 13–23.

67. Peter G. Bourne, ed., *The Psychology and Physiology of Stress* (New York: Academic Press, 1969), 10.

68. Ibid., xiii.

69. Ibid., 226.

70. Ibid., xxvi; Colbach and Parrish, "Army Mental Health Activities in Vietnam," III–39.

71. Bourne, *The Psychology and Physiology of Stress*, 5.

72. Bourne, *Men, Stress, and Vietnam*, 78–79.

73. Turner, *Echoes of Combat*, 18.

74. Horowitz, *Stress Response Syndromes*, 41–42.

75. Chaim F. Shatan, "The Grief of Soldiers: Vietnam Combat Veterans Self-Help Movement," *American Journal of Orthopsychiatry* 43 (July 1973): 645–646.

76. "Release of McCain's Medical Records Provides Unusually Broad Psychological Profile," *New York Times*, 6 December 1999. On reintegration, see Richard C. W. Hall and Patrick T. Malone, "Psychiatric Effects of Prolonged Asian Captivity: A Two-Year Follow-Up," *American Journal of Psychiatry* 133, no. 7 (1976): 786–790.

77. See Charles R. Figley and Seymour Leventman, eds., *Strangers at Home: Vietnam Veterans since the War* (1980; repr., New York: Praeger, 1990), xxvi–xxxi, 275–276. A comparable example is Fred Cherry, the African American colonel who underwent intense mental and physical stress as a POW in Hanoi. After the war, he continued to suffer from muscle spasms and he never fully recovered his sight or hearing, but he did not mention any lingering psychological symptoms. See Wallace Terry, *Bloods* (New York: Random House, 1984), 266–291.

78. "From Dakto to Detroit: Death of a Troubled Hero," *New York Times*, 26 May 1971; "New Public Enemy No. 1," *Time*, 28 June 1971, 20. For analysis, see Lifton, *Home from the War*, 39; Shatan, "The Grief of Soldiers," 643–644; Turner, *Echoes of Combat*, 50–51; Lembcke, *The Spitting Image*, 107–108.

79. "Viet Veteran Holds 3 at Gunpoint in Park before Surrendering," *Los Angeles Times*, 5 August 1974; "Vietnam Vets—How Many Time Bombs?," *Los Angeles Times*, 9 August 1974. See also "When Johnny Came Marching Home," *Los Angeles Times*, 28 March 1976.

80. Lembcke discusses the *New York Times* piece "Postwar Shock Is Found to Beset Veterans Returning from the War in Vietnam" (21 August 1972) that coincided with Kovic's disruption of the Republican National Convention; see Lembcke, *The Spitting Image*, 107–108.

81. Jimmy Carter, "Proclamation 4483—Granting Pardon for Violations of the Selective Service Act, August 4, 1964 to March 28, 1973," 21 January 1977, *The American*

Presidency Project, accessed 8 December 2016, www.presidency.ucsb.edu/ws/index.php?pid=7255&st=&st1=; Jimmy Carter, "Address to the American Legion Convention," 24 August 1976, in *The Presidential Campaign 1976*, vol. 1, part 1, 515–517.

82. Memo from Stuart Eizenstat to President Carter, 21 January 1977, Box 39, Folder 2, Office of Council to the President, Jimmy Carter Presidential Library.

83. Carter, "Address to the American Legion Convention," 589.

84. Stuart F. Feldman, "Vietnam Veterans Need Presidential Attention When the Pardon Is Announced," 7 December 1976, Box 39, Folder 2, Office of Council to the President, Jimmy Carter Presidential Library; "The Invisible Vietnam Veteran," *Washington Post*, 4 August 1976.

85. "Vietnam Era Veterans Update."

86. Jimmy Carter, "Vietnam Era Veterans," *Public Papers of the Presidents, Jimmy Carter, 1978*, Book 2, 1741.

87. "Vietnam Veterans Still Feel Chill from the White House," Washington Post, 28 April 1979.

88. Lifton, *Home from the War*, 78.

89. Ibid., 81. See Arthur Egendorf, "Vietnam Veteran Rap Groups and Themes of Postwar Life," *Journal of Social Issues* 31, no. 4 (Fall 1975): 111–124; Arthur Egendorf, *Healing from the War: Trauma and Transformation after Vietnam* (Boston: Houghton Mifflin, 1985).

90. Jacob Katzman, "From Outcast to Cliché: How Film Shaped, Warped and Developed the Image of the Vietnam Veteran, 1967–1990," *Journal of American Culture* 16 (Spring 1993): 7.

91. See Joel Brende and Erwin Parson, *Vietnam Veterans: The Road to Recovery* (New York: Plenum, 1985); Wilbur J. Scott, *The Politics of Readjustment: Vietnam Veterans Since the War* (1993; repr., New Brunswick, NJ: Transaction, 2012).

92. *Diagnostic and Statistical Manual of Mental Disorders*, 3rd rev. ed. (Washington, DC: American Psychiatric Association, 1987), 250. Flashbacks were included in this edition for the first time.

93. Figley and Leventman, *Strangers at Home*, 87.

94. Arthur Egendorf, *Legacies of Vietnam: Comparative Adjustment of Veterans and their Peers: A Study* (Washington, DC: U.S. Government Printing Office, 1981). For a skepticism about the PTSD construct, see Allan Young, *The Harmony of Illusions: Inventing Post-Traumatic Stress Disorder* (Princeton, NJ: Princeton University Press, 1997).

95. "Vietnam as a Metaphor," *Hospital and Community Psychiatry* 35 (July 1984): 655.

96. Reagan, *An American Life*, 451.

97. "The CIA's Murder Manual," *Washington Post*, 21 October 1984.

98. "1980 Republican Platform Text," *Congressional Quarterly*, 19 July 1980, 2032.

99. Peter Marin, "Coming to Terms with Vietnam: Settling Our Moral Debts," *Harper's*, December 1980, 41.

100. Gloria Emerson, *Winners and Losers*, rev. ed. (1985; repr., New York: Norton, 1992), xi.

101. Shatan, "The Grief of Soldiers," 650.

102. "After Vietnam: Voices of a Wounded Generation," *Washington Post*, 25 May 1980.

103. O'Brien, *The Things They Carried*, 68.

104. See Maria S. Bonn, "Can Stories Save Us? Tim O'Brien and the Efficiency of the Text," *Critique: Studies in Contemporary Fiction* 36 (Fall 1994): 2–15.

105. "What Are We Doing to Ourselves?," Winter Soldier Investigation: Testimony Given in Detroit, Michigan, on 31 January 1971 and 1 and 2 February 1971, accessed 8 December 2016, www2.iath.virginia.edu/sixties/HTML_docs/Resources/Primary/Winter_Soldier/WS_18_Ourselves.html.

106. O'Brien, *The Things They Carried*, 78.

107. Philip Caputo, *Indian Country* (London: Arrow, 1987), 131.

108. Ibid., 77.

109. Thomas Myers, *Walking Point: American Narratives of Vietnam* (New York: Oxford University Press, 1988), 225.

110. Caputo, *Indian Country*, 389.

111. Ibid., 390. See Peter M. Hayman, Rita Sommers-Flanagan, and John P. Parsons, "Aftermath of Violence: Posttraumatic Stress Disorder among Vietnam Veterans," *Journal of Counseling and Development* 65 (March 1987): 363–366.

112. Caputo, *Indian Country*, 391.

113. Ibid., 392.

114. Ibid., 414. For related clinical research, see Hillel Glover, "Survival Guilt and the Vietnam Veteran," *Journal of Nervous Mental Disorders* 172 (July 1984): 393–397.

115. Caputo, *Indian Country*, 495.

116. Ibid., 503.

117. Ibid., 504.

118. On post-combat dreams, see the Jungian analyst Harry A. Wilmer's article "Vietnam and Madness: Dreams of Schizophrenic Veterans," *Journal of the American Academy of Psychoanalysis* 10 (January 1982): 46–65.

119. Ronald Reagan, "Remarks at the Veterans Day Ceremony at the Vietnam Veterans Memorial," 11 November 1990, in *Public Papers of the Presidents of the United States: Ronald Reagan, 1988–89*, Book 2 (Washington, DC: U.S. Government Printing Office, 1991), 1496.

120. Bruce Joel Rubin, *Jacob's Ladder Screenplay* (New York: Applause, 1990), 179.

121. Robin Wood, *Hollywood from Vietnam to Reagan* (New York: Columbia University Press, 1986), 41–62.

122. "Text of Radio Address by President Bush," *New York Times*, 6 January 1991; George H. W. Bush, "Inaugural Address," 20 January 1989, in *Public Papers of the Presidents of*

the United States: George Bush, 1988–89, Book 1 (Washington DC: U.S. Government Printing Office, 1991), 3.

123. Ibid.

124. Cleveland Jordan, National Commander of Disabled American Veterans, to George Bush, 2 August 1991, OA/ID 06025, White House Office of Advance, Peggy Hazelrigg Files, George Bush Presidential Library, College Station, Texas.

125. The condensed report was published as Richard A. Kulka, William E. Schlenger, John A. Fairbanks, Richard L. Hough, B. Kathleen Jordan, Charles R. Marmar, and Daniel S. Weiss, *Trauma and the Vietnam War Generation: Report of Findings from the National Vietnam Veterans Readjustment Study* (New York: Brunner/Mazel, 1990). For clinical trials at the headquarters of the National Center for PTSD, see Matthew C. Weincke, "Escaping the Grip of PTSD," *Dartmouth Medicine*, Fall 2013, 37–43.

126. Richard A. Kulka, *Contractual Report of the Findings from the National Vietnam Readjustment Study*, vol. 1 (Research Triangle Park, NC: Research Triangle Institute, 1988), 1–4.

127. Eric T. Dean Jr., "'A Scene of Surpassing Terror and Awful Grandeur': The Paradoxes of Military Service in the American Civil War," *Michigan Historical Review* 21 (Fall 1995): 42.

128. Early media coverage included "Coming Home to Pain: Why Are So Many Gulf War Veterans So Sick?," *Newsweek*, 28 June 1993, 58–59; and "Tracking the Second Storm," *Newsweek*, 16 May 1994, 56–57. The first systematic report of Gulf War syndrome was in Research Advisory Committee on Gulf War Veterans' Illnesses, *Gulf War Illness and the Health of Gulf War Veterans* (Washington, DC: U.S. Government Printing Office, 2008). That study drew upon Robert J. Ursano and Ann E. Norwood, eds., *Emotional Aftermath of the Persian Gulf War* (Washington, DC: American Psychiatric Press, 1996).

129. Jay Himmelstein to Atul Gawandi, 16 September 1992, Box 205, Gulf War Veterans Health, White House Interdepartmental Working Group, William J. Clinton Presidential Library, Little Rock, Arkansas.

130. Jenna Pitchford, "From One Gulf to Another: Reading Masculinity in American Narratives of the Persian Gulf and Iraq Wars," *Literature Compass* 9, no. 5 (2012): 357–370.

131. See Patricia Sutker, Madeline Uddo, Kevin Brailey, and Albert N. Allain Jr., "War-Zone Trauma and Stress-Related Symptoms in Operation Desert Shield/Storm (ODS) Returnees," *Journal of Social Issues* 49 (Winter 1993): 33–49.

132. Gabe Hudson, *Dear Mr. President* (New York: Knopf, 2002), 41–57.

133. Anthony Swofford, *Jarhead* (New York: Scribner's, 2003), 40–41.

134. Ibid., 239, 135.

135. Ibid., 182–183. On PB pills, see Jenna Pitchford-Hyde, "Invisible Warriors: Trauma and Ethics in the Narratives of the Iraq Wars," in *America: Justice, Conflict, War*, ed. Amanda Gilroy and Marietta Messmer (Heidelberg: Verlag, 2016), 13–29.

136. Swofford, *Jarhead*, 251. See also Walter H. Capps, *The Unfinished War: Vietnam and the American Conscience*, 2nd ed. (1982; repr., Boston: Beacon, 1990); Appy, *Working-Class War*, 9–10.

CHAPTER 3 — ADDICTION AND THE WAR ON DRUGS

1. Edward M. Brecher, *Licit and Illicit Drugs* (Boston: Little, Brown, 1972), 183–186.

2. "Drug Abuse and Society: The 'Chemical Cop-Out,'" *New Pittsburgh Courier*, 3 November 1973.

3. "Progress Report of an Ad Hoc Panel on Drug Abuse" (7 September 1962), OA/ID 18188, War on Drugs (2), Nancy Kennedy Collection, Ronald Reagan Library, Simi Valley, California. This "moral deficiency" model persisted despite the *Robinson vs. California* case of 1962, which provided a constitutional framework for treating drug addiction as a disease rather than a criminal offense. See Robert G. Meyer and Christopher M. Weaver, *Law and Mental Health: A Case-Based Approach* (New York: Guilford Press, 2006), 208–212.

4. Richard M. Nixon, "Remarks about an Intensified Program for Drug Abuse Prevention and Control," 17 June 1971, *Public Papers of the Presidents, Richard Nixon, 1971* (Washington, DC: U.S. Government Printing Office, 1972), 738.

5. See Harold Kolansky and William T. Moore, "Effects of Marihuana on Adolescents and Young Adults," *Journal of the American Medical Association* 216, no. 3 (1971): 486–492. For an overview of the article, see "The Polemics of Pot," *Newsweek*, 3 May 1971, 109–110.

6. Peter Conrad, "Types of Medical Social Control," *Sociology of Health and Illness* 1, no. 1 (1979): 1–11; Robert Crawford, "Healthism and the Medicalization of Everyday Life," *International Journal of Health Services* 10, no. 3 (1980): 365–388. See also Peter Conrad and Joseph Schneider, *Deviance and Medicalization*, 110–145.

7. Peter G. Bourne and Ruth Fox, eds., *Alcoholism: Progress in Research and Treatment* (New York: Academic Press, 1973), xiii. The Department of Health, Education, and Welfare recorded the statistics of 23 deaths per 100,000 in 1950 from cirrhosis compared to 45 deaths per 100,000 in 1973: *Health, United States, 1975* (Washington, DC: U.S. Government Printing Office, 1976), 166.

8. James D. Isbister, "The National Alcohol Program: A Vital Component of the Alcohol, Drug Abuse, and Mental Health Administration," no date, www.ncbi.nlm.nih.gov/pmc/articles/PMC1437869/pdf/pubhealthrep00158-0002a.pdf.

9. *Alcohol and Health: Report from the Secretary of Health, Education, and Welfare* (New York: Scribner, 1973). On controlled drinking, see Mark B. Sobell and Linda C. Sobell, *Behavioral Treatment of Alcohol Problems: Individualized Therapy and Controlled Drinking* (New York: Plenum, 1978) and Mark B. Sobell and Linda C. Sobell, "Controlled Drinking after 25 Years: How Important Was the Great Debate?" *Addiction* 90, no. 9 (1995): 1149–1153.

10. Cited in Carolyn Wiener, *The Politics of Alcoholism: Building an Arena Around a Social Problem* (New York: Transaction, 1981), 1. Senator Harold Hughes chaired a Special Sub-Committee on Alcoholism and Narcotics in 1969. For statistics on dependency, see Ronald C. Kessler, Katherine A. McGonagle, Shanyang Zhao, Christopher B. Nelson, Michael Hughes, Suzann Eschleman, Hans-Ulrich Wittchen, and Kenneth S. Kendler, "Lifetime and 12-Month Prevalence of DSM-III-R Psychiatric Disorders in the United States: Results from the National Comorbidity Survey," *Archives of General Psychiatry* 51, no. 1 (1994): 8–19.

11. See Richard Nixon, "Address Accepting the Presidential Nomination at the Republican National Convention in Miami Beach, Florida," *The American Presidency Project*, accessed 8 December 2016, www.presidency.ucsb.edu/ws/index.php?pid=25968&st=&st1=.

12. See David E. Smith and George R. Gay, eds., *"It's So Good, Don't Even Try It Once": Heroin in Perspective* (Englewood Cliffs, NJ: Prentice-Hall, 1972).

13. Operation Intercept was initially successful in stopping the importation of marijuana from Mexico, but one consequence was the rise of heroin use among white high-school pupils in border towns.

14. For the racial implications of Nelson Rockefeller's campaign, see Michael Javen Fortner, *Black Silent Majority: The Rockefeller Drug Laws and the Politics of Punishment* (Cambridge, MA: Harvard University Press, 2015).

15. On fearmongering, see Edward Jay Epstein, *Agency of Fear: Opiates and Political Power in America* (1977; repr., London: Verso, 1990), 138–140.

16. See Kathleen J. Frydl, *The Drug Wars in America, 1940–1973* (Cambridge: Cambridge University Press, 2013), 362–364.

17. Dan Baum, *Smoke and Mirrors: The War on Drugs and the Politics of Failure* (Boston: Little, Brown, 1996), 5.

18. "Blacks Declare War on Dope," *Ebony*, June 1970, 31.

19. Donald Goines, *Dopefiend* (1971; repr., New York: Holloway House, 1999), 15.

20. See "King Heroin," *Ebony*, June 1971, 56–61; "Do You Know Any 12-Year Old Junkies?" *New York Times*, 4 January 1972.

21. Nixon, "Remarks about an Intensified Program for Drug Abuse Prevention and Control," 738.

22. For drug pushing in VA hospitals, see Jeff Donfeld to Egil Krogh, memo, 1 November 1971, Box 3, SAO–Veterans Administration, Geoffrey Shepherd Collection, White House Special Files, Richard Nixon Presidential Library, Yorba Linda, California. See also "Addict Runs Amuck with Rifle in Clinic," *New York Times*, March 31, 1973.

23. Lifton, *Home from the War*, 125–126.

24. Kuzmarov, *The Myth of the Addicted Army*, 44. See also Morgan F. Murphy and Robert H. Steele, *The World Heroin Problem* (Washington, DC: U.S. Government Printing Office, 1971); David J. Bentel and David E. Smith, "Drug Abuse in Combat: The Crisis of Drugs and Addiction among American Troops in Vietnam," *Journal of Psychedelic Drugs* 4, no. 1 (1971): 23–24.

25. Stewart Alsop, "Worse than My Lai," *Newsweek*, 24 May 1971, 108. This is critiqued in Starr, *The Discarded Army*, 115. See also "Vietnam Aftershocks," *Washington Post*, 24 March 1981.

26. Bental and Smith, "Drug Abuse in Combat," 24; Kuzmarov, *The Myth of the Addicted Army*, 45.

27. See Robert L. DuPont, "The Evolving Federal Substance Abuse Organization," *American Journal of Drug and Alcohol Abuse* 1, no. 1 (1974): 1.

28. For Nixon's opinion of Jaffe, see "The President: War on Drugs," *Newsweek*, 28 June 1971, 32–36.

29. See *Community Implications of Methadone Use in Treating Heroin Addiction* (Washington, DC: Public Technology, Inc., 1973), 24. Claudio Naranjo discussed the therapeutic properties of ibogaine in *The Healing Journey: New Approaches to Consciousness* (New York: Pantheon, 1974), but its anti-addiction properties were not widely understood until the 1980s.

30. See "Methadone Linked to Addict Deaths," *New York Times*, 2 February 1982. On methadone treatment, see Brecher, *Licit and Illicit Drugs*, 135–182; Jerome J. Platt and Christina Labate, *Heroin Addiction: Theory, Research, and Treatment* (New York: Wiley, 1976), 260–307. See also Eric C. Schneider, *Smack: Heroin and the American City* (Philadelphia: University of Pennsylvania Press, 2008), 159–181.

31. Gerald R. Ford, "Special Message to the Congress on Drug Abuse," 27 April 1976, in *Public Papers of the Presidents of the United States: Gerald R. Ford, 1976–77*, Book 2 (Washington, DC: U.S. Government Printing Office, 1979), 1218.

32. Ibid.

33. Ibid.

34. *Newsweek* covered the 32-part report in the period 1 February–4 March 1973. It was republished as *The Heroin Trail* (New York: New American Library, 1974).

35. *White Paper on Drug Abuse: A Report to the President from the Domestic Council Drug Abuse Task Force* (Washington, DC: U.S. Government Printing Office, 1975), 2.

36. Ibid., 6.

37. See Robert E. Shute, "The Impact of Peer Pressure on the Verbally Expressed Drug Attitudes of Male College Students," *American Journal of Drug and Alcohol Abuse* 2, no. 2 (1975): 231–243.

38. See Stewart L. Baker, "Drug Abuse in the United States Army," *Bulletin of the New York Academy of Medicine* 47, no. 6 (1971): 541, cited in Bentel and Smith, "Drug Abuse in Combat," 23.

39. "Kids and Heroin: The Adolescent Epidemic," *Time*, 16 March 1970, 16.

40. "The Heroin Plague: What Can Be Done?" *Newsweek*, 5 July 1971, 27–32.

41. William S. Burroughs, *Junky* (1953; repr., London: Penguin, 1977), 43.

42. Burroughs thought that apomorphine (a non-addictive dopamine receptor stimulant) was a better cure for heroin addiction than methadone.

43. William S. Burroughs Jr., *Speed* and *Kentucky Ham* (New York: Overlook Press, 1993).

44. Mark Vonnegut, *The Eden Express: A Memoir of Insanity* (1975; repr.; New York: Seven Stories Press, 2002), 276. See also Chares J. Shields, *And So It Goes: Kurt Vonnegut: A Life* (New York: St Martin's Griffin, 2011), 266–268, 329–330.

45. An example of a longitudinal study is Lloyd Johnston, *Drugs and American Youth* (Ann Arbor, MI: Institute for Social Research, 1973), 21–27.

46. These concerns were voiced in 1977 by the director of the Baltimore outpatient center Man Alive: "Low-Grade Heroin Gives Rise to Addicts on Several Drugs Simultaneously," *The Baltimore Sun*, 8 May 1977. Low-grade Mexican heroin was also causing addiction problems in towns on the border between Mexico and the United States.

47. An influential study of child control is Peter Schrag and Diane Divoky, *The Myth of the Hyperactive Child* (New York: Pantheon, 1975).

48. Mark Lieberman, *The Dope Book: All about Drugs* (New York: Praeger, 1971), 134.

49. See the first lady's remarks at an Advertising Council Luncheon, 23 April 1982, Box 57, Mrs. Reagan (1), Carlton E. Turner Files, 1981–87, Ronald Reagan Presidential Library, Simi Valley, California.

50. Anonymous, *Go Ask Alice* (1971; repr., New York: Aladdin, 1998), 42.

51. Ibid., 68.

52. Ibid., 99.

53. Ibid., 157–158.

54. Ibid., 185.

55. See Allen Pace Nilsen, "The House that Alice Built," *School Library Journal* 26, no. 2 (1979): 109–112.

56. Unstable homes were thought to be a major factor in teenage drug use. See Nathan Straus III, *Addicts and Drug Abusers: Current Approaches to the Problem* (New York: Twayne, 1971) and Herbert S. Anhalt, "Drug Abuse in Junior High School Populations," *American Journal of Drug and Alcohol Abuse* 3, no. 4 (1976): 589–603.

57. J. Maurice Rogers, "Drug Abuse: Just What the Doctor Ordered," *Psychology Today*, September 1971, 16–24.

58. "Firms Expand Their Markets by Understating Drug Risks," *Washington Post*, 29 June 1976; "Board Acts to Weed Out the Doctors Who Push Drugs," *New York Times*, 6 April 1977.

59. Lois Armstrong, "Not So Funny Reality," *People*, 1 October 1979, 82–85; Andrea Tone, "Tranquilizers on Trial: Psychopharmacology in the Age of Anxiety," in *Medicating Modern America: Prescription Drugs in History*, ed. Andrea Tone and Elizabeth Siegel Watkins (New York: New York University Press, 2007), 156.

60. Tone, "Tranquilizers on Trial," 170. See also Milton Silverman and Philip R. Lee, *Pills, Profits, and Politics* (Berkeley: University of California Press, 1974), 168.

61. See David Herzberg, *Happy Pills in America: From Miltown to Prozac* (Baltimore, MD: Johns Hopkins University Press, 2009), 122–149.

62. Ruth Cooperstock and Henry L. Lennard, "Some Social Meanings of Tranquilizer Use," *Sociology of Health and Illness* 1, no. 3 (1979): 335, 344.

63. See "Danger Ahead! Valium: The Pill You Love Can Turn on You," *Vogue*, February 1975, 152–153. See also "Women and Tranquilizers," *Ladies' Home Journal*, November 1976, 164–167.

64. Richard Hughes and Robert Brewin, *The Tranquilizing of America: Pill Popping and the American Way of Life* (New York: Harcourt Brace Jovanovich, 1978), 8.

65. Barbara Gordon, *I'm Dancing as Fast as I Can* (1978; repr., New York: Beaufort, 2011), 34.

66. Ibid., 52.

67. Ibid., 94.

68. Ibid., 134.

69. Ibid., 148, 176.

70. Ibid., 289–290.

71. Mark Vonnegut was initially enthusiastic about vitamin pills to aid his recovery but tempered his view in the mid-1990s: Vonnegut, *Eden Express*, 275. It is perhaps surprising that Gordon does not cite accounts like *Eden Express* (especially as Vonnegut takes Thorazine after his breakdown); she only mentions her own documentary work with mental health patients.

72. Gordon, *I'm Dancing as Fast as I Can*, 309–310.

73. Anton Holden, *Prince Valium* (New York: Stein and Day, 1982), 179.

74. Ibid., 266.

75. William White, *Slaying the Dragon: The History of Addiction Treatment and Recovery in America* (Bloomington, IL: Chestnut Health Systems, 1998), 267–268.

76. "Woman of the Year," *Newsweek*, 29 December 1975, 19–23.

77. See Ford, *A Time to Heal*, 306–307.

78. Maryanne Borrelli, "Competing Conceptions of the First Ladyship: Public Responses to Betty Ford's '60 Minutes' Interview," *Presidential Studies Quarterly* 31, no. 3 (2001): 402, 409–410. See also Leesa Tobin, "Betty Ford as First Lady: A Woman for Women," *Presidential Studies Quarterly* 20, no. 4 (1990): 761–767.

79. National Symphony Orchestra Concert Invitation, 6 April 1976, Box 6, Hospital for Sick Children Benefit Performance, Betty Ford Papers, Gerald R. Ford Presidential Library, Ann Arbor, Michigan.

80. Betty Ford, "I Feel Like I've Been Reborn," *McCall's*, February 1975, 142. The Breast Cancer Conference on 22 November 1976 was held in collaboration with the National Cancer Institute and the American Cancer Society, but Mrs. Ford had to cancel her appearance. See John Robert Greene, *Betty Ford: Candor and Courage in the White House* (Lawrence: University Press of Kansas, 2004), 49–50.

81. Betty Ford, *The Times of My Life* (New York: HarperCollins, 1978), 127.

82. "The Strain on Betty," *Newsweek*, 18 August 1975, 21.

83. Myra MacPherson, "The Blooming of Betty Ford," *McCall's*, September 1975, 93. The piece noted the "rumors" that Mrs. Ford was "at times overly drugged" (120–121).

84. Hazelden expanded its operations to Florida in 1983, and in early 2014 it merged with the Betty Ford Center to form the Hazelden Betty Ford Foundation.

85. Betty Ford, *Betty: A Glad Awakening* (Garden City, NY: Doubleday, 1987), 61; Ford, *The Times of My Life*, 280–281.

86. Ford, *The Times of My Life*, 285.

87. Ibid., 292.

88. Ibid., 292–293. John Berryman satirized group therapy in his posthumously published semi-autobiographical novel *Recovery* (1973).

89. Ford, *Betty: A Glad Awakening*, 26.

90. Ibid., 128.

91. Ibid., 163.

92. Ibid., 164–165

93. Ibid., 166.

94. Ibid., 217. For analysis of Ford's and Gordon's narratives, see Herzberg, *Happy Pills in America*, 143–144.

95. See Mick Brown, "Stevie Nicks: A Survivor's Story," *The Telegraph*, 8 September 2007; Zoe Howe, *Stevie Nicks: Visions, Dreams and Rumours* (New York: Omnibus, 2014).

96. David Crosby and Carl Gottlieb, *David Crosby: Long Time Gone* (1988; repr., New York: Dell, 2007), 293–295, 358–360.

97. On the rise in cocaine use, see Susan Schober and Charles Schade, eds., *The Epidemiology of Cocaine Use and Abuse* (Washington, DC: Department of Health and Human Services, 1991), 8–9. On cocaine addiction in this period, see James A. Inciardi, *The War on Drugs: Heroin, Cocaine, Crime, and Public Policy* (Palo Alto, CA: Mayfield, 1986), 78–85.

98. Reagan, "Address to the Nation on the Campaign against Drug Abuse," 14 September 1986, in *Public Papers of the Presidents of the United States: Ronald Reagan, 1986*, Book 2 (Washington, DC: U.S. Government Printing Office, 1989), 1178. For spikes in media reports of crack during the period 1984–1992, see Steven R. Belenko, *Crack and the Evolution of Anti-Drug Policy* (Westport, CT: Greenwood Press, 1993), 23–31; Craig Reinarman and Harry G. Levine, *Crack in America: Demon Drugs and Social Justice* (Berkeley: University of California Press, 1997), 18–24.

99. Martha A. Morrison, *White Rabbit: A Doctor's Own Story of Addiction, Survival and Recovery* (1989; repr., New York: Berkeley, 1991), 248. See also Joanne Muzak, "'They Say the Disease Is Responsible': Social Identity and the Disease Concept in Drug Addiction," in *Unfitting Stories: Narrative Approaches to Disease, Disability, and Trauma*, ed. Valerie Raoul, Connie Canam, and Carla Peterson (Waterloo, Ontario: Wilfred Laurier University Press, 2007), 255–264.

100. Gordon, *I'm Dancing as Fast as I Can*, 313.

101. See Drug Abuse Policy Office Communication Implementation Strategies 1982–1986 (3), OA/ID 19043, Neil Romano Files, Ronald Reagan Presidential Library.

102. Carter argued that federal criminal penalties should be lifted for the possession of up to one ounce of marijuana. See Jimmy Carter, "Drug Abuse Message to the Congress,"

2 August 1977, in *Public Papers of the Presidents of the United States: Jimmy Carter, 1977*, Book 2 (Washington, DC: U.S. Government Printing Office, 1978), 1404.

103. Reagan, "Address to the Nation on the Campaign against Drug Abuse."

104. See James G. Benze Jr., *Nancy Reagan: On the White House Stage* (Lawrence: University Press of Kansas, 2005), 58–64; Kitty Kelley, *Nancy Reagan: The Unauthorized Biography* (New York: Simon and Schuster, 1991), 368–371, 389–395.

105. Benze, *Nancy Reagan*, 59.

106. For Carlton Turner's formative role in the Just Say No campaign, see Michael Massing, *The Fix* (1998; repr., Berkeley: University of California Press, 2000), 158–164.

107. "Takes 'Just Say No' Campaign to Oakland," *Los Angeles Times*, 27 November 1985.

108. Nancy Reagan's appearance on *Diff'rent Strokes* turned out to be ironic: Todd Bridges, one of the two African American leads, developed a crack habit in the mid-1980s, and Dana Plato, who played the daughter of white middle-class do-gooder Mr. Drummond, overdosed on Valium in 1978 as a fourteen-year-old and served a prison sentence after forging a prescription in 1992. (She died from an overdose in 1999 at the age of 34.)

109. Carlton Turner spoke on behalf of President Reagan at the Health Care Expo press conference, 29 November 1984, Box 30, Health Care Expo 1985, Washington, DC, Carlton E. Turner Files, Ronald Reagan Presidential Library.

110. Mrs. Reagan's remarks during President Reagan's "Address to the Nation on the Campaign against Drug Abuse," 1179.

111. Ibid., 1180. Mrs. Reagan stressed "The Need for Intolerance" in an op-ed piece in *The Washington Post*, 21 July 1986. On addiction and pregnancy, see Richard Brotman, David Hutson, and Frederic Suffet, eds., *Pregnant Addicts and their Children: A Comprehensive Care Approach* (New York: Center for Comprehensive Health Practice, 1985).

112. Barbara Shook Hazen's *Just Say No* (New York: Western, 1990) is more effective in involving the reader than earlier anti-drug books written for children.

113. See, for example, "Kids and Cocaine," *Newsweek*, 17 March 1986, 58–65; "In State-Funded Project, Ex-Drug Addicts take AIDS Warnings to the Streets," *Baltimore Sun*, 15 April 1986; "Spread of AIDS Virus Is Unabated among Intravenous Drug Takers," *New York Times*, 4 June 1987. The link between drugs and AIDS proved embarrassing for Reagan when in the fall of 1986 Carlton Turner proclaimed a direct connection between marijuana and AIDS and argued that extensive use weakens the immune system. Turner resigned when *Newsweek* covered the story: "Reagan Aide: Pot Can Make You Gay," *Newsweek*, 27 October 1986, 95. In 1988, Vice-President Bush was still claiming that "the AIDS crisis and the drug crisis are intertwined": Statement by the Vice-President on the AIDS Commission Report, 28 June 1988, OA/ID 23344, Emily Mead Files, George Bush Presidential Library, College Station, Texas.

114. See *A Woman Like You: Life Stories of Women Recovering from Alcoholism and Addiction* (San Francisco: Harper and Row, 1985); Nancy Dudley, "A Million Dollar Habit," *The*

Washingtonian, June 1987, 98–163; and Carrie Fisher, *Postcards from the Edge* (1987; repr., New York: Simon and Schuster, 2010).

115. Dudley, "A Million Dollar Habit," 100, 163.

116. Reagan, "Address to the Nation on the Campaign against Drug Abuse," 1181.

117. Kelley, *Nancy Reagan*, 523–524.

118. Todd Gold, "The Secret Drew Barrymore," *People*, 13 January 1989; Drew Barrymore and Todd Gold, *Little Girl Lost* (New York: Pocket Books, 1990).

119. George H. W. Bush, "Inaugural Address," 20 January 1989, in *Public Papers of the Presidents of the United States: George Bush, 1989*, Book 1 (Washington, DC: U.S. Government Printing Office, 1990), 3.

120. *Understanding Drug Treatment* (Washington, DC: Office of National Drug Control Policy, 1990); George Bush, "Remarks to the Academy of Television Arts and Sciences in Los Angeles, California," 2 March 1990, in *Public Papers of the Presidents of the United States: George Bush, 1990*, Book 1 (Washington, DC: U.S. Government Printing Office, 1991), 300.

121. See William N. Elwood, *Rhetoric in the War on Drugs: The Triumphs and Tragedies of Public Relations* (Westport, CT: Praeger, 1994), 27.

122. Bush, "Address to the Nation on the National Drug Control Strategy," 5 September 1989, in *Public Papers of the Presidents of the United States: George Bush, 1989*, Book 2, 1136. The National Drug Control Strategy document is available at: www.ncjrs.gov/pdffiles1/ondcp/119466.pdf

123. "Heroin Is Making Comeback in Lethal Tandem with Crack," *New York Times*, 21 July 1990; "From the Front Lines of the War on Drugs, A Few Small Victories," *New York Times*, 24 February 1991). See also Treaster's piece "20 Years of War on Drugs, and No Victory Yet," *New York Times*, 14 June 1992.

124. "Heroin and AIDS: Deadly Mix for Blacks," *Washington Post*, 10 January 1989. African Americans represented 22 percent of drug arrests in 1976, a figure that had increased to 41 percent in 1990. See Stephanie R. Bush-Baskette, "The War on Drugs as a War against Black Women," in *Crime Control and Women: Feminist Implications of Criminal Justice Policy*, ed. Susan L. Miller (Thousand Oaks, CA: Sage, 1998), 114. An estimated 25 percent of prisoners in 1980 was convicted for drug-related crimes, rising to 58 percent by 1992. See Michael Tonry, *Malign Neglect: Race, Crime, and Punishment in America* (Oxford: Oxford University Press, 1995), 81–82.

125. David T. Courtwright, *Forces of Habit: Drugs and the Making of the Modern World* (Cambridge, MA: Harvard University Press, 2001), 201–202.

126. On 25 January 1996, at Keene State College in New Hampshire, Hillary Clinton used the term "super-predator" to refer to perpetrators of drug-related violent crime who have no empathy for their victims. This term was seized upon as a covert criticism of crime in African American communities.

127. See John J. Dilulio Jr., "The Next War on Drugs: Targeting the Inner Cities," *The Brookings Review* 11, no. 3 (1993): 28–33. On MDMA, see "The Lure of Ecstasy," *Time*,

28 May 2000. These new voices include director Lisa McElaney, *Straight from the Heart: Stories of Mothers Recovering from Addiction* (1991); Jefferson A. Singer, *Message in a Bottle: Stories of Men and Addiction* (New York: Free Press, 1997); the Columbia University Health Department's *Go Ask Alice!* website (launched in 1993 as a forum for health issues, including addiction); and the Faces and Voices of Addiction Support Group, founded in 1991 by the Johnson Institute in collaboration with the Hazelden Foundation.

CHAPTER 4 — DEMENTIA AND THE LANGUAGE OF AGING

1. Gerald Ford, "Proclamation 4405, Thanksgiving Day, 1975," 4 November 1975, *The American Presidency Project*, 9 December 2016, www.presidency.ucsb.edu/ws/index.php?pid=72481&st=&st1=.

2. Robert N. Butler received the 1976 Pulitzer Prize for *Why Survive? Being Old in America* (New York: Harper and Row, 1975).

3. Richard Nixon, "Proclamation 4021: Thanksgiving Day, 1970," 5 November 1970, *The American Presidency Project*, accessed 9 December 2016, www.presidency.ucsb.edu/ws/index.php?pid=72476&st=&st1=. For proceedings, see White House Conference on Aging, Boxes 1–7, White House Central Files, Richard Nixon Presidential Library, Yorba Linda, California. See also the conference report, *Towards a National Policy on Aging*, vols. 1–2 (Washington, DC: U.S. Government Printing Office, 1971).

4. Press Release, 20 November 1975, Box 5, Senior Citizen Dinner, Betty Ford Papers, Gerald R. Ford Presidential Library, Ann Arbor, Michigan.

5. In fact, while the U.S. population grew by 4 percent from 1970 to 1974, the population over 65 grew by 9.2 percent in this period, from 20 to 22 million: William C. Martin and Albert J. E. Wilson III, ed., *Aging and Total Health* (St. Petersburg, FL: Eckerd College Gerontology Center, 1976), 3.

6. The criticism that Nixon entirely ignored the elderly is debatable because he extended the Older Americans Act in 1972. See *Public Papers of the Presidents of the United States: Richard M. Nixon, 1972* (Washington, DC: U.S. Government Printing Office, 1974), 461–485.

7. On the June 1974 AMA Conference, see Roger Sanjek, *Gray Panthers* (Philadelphia: University of Pennsylvania Press, 2009), 39–40. For policies on the elderly in the mid-1970s, see Carroll Estes, *The Aging Enterprise* (San Francisco: Jossey-Bass, 1979), 76–78.

8. Butler, *Why Survive?* 331. On Butler's response to the 1971 conference and the genesis of *Why Survive?*, see W. Andrew Achenbaum, *Robert N. Butler, MD: Visionary of Healthy Aging* (New York: Columbia University Press, 2013), 81–89.

9. For a summary of related research, see *Research on the Mental Health of Aging, 1960–1976* (Rockville, MD: National Institute of Mental Health, 1977), ix–xii. See also Television Commercial "Aged Health Care," 12 October 1976, Box E40, Ford Campaign Scripts, Campaign '76 Office: General Election, President Ford Committee Records, 1975–77, Gerald R. Ford Presidential Library.

10. Mickey C. Smith, "Portrayal of the Elderly in Prescription Drug Advertising," *The Gerontologist* 16, no. 4 (1976): 333; Butler, *Why Survive?* 255.

11. Memo on Health Care, September 1976, Box 5, Health Care, David Gergen Files, Gerald R. Ford Presidential Library.

12. For Kennedy's criticism of Ford's catastrophic care plan, see news article UP-081, Box 5, Health Care, David Gergen Files, Gerald R. Ford Presidential Library.

13. *Aging in America: The Federal Government's Role* (Washington, DC: Congressional Quarterly, 1989), 65, 74. A 1985 report recommended that the federal government "should be careful to avoid committing additional funding to long-term care," despite the estimation that 60 to 80 percent of long-term care was being provided by families or local communities. See "Report of the White House Working Group on Health Policy and Economics," 56–58, Health Policy [1985] (2) OA15701, Richard A. Davis Collection, Ronald Reagan Library, Simi Valley, California. Reagan sometimes mentioned the elderly, as he did in his "Message on the Observance of Grandparents Day" on 5 September 1986, in which he stressed that "grandparents are the backbone of voluntarism and charity": *Public Papers of the Presidents of the United States: Ronald Reagan, 1986*, Book 2 (Washington, DC: U.S. Government Printing Office, 1989), 1138.

14. See R. L. McNeely and John L. Colen, eds., *Aging and Minority Groups* (Beverly Hills, CA: Sage, 1983), 161–173.

15. Maggie Kuhn, *No Stone Unturned: The Life and Times of Maggie Kuhn* (New York: Ballantine, 1991), 151–153.

16. "A Clue to Senility," *Newsweek*, 23 August 1971, 40; Ewald W. Busse, "Duke Longitudinal Study 1: Senescence and Senility," in *Alzheimer's Disease: Senile Dementia and Related Disorders*, ed. Robert Katzman, Robert D. Terry, and Katherine L. Bick (New York: Raven Press, 1978), 67. It is important to recognize other pockets of research, such as the focus on middle-aged women at the University of Maryland's Center on Aging. This led to the 1978 volume *Uncharted Territory: Issues and Concerns of Women over 40*, which was updated twice in the 1980s.

17. "A Clue to Senility," 39; Butler, *Why Survive?* 259.

18. These figures were complicated by the fact that death certificates rarely gave organic brain disease as the primary cause of death.

19. Donald B. Tower, "Alzheimer's Disease—Senile Dementia and Related Disorders: Neurobiological Status," in *Alzheimer's Disease: Senile Dementia and Related Disorders*, ed. Robert Katzman, Robert D. Terry, and Katherine L. Bick (New York: Raven Press, 1978), 1.

20. Stephen Katz, *Disciplining Old Age: The Formation of Gerontological Knowledge* (Charlottesville, VA: University Press of Virginia, 1996).

21. Christopher Lasch, *The Culture of Narcissism: American Life in an Age of Diminishing Expectations* (New York: Norton, 1979), 207–217.

22. For unreliability in dementia stories, see Naomi Kruger, "The 'Terrifying Question Mark': Dementia, Fiction, and the Possibilities of Narrative," in *Popularizing Dementia: Public Expressions and Representations of Forgetfulness*, ed. Aagie Swinnen and Mark Schweda (Bielefeld: Transcript-Verlag 2015), 109–133.

23. "Presidential Candidates Respond to NCOA Queries for Their Stands on Major Issues for the Aging," *Perspectives on Aging* 5 (September–October 1976): 34.

24. Butler, *Why Survive?* 225. See also Gail Sheehy, *Passages: Predictable Crises of Adult Life* (New York: Dutton 1976). In 1995 Sheehy wrote a sequel, *New Passages: Mapping Your Life across Time*, which focused on the 40-plus age groups.

25. *The Fitness Challenge in the Later Years: An Exercise Program for Older Americans* (1968; repr., Washington, DC: U.S. Government Printing Office, 1975), 1. For the report on West Germany see David Gergen to Richard S. Brannon, 3 September 1976, Box 5, Heath Care, David Gergen Files, Gerald R. Ford Presidential Library. In 1982, the Reagan administration established a Council on Physical Fitness and Sports under the governance of the Department of Health and Human Services.

26. The Gerontological Society of America had been exploring these issues since the first White House Conference on Aging in 1961.

27. Jesse F. Ballenger, *Self, Senility, and Alzheimer's Disease in Modern America: A History* (Baltimore, MD: Johns Hopkins University Press, 2006), 128. For the WNBC-TV interview with Katzman, see "Robert Katzman–Faculty Collection," Samuel Gottesman Library, The Bronx, New York. In the mid-1980s, Katzman became the founding director of the Shiley-Marcos Alzheimer's Disease Research Center at University of California, San Diego.

28. By 1981, the elderly represented 12 percent of the population and more than 15 percent of them were living under the poverty line; Ted Tedrick, ed., *Aging: Issues and Policies for the 1980s* (New York: Praeger, 1985), 4.

29. See Ewald W. Busse and Dan G. Blazer, eds., *Handbook of Geriatric Psychiatry* (New York: Van Nostrand Reinhold, 1980), cited in Tedrick, *Aging*, 39.

30. Richard S. Schweiker to Jacob Clayman, president of the National Council of Senior Citizens, 27 November 1981, MC003 (050800–051999), White House Office of Records Management Subject Files, Box 12, Ronald Reagan Library. See *Toward an Independent Old Age: A National Plan for Research on Aging* (Bethesda, MD: U.S. Department of Health and Human Services, 1982); and "Healthy Older Adults" in *Healthy People: The Surgeon General's Report on Health Promotion and Disease Prevention* (Washington, DC: U.S. Public Health Service, 1979).

31. "White House Conference on Aging Reports", MC003 (050766) (4), White House Office of Records Management Subject Files, Box 12, Ronald Reagan Library.

32. On Alzheimer's advocacy, see Patrick Fox, "From Senility to Alzheimer's Disease: The Rise of the Alzheimer's Disease Movement," *The Milbank Quarterly* 67 (March 1989): 58–102.

33. Robert Katzman and Katherine Bick, *Alzheimer Disease: The Changing View* (San Diego, CA: Academic Press, 2000), xi.

34. See Margaret Lock, *The Alzheimer Conundrum: Entanglements of Dementia and Aging* (Princeton, NJ: Princeton University Press, 2013), 7, 37.

35. Katzman and Bick, *Alzheimer Disease*, 7.

36. Lock, *The Alzheimer Conundrum*, 10. See also Donald G. Stein, "Neurobehavioral Plasticity in the Aging Brain," in *Aging of the Brain*, ed. David Samuel (New York: Raven Press, 1983), 155–163.

37. Tower, "Alzheimer's Disease—Senile Dementia and Related Disorders," 5–6.

38. Ibid., 36.

39. Ibid., 35.

40. Butler, *Why Survive?* 231. A November 1983 symposium on this topic at the National Institute on Alcohol Abuse and Alcoholism at Washington University in St. Louis was published as *Nature and Extent of Alcohol Problems among the Elderly* (Washington, DC: U.S. Department of Health and Human Services, 1983).

41. Butler, *Why Survive?* 420. A more positive take on the opportunities available to late-century seniors is Harry R. Moody, *Abundance of Life: Human Development Policies of an Aging Society* (New York: Columbia University Press, 1988).

42. Sally Chivers, *The Silvering Screen: Old Age and Disability in Cinema* (Toronto: University of Toronto Press, 2011), 60. On Butler's aversion to seeing geriatrics as a discrete medical field, see Betty Friedan, *The Fountain of Age* (New York: Simon & Schuster, 1993), 422–423.

43. Janet Majerus, *Grandpa and Frank* (Philadelphia: Lippincott, 1976), 10, 181.

44. Andrea B. O'Connor, *Nursing: The Older Adult* (New York: American Journal of Nursing, 1978), 8.

45. See Derek Parker Royal, ed., *Philip Roth: New Perspectives on an American Author* (Westport, CT: Praeger, 2005), 130; David Brauner, *Philip Roth* (Manchester: Manchester University Press, 2007), 82.

46. For the zombie metaphor, see Susan Behuniak, "The Living Dead? The Construction of People with Alzheimer's Disease as Zombies," *Ageing and Society* 31 (January 2011): 70–92.

47. Robert E. Gard, *Beyond the Thin Line* (Madison, WI: Prairie Oak Press, 1992), 3.

48. On assisted identity, see Amelia DeFalco, *Uncanny Subjects: Aging in Contemporary Narrative* (Columbus: Ohio State University Press, 2010), 59.

49. Oliver Sacks, "The Great Awakening," *The Listener*, 25 October 1972, 522.

50. Oliver Sacks, *Awakenings* (1973; repr., London: Picador, 1991), xviii.

51. Ibid. xviii.

52. Falco, *Uncanny Subjects*, 59.

53. Roy Shafer, *Retelling a Life: Narration and Dialogue in Psychoanalysis* (New York: Basic Books, 1992), 10.

54. Sacks, *Awakenings*, 67.

55. Ibid, 62.

56. Ibid., 43.

57. Ibid., 55.

58. Ibid., 57. Sacks might have explored the psychoactive properties of L-DOPA more deeply as its side effects had been described as being similar to a bad LSD trip. See "Bush Abandons Victims of Parkinson's Disease," *New York Times*, 18 November 1989.

59. Sacks, *Awakenings*, 59.

60. Frank, *The Wounded Storyteller*, 75–96.

61. Sacks, *Awakenings*, 207.

62. Ibid., 202.

63. Ibid., 213.

64. Ibid., 219.

65. Oliver Sacks, *The Man Who Mistook His Wife for a Hat* (London: Picador, 1985), 106. For a fuller discussion, see Martin Halliwell, *Romantic Science and the Experience of Self: Transatlantic Crosscurrents from William James to Oliver Sacks* (1999; repr., London: Routledge, 2016).

66. On Korsakoff syndrome, see Maurice Victor and Betty Q. Banker, "Alcohol and Dementia," in *Alzheimer's Disease: Senile Dementia and Related Disorders*, 149–170.

67. Sacks, *The Man Who Mistook His Wife for a Hat*, 106.

68. Reagan, *An American Life* (1990; repr., New York: Simon and Schuster, 2011), 25, 130.

69. Ibid., 391.

70. Nancy Reagan, *My Turn: The Memoirs of Nancy Reagan* (New York: Random House, 1989), 112.

71. Ron Reagan, *My Father at 100: A Memoir* (New York: Viking, 2011), 205.

72. Nancy Reagan, *I Love You Ronnie: The Letters of Ronald Reagan to Nancy Reagan* (New York: Random House, 2000), 180; George Bush, "Building a Better America," 9 February 1989, in *Public Papers of the Presidents: George Bush, 1989*, Book 1 (Washington, DC: U.S. Government Printing Office, 1990), 78. *Newsweek* ran a cover story on Alzheimer's that year: "The Brain Killer," *Newsweek*, 18 December 1989, 54–56.

73. For Reagan's final public letter of 5 November 1994, see Lou Cannon, *President Reagan: The Role of a Lifetime* (1991; repr., New York: Public Affairs, 2000), xv.

74. Patti Davis, *The Long Goodbye* (New York: Plume, 2004), xi.

75. Patti Davis, *The Way I See It: An Autobiography* (New York: Putnam, 1992), 262.

76. Davis, *The Long Goodbye*, xii.

77. Davis, *The Way I See It*, 4, 21.

78. Davis, *The Long Goodbye*, 54.

79. Ibid., 55.

80. Ibid., 4.

81. Ibid., 180.

82. Ibid., 72.

83. Ibid., 43, 37.

84. Ibid, 63.

85. Ronald Reagan, "Remarks at the Republican National Convention in New Orleans, Louisiana," 15 August 1988, in *Public Papers of the Presidents of the United States: Ronald Reagan, 1988–89*, Book 2 (Washington, DC: U.S. Government Printing Office, 1991), 1085.

86. Davis, *The Long Goodbye*, 17, 25.

87. Ibid., 95.

88. Ibid., 51.

89. Ibid., 18.

90. Davis, *The Way I See It*, 294.

91. See Diana Friel McGowin, *Living in the Labyrinth: A Personal Journey through the Maze of Alzheimer's* (New York: Delacorte, 1993); Larry Rose, *Show Me the Way to Go Home* (Forest Knolls, CA: Elder Books, 1996); J. Bernlef, *Out of Mind*, trans. Adrienne Dixon (Boston: David R. Godine, 1989).

92. Jonathan Franzen, *How to Be Alone* (2002; repr., London: Harper, 2004), 11. See also Esther Strauss Smoller, *I Can't Remember: Family Stories of Alzheimer's Disease* (Philadelphia, PA: Temple University Press, 1997).

93. Roth, *Patrimony*, 189.

94. Ibid., 191.

95. Ibid., 173. See also Brauner, *Philip Roth*, 163–164.

96. Roth, *Patrimony*, 230.

97. Ibid., 233.

98. Ibid., 232.

99. Ibid., 237, 238.

100. Michael Ignatieff, *Scar Tissue* (London: Vintage, 1993), 95.

101. Ibid., 17, 20.

102. Ibid., 149.

103. Ibid., 47

104. Ibid., 101, 58.

105. John Wiltshire, "Biography, Pathography, and the Recovery of Meaning," *The Cambridge Quarterly* 29, no. 4 (2000): 419.

106. Ignatieff, *Scar Tissue*, 125.

107. Ibid., 130.

108. On loss of self, see Lock, *The Alzheimer Conundrum*, 25. See also Annette Leibling and Lawrence Cohen, eds., *Thinking about Dementia: Culture, Loss, and the Anthropology of Senility* (New Brunswick, NJ: Rutgers University Press, 2006).

109. Ignatieff, *Scar Tissue*, 168.

110. Ibid., 170.

111. Jimmy Carter, "Comprehensive Older Americans Act Amendments of 1978: Statement on Signing H.R. 12255 into Law," 18 October 1978, in *Public Papers of the Presidents of the United States: Jimmy Carter, 1978*, Book 2 (Washington, DC: U.S. Government Printing Office, 1979), 1794. For criticism of the Administration on Aging, see William Bechill, "Politics of Aging and Ethnicity," in *Ethnicity and Aging: Theory, Research, and Policy*, ed. Donald E. Gelfand and Alfred J. Kutzik (New York: Springer, 1979), 137–148.

112. Ballenger, *Self, Senility, and Alzheimer's Disease in Modern America*, 114.

113. E. Percil Stanford, Shirley A. Lockery, and Susan A. Schoenrock, *Ethnicity and Aging: Mental Health Issues* (San Diego, CA: San Diego State University, 1990), 2.

114. See Deborah K. Padgett, ed., *Handbook on Ethnicity, Aging, and Mental Health* (Westport, CT: Greenwood, 1995), 116–117.

115. Stanford, Lockery, and Schoenrock, *Ethnicity and Aging*, 35, 38.

116. Amy Tan, *The Bonesetter's Daughter* (2001; repr., London: Harper, 2004), 43.

117. See Stanley Sue and Herman McKinney, "Asian Americans in the Community Mental Health Care System," *American Journal of Orthopsychiatry* 45 (January 1975): 111–118; Stanley Sue and James K. Morishima, *The Mental Health of Asian Americans* (San Francisco: Jossey-Bass, 1982); Karen S. Kurasaki, Sumie Okazaki, and Stanley Sue, eds., *Asian American Mental Health* (New York: Kluwer/Plenum, 2002).

118. Tan, *The Bonesetter's Daughter*, 142–143.

119. On translation and ghosts, see Ken-fang Lee, "Cultural Translation and the Exorcist: A Reading of Kingston's and Tan's Ghost Stories," *MELUS* 29 (Summer 2004): 105–127.

120. See Padgett, *Handbook on Ethnicity, Aging, and Mental Health*, 276–279.

121. *The Road to an Aging Policy for the 21st Century: Executive Summary* (Washington, DC: n.p., 1996), 50. Annual investment prior to this injection of funds was estimated to be less than $78 per U.S. citizen with Alzheimer's.

122. Donna E. Shalala to President Clinton, February 1996, in *The Road to an Aging Policy for the 21st Century: Executive Summary* (Washington, DC: n.p., 1996), frontispiece.

123. Key texts in establishing Age Studies include Kathleen Woodward, *Aging and Its Discontents* (Bloomington: Indiana University Press, 1991); Margaret Morganroth Gullette, *Declining to Decline: Cultural Combat and the Politics of the Midlife* (Charlottesville: University of Virginia Press, 1997); Kathleen Woodward, ed., *Figuring Age: Women, Bodies, Generations* (Bloomington: Indiana University Press, 1999).

CHAPTER 5 — DEVELOPMENTAL DISABILITIES BEYOND THE EMPTY FORTRESS

1. "Notes on Briefing of Commissioners-Designate of President's Commission on Mental Health," 29 March 1977, Box 1, Gathering at the White House, 3/29/77, Federal Records–President's Commission on Mental Health, Jimmy Carter Presidential Library, Atlanta, Georgia.

2. These workshops were reflected in George Tarjan, ed., *The Physician and the Mental Health of the Child*, 2 vols. (Monroe, WI: American Medical Association, 1979). See also

Julius B. Richmond, George Tarjan, and Robert S. Mendelsohn, *Mental Retardation: A Handbook for the Primary Physician*, 3rd ed. (1965; repr., Chicago: American Medical Association, 1976).

3. "Notes on Briefing of Commissioners-Designate of President's Commission on Mental Health," 10–11.

4. President Reagan, "Remarks on Signing the National Decade of Disabled Persons Proclamation," 28 November 1983, in *Public Papers of the Presidents of the United States: Ronald Reagan, 1983*, Book 2 (Washington, DC: U.S. Government Printing Office, 1984), 1627–1629.

5. For discussion of this funding cut and the block grant system, see Judith Feder, John Holahan, Randall R. Bovbjerg, and Jack Hadley, "Health," in *The Reagan Experiment: Examination of Economic and Social Policies under the Reagan Administration*, ed. John L. Palmer and Isabel V. Sawhill (Washington, DC: Urban Institute Press, 1982), 291–296.

6. Committee on Assuring the Health of the Public in the 21st Century, *The Future of Public Health* (Washington, DC: National Academy Press, 1988). For a more affirmative summary of mental health reform in the 1980s, see Gerald N. Grob and Howard H. Goldman, *The Dilemma of Federal Mental Health Policy: Radical Reform or Incremental Change?* (New Brunswick, NJ: Rutgers University Press, 2006), 146–147.

7. In early 1984, Reagan made passing mention of equal medical treatment for those with a "mental and physical handicap"; President Reagan, "Remarks at the Annual Convention of the National Religious Broadcasters," 30 January 1984, in *Public Papers of the Presidents of the United States: Ronald Reagan, 1984*, Book 1 (Washington, DC: U.S. Government Printing Office, 1987), 119. Reagan used the phrase "mental problems" to encompass "retardation" in a news conference on 12 August 1986: *Public Papers of the Presidents of the United States: Ronald Reagan, 1986*, Book 2 (Washington, DC: U.S. Government Printing Office, 1987), 1089.

8. Dwight Fee, ed., *Pathology and the Postmodern: Mental Illness as Discourse and Experience* (London: Sage, 2000), 4.

9. Ibid., 3.

10. See *Action Against Mental Disability: The Report* (Washington, DC: U.S. Government Printing Office, 1970).

11. "Statement about Mental Retardation," 16 November 1971, in *Public Papers of the Presidents of the United States: Richard M. Nixon, 1971* (Washington, DC: U.S. Government Printing Office, 1972), 1112.

12. The zeal of the early Reagan Revolution softened in the second half of the 1980s; see Eric J. Schmertz, *Ronald Reagan's America* (Greenwood, CT: Praeger), 263–275.

13. George Bush, "Remarks to the President's Committee on Employment of the Handicapped, Washington Hilton Hotel, Washington, DC, May 5 1983," OA/ID 14876, Press Office, Speechwriter Files, George Bush Presidential Library, College Station, Texas.

14. *Mental Retardation: Prevention, Amelioration, and Service Delivery* (Brussels: Joint Commission on International Aspects of Mental Retardation, 1980).

15. Hannah S. Decker, *The Making of DSM-III: A Diagnostic Manual's Conquest of American Psychiatry* (Oxford: Oxford University Press, 2013), 57–58. For this group's philosophy, see Robert A. Woodruff, Donald W. Goodwin, and Samuel B. Guze, *Psychiatric Diagnosis* (New York: Oxford University Press, 1974).

16. *Diagnostic and Statistical Manual of Mental Disorders*, 3rd ed. (Washington, DC: American Psychiatric Association, 1980), 40.

17. Ibid., 36.

18. Ibid., 94. Reagan said nothing positive about mental health support in his "Statement on Signing of the State Comprehensive Mental Health Plan Bill," 14 November 1986, in *Public Papers of the Presidents: Ronald Reagan, 1986*, Book 2, 1553–1554.

19. *The President's Committee on Mental Retardation, 1987: Report to the President* (Washington, DC: U.S. Department of Health and Human Services, 1987), 13–14. In 1991, on the twenty-fifth anniversary of the committee, President Bush's secretary of health and human services, Louis Wade Sullivan, talked about the need for prevention and personal responsibility. He also contributed to *Report to the President: Citizens with Mental Retardation and the Criminal Justice System* (Washington, DC: U.S. Department of Health and Human Services, 1991).

20. See Rick Mayes, Catherine Bagwell, and Jennifer Erkulwater, *Medicating Children: ADHD and Pediatric Mental Health* (Cambridge, MA: MIT Press, 2009), 4.

21. Evidence that this shift was occurring prior to 1990 is found in the proceedings of the National Conference on State Planning for the Prevention of Mental Retardation and Related Developmental Disabilities, held in Washington, DC, 11–12 February 1987; *The President's Committee on Mental Retardation, 1987*, 13–14.

22. An important sociological account of the medical and social models is Michael Oliver's *The Politics of Disablement: A Sociological Approach* (London: Macmillan, 1990).

23. Bruno Bettelheim, *The Empty Fortress: Infantile Autism and the Birth of the Self* (New York: Free Press 1967), 11.

24. Ibid., 9. For commentary, see Richard Pollak's critical take on Bettelheim, *The Creation of Dr. B: A Biography of Bruno Bettelheim* (New York: Simon & Schuster, 1997), 261–272: Pollak's autistic brother Stephen was a pupil at the Sonia Shankman Orthogenic School but died suddenly on a visit home. Bettelheim insisted that Pollak's brother's death was a suicide.

25. Bettelheim, *The Empty Fortress*, 364.

26. Ibid., 7. See also Bettelheim's essay "Schizophrenia as a Reaction to Extreme Situations," *American Journal of Orthopsychiatry* 26 (July 1956): 507–518.

27. Disagreement about Bettelheim's legacy played out in the pages of the *New York Review of Books* in 2003. Reviewing a number of studies (including Pollak's *The Creation of Dr. B*), Robert Gottlieb assessed the damage to Bettelheim's reputation since his suicide in 1990. In response, Jacquelyn Sanders, Bettelheim's co-worker and his successor as director of the Sonia Shankman Orthogenic School, defended his methods, although she acknowledged that he was wrong about autism on some counts: Robert Gottlieb, "The Strange

Case of Dr. B.," *New York Review of Books*, 27 February 2003; Jacquelyn Seevak Sanders, "Defending Bruno Bettelheim," *New York Review of Books*, 20 November 2003.

28. Bettelheim, *The Empty Fortress*, 344.

29. "Medicine: The Child Is the Father," *Time*, 25 July 1960. Kanner's July 1969 comments were to the National Society for Autistic Children, cited in Clara Claiborne Park, *Exiting Nirvana: A Daughter's Life with Autism* (New York: Little Brown, 2001), 11.

30. Clara Claiborne Park, *The Siege: The Battle for Communication with an Autistic Child* (1967; repr., London: Penguin, 1972), 186. For commentary, see Pollak, *The Creation of Dr. B*, 276–277.

31. Park, *The Siege*, 1, 17

32. Ibid., 17.

33. *DSM-III*, 89.

34. Park, *The Siege*, 76.

35. Ibid., 84.

36. Ibid., 103.

37. Ibid., 186.

38. Joan Beck, *How to Raise a Brighter Child: The Case for Early Learning* (1967; repr., London: Fontana, 1970), 271.

39. Ibid., 273.

40. Ibid., 249.

41. See Paula J. Caplan and Ian Hall-McCorquodale, "Mother-Blaming in Major Clinical Journals," *American Journal of Orthopsychiatry* 55 (July 1985): 348–353; Eric Shopler, "Parents of Psychotic Children as Scapegoats," in *Classic Readings in Autism*, ed. Anne M. Donnellan (New York: Teacher's College Press, 1985), 236–241. A response to Shopler's essay is Jane Taylor McDonnell, "On Being the 'Bad' Mother of an Autistic Child," in *"Bad" Mothers: The Politics of Blame in Twentieth-Century America*, ed. Molly Ladd-Taylor and Lauri Umansky (New York: New York University Press, 1998), 220–229.

42. E. James Anthony and Cyrille Koupernik, *The Child in His Family: Children at Psychiatric Risk* (New York: Wiley, 1974), 42.

43. "President Nixon Meets 1972 Poster Child," *Mental Retardation News* 21, no. 4 (1972).

44. Dorothy J. Beavers to John Ehrlichman, Assistant to the President for Domestic Affairs, 6 March 1970, Box 11, HE 1–5 Mental Disorders, White House Central Files, Richard Nixon Presidential Library, Yorba Linda, California.

45. See Eric Schopler and Gary B. Mesibov, eds., *Neurobiological Issues in Autism* (New York: Plenum, 1987), 389–405.

46. Gil Eyal, Brendan Hart, and Emine Onculer, *The Autism Matrix: The Social Origins of the Autism Epidemic* (Oxford: Polity Press, 2010), 163.

47. "Justices Restrict a 'Bill of Rights' for the Retarded," *New York Times*, 21 April 1981.

48. Barry Neil Kaufman, *A Miracle to Believe In* (New York: Doubleday, 1981), 14.

49. Ibid., 15.

50. Sally L. Smith, *No Easy Answers: The Learning Disabled Child at Home and at School* (1978; repr., New York: Bantam Books, 1981), 4.

51. Barry Neil Kaufman, *Son-Rise* (New York: Harper & Row 1976), 2.

52. Kaufman, *A Miracle to Believe In*, 16.

53. Kaufman, *Son-Rise*, 151. Kaufman details his Option Process philosophy in his books *To Love Is to Be Happy With* (1977) and *Giant Steps* (1979).

54. Kaufman, *A Miracle to Believe In*, 25–26.

55. Ibid., 86.

56. Ibid., 135.

57. Kaufman, *Son-Rise*, 146.

58. Kaufman, *A Miracle to Believe In*, 359.

59. Ibid., 377–379.

60. See Glenn Doman, *What to Do about Your Brain-Injured Child* (New Hyde Park: Square One, 1974); Glenn Doman, Gretchen Kerr, and Maxwell Britt, *Babies, Mobility, and Intelligence* (Philadelphia: Better Baby Press, 1980).

61. For a critique of Doman's theories, see Herman Spitz, *The Raising of Intelligence* (London: Routledge, 1986), 83–87; Larry B. Silver, "The 'Magic Cure': A Review of the Current Controversial Approaches to Treating Learning Disabilities," *Journal of Learning Disabilities* 20 (October 1987): 498–504.

62. This description is by speech pathologist Holly Hamilton in *The Bridge School Story*, a documentary included on the 2011 DVD *Bridge School Benefit: 25th Anniversary Edition*.

63. Fredric Jameson, *Postmodernism, or the Cultural Logic of Late Capitalism* (London: Verso, 1991), 26.

64. "The Fight of Sly Stallone's Life," *People*, 3 June 1985, 95–96.

65. Eyal, Hart, and Onculer, *The Autism Matrix*, 141–142.

66. See George Victor, *The Riddle of Autism: A Psychological Analysis* (Lexington, MA: Lexington Books, 1983) and Institute of Medicine, *Research on Mental Illness and Addictive Disorders: Progress and Prospects* (Washington, DC: National Academy Press, 1984), 34–35.

67. See Martin F. Norden, *The Cinema of Isolation: A History of Physical Disability in the Movies* (New Brunswick, NJ: Rutgers University Press, 1994) and Martin Halliwell, *Images of Idiocy: The Idiot Figure in Modern Fiction and Film* (Burlington, VT: Ashgate, 2004).

68. See *The Real Rain Man*, a documentary film that aired on the Discovery Health Channel on 26 November 2006. For the genesis of *Rain Man*, see Steve Silberman, *Neurotribes* (London: Allen and Unwin, 2015), 354–380.

69. It was not until twenty years after the film that Peek was diagnosed as having a rare genetic syndrome that accounted for a least some of his physical and cognitive traits.

70. Sherri Dalphonse, "Dustin and Me," *Washingtonian Magazine*, 1 July 1992, 50–55, 136–138. See also Ruth C. Sullivan, "Rain Man and Joseph," in *High-Functioning Individuals with Autism*, ed. Eric Schopler and Gary B. Mesibov (New York: Plenum, 1992), 243–250.

71. Stuart Murray, *Representing Autism: Culture, Narrative, Fascination* (Liverpool: Liverpool University Press, 2008), 85.

72. Leonore Fleischer, *Rain Man* (London: Penguin, 1989), 66.

73. Stuart Murray gives the example of Rich Shull's book *Autism, Pre Rain Man* (New York: iUniverse, 2003).

74. Oliver Sacks, *An Anthropologist on Mars: Seven Paradoxical Tales* (New York: Knopf, 1995), 247.

75. Fleisher, *Rain Man*, 88.

76. See Darold Treffert, *Extraordinary People: Understanding "Idiot Savants"* (New York: Harper & Row, 1989), xviii, 197. For commentary on Treffert, see Murray, *Understanding Autism*, 67. On remarkable abilities in word recognition, numeracy, memory, and music, see Loraine K. Obler and Deborah Fein, eds., *The Exceptional Brain: Neuropsychology of Talent and Special Abilities* (New York: Guilford Press, 1988).

77. Cited in "Rain Man Touches Home," *Washington Post*, 29 March 1989; and "Rain Man Puts Autism on the Map," *Orlando Sentinel*, 22 December 1988. Bernard Rimland's 1964 book *Infantile Autism: The Syndrome and Its Implications for a Neural Theory of Behavior* was one of the founding texts for considering the genetic implications of autism.

78. "Rain Man Touches Home."

79. "Let Down by Rain Man," *St Louis Post-Dispatch*, 23 January 1993.

80. See Francis Peek with Lisa L. Hanson, *The Life and Message of The Real Rain Man: The Journey of a Mega-Savant* (Port Chester, NY: Dude Publishing, 2007). For a recycling of the phrase, see the UK Channel 5 documentary *The Rain Man Twins*, 23 July 2008, about twin female identical autistic savants.

81. Temple Grandin and Margaret M. Scariano, *Emergence: Labeled Autistic* (1986; repr., New York: Warner, 1996), 8.

82. Ibid., 9.

83. Temple Grandin, *The Way I See It: A Personal Look at Autism and Asperger's*, rev. ed. (Arlington, TX: Future Horizons, 2011), xiv. See also the BBC documentary *The Woman Who Thinks Like a Cow*, aired 8 June 2006.

84. See "Rain Man Illuminates Autism," *Boston Globe*, 23 December 1988.

85. Grandin, *The Way I See It*, 185–187.

86. Temple Grandin, "How Does Visual Thinking Work in the Mind of a Person with Autism? A Personal Account," in *Autism and Talent*, ed. Francesca Happé and Uta Frith (Oxford: Oxford University Press, 2010), 140, 144.

87. See Temple Grandin, *Thinking in Pictures and Other Reports from My Life with Autism* (New York: Doubleday, 1995), 1; and Temple Grandin, "Nurturing the Ways in Which

We See the World," in Jill Mullin, *Drawing Autism* (2009; repr., New York: Akashic Books, 2014), 7.

88. Ruud Hendriks, *Autistic Company*, rev. ed., trans. Lynne Richards (Amsterdam: Rodopi, 2012), 86, 90.

89. On the squeeze machine and medication, see Temple Grandin, "An Inside View of Autism," in *High-Functioning Individuals with Autism*, ed. Eric Schopler and Gary B. Mesibov (New York: Plenum, 1992), 109–112.

90. Sacks, *An Anthropologist on Mars*, 256. See also Silberman, *Neurotribes*, 429–431.

91. Ibid., 270. For Grandin's language development, see *Thinking in Pictures*, 14–15.

92. Grandin, *Thinking in Pictures*, 20–21.

93. Judy Barron and Sean Barron, *There's a Boy in Here* (New York: Simon & Schuster, 1992); Catherine Maurice, *Let Me Hear Your Voice: A Family's Triumph over Autism* (New York: Fawcett Columbine, 1993).

94. Rimland was an advocate of megadoses of vitamin B-6 for individuals with autism. See Chloe Silverman, *Understanding Autism: Parents, Doctors, and the History of a Disorder* (Princeton, NJ: Princeton University Press, 2012), 171–178.

95. See Sherry Turkle, *Life on the Screen: Identity in the Age of the Internet* (1995; repr., New York: Simon & Schuster, 2011), 70.

96. Steven R. Rothman, "Support for Autism Funding," House of Representatives, 105th Congress, *Congressional Record*, 5 June 1997, accessed 22 December 2016, https://www.congress.gov/crec/1997/06/05/CREC-1997-06-05-pt1-PgE1123.pdf.

97. A 1996 longitudinal study based in Atlanta, Georgia, gave strong evidence of increased rates of autism. See Marshalyn Yeargin-Allsopp, Catherine Rice, Tanya Karapurkar, Nancy Doernberg, Coleen Boyle, and Catherine Murphy, "Prevalence of Autism in a US Metropolitan Area," *Journal of the American Medical Association* 289 (January 2003): 49–55. The Centers for Disease Control and Prevention investigated the rise of autism in Brick Township, New Jersey, where a spike in the number of cases was thought to be linked to air and water quality and the proximity of toxic waste sites: "Autism has a Town Struggling with Fear," *New York Times*, 30 January 1999.

98. David Kirby, *Evidence of Harm: Mercury in Vaccines and the Autism Epidemic: A Medical Controversy* (New York: St Martin's Press, 2005), 81. See also Roy Grinker, *Unstrange Minds: Remapping the World of Autism* (New York: Basic Books, 2007); Seth Mnookin, *The Panic Virus: A True Story of Medicine, Science, and Fear* (New York: Simon & Schuster, 2011). In 2003, the NIMH estimated that between 1 in 500 and 1 in 1,000 Americans had autism.

99. George Bush, "Proclamation 6476: National Disability Employment Awareness Month," 23 September 1992, *The American Presidency Project*, accessed 22 December 2016, www.presidency.ucsb.edu/ws/index.php?month=09&year=1992.

100. After receiving over twenty letters in the fall of 1988 that asked her to make mental illness her special project, Barbara Bush said that this "is a very serious issue facing our country today" but that her focus would be on literacy. See Barbara Bush to Vita Beckman, 2 November 1988, OA/ID 28719, George H. W. Bush Vice Presidential Records,

HE 1–5 [Health: Disease: Physically Handicapped], Mrs. Bush's Office, George Bush Presidential Library.

101. In December 1991, Mrs. Bush hosted Eric Apple, a 25-year-old from Ohio who had been diagnosed with autism at age three and specialized in facts about presidents and first ladies. See "Photo with Eric Apple (disabled)–State Floor, OA/ID 04878, First Lady, Office of Scheduling–Ann Brock Files, George Bush Presidential Library.

102. Charles W. Schmidt, "A Growth Spurt in Children's Health Laws," *Environmental Health Perspectives* 109, no. 6 (2001): A270–A273. See also Trudy Steuernagel, "Increases in Identified Cases of Autism Spectrum Disorders: Policy Implications," *Journal of Disability Policy Studies* 16 (Winter 2005): 138–146.

103. Mohammad Ghaziuddin, *Mental Health Aspects of Autism and Asperger's Syndrome* (London: Jessica Kingsley, 2005), 9.

104. Ibid., 10.

105. Ibid., 106–107.

106. On the genetic vulnerability of individuals with autism, see "New Theories Help Explain Mysteries of Autism," *New York Times*, 28 December 1999.

107. See Ian Hacking's inquiry into the "sciences of memory" in *Rewriting the Soul* (Princeton, NJ: Princeton University Press, 1995) and French actor and journalist Jean-Dominique Bauby's memoir of his locked-in syndrome in *The Diving Bell and the Butterfly* (Paris: Éditions Robert Laffont, 1997).

108. The character of Simon Lynch obliquely recalls science fiction writer Philip K. Dick's interest in developmental disabilities, for example the child character Manfred Steiner in his 1964 novel *Martian Time-Slip*.

109. Mark Osteen, "Narrating Autism," in *Worlds of Autism: Across the Spectrum of Neurological Difference*, ed. Joyce Davidson and Michael Orsini (Minneapolis: University of Minnesota Press, 2013), 261–263.

110. Jonathan Lethem, *Motherless Brooklyn* (New York: Vintage, 1999), 110.

111. James Berger, *The Disarticulate: Language, Disability, and the Narratives of Modernity* (New York: New York University Press, 2014), 211, 218.

112. For facilitated communication, see "New Treatments for Autism Arouse Hope and Skepticism," *New York Times*, 13 July 1993 and "Shattering the Silence of Autism," *New York Times*, 12 February 1994. On secretin and vaccines, see Michael Fitzpatrick, *Defeating Autism: A Damaging Delusion* (London: Routledge, 2009), xi–xv.

113. Clara Claiborne Park, *Exiting Nirvana* (Boston: Little, Brown, 2001), 28. *Exiting Nirvana* includes a preface by Oliver Sacks that comments on the allegorical nature of Parks's title. See also Park's "Epilogue: Fifteen Years After," in Clara Claiborne Park, *The Siege: A Family's Journey into the World of an Autistic Child* (1967; repr., Boston: Little, Brown, 1982), 278–320.

114. Park, *Exiting Nirvana*, 208.

115. Ibid., 122.

116. Ibid., 126.

117. Raun K. Kaufman, *Autism Breakthrough* (New York: St Martin's Press, 2014), 19.

CHAPTER 6 — BODY IMAGE, ANOREXIA, AND THE MASS MEDIA

1. Carlton E. Turner, "Remarks at the Health Care Expo '85," Washington, DC, Box 30, Folder 2, Carlton E. Turner Files, Ronald Reagan Library, Simi Valley, California. For the scope and limitations of the Expo, held at the Washington Convention Center on 18–24 August 1985, see Milan Korcok, "HealthCare Expo '85: County Fair, Medical Meeting and Marathon," *Canadian Medical Association Journal* 133 (December 1985): 1162–1167.

2. For an extended account of megavitamins, see the four-part series "Megavitamin Controversy" in the *Los Angeles Times*, 26–29 November 1972. In 1981, the California-based company Bronson Pharmaceutical marketed a "smart pill" based on nineteen vitamins and minerals.

3. Eric Schlosser estimates spending on fast food in the United States increased from $6 billion in 1970 to $110 billion in 2001: Schlosser, *Fast Food Nation* (London: Penguin, 2001). For data on the rise of obesity levels, see Kelly D. Brownell and Mark S. Gold, *Food and Addiction: A Comprehensive Handbook* (Oxford: Oxford University Press, 2012), 69–80. For a consideration of related nutritional issues, see Andrea Freeman, "Fast Food: Oppression through Poor Nutrition," *California Law Review* 95 (December 2007): 2221–2259. For children at risk, see Sue Palmer, *Toxic Childhood* (London: Orion, 2006).

4. "Message from Donna E. Shalala," in *Physical Activity and Health: A Report of the Surgeon General* (Washington, DC: U.S. Department of Health and Human Services, 1996). See also *Surgeon General's Report on Nutrition and Health* (Washington, DC: U.S. Department of Health and Human Services, 1988).

5. See Elizabeth Stark, "Forgotten Victims: Children of Alcoholics," *Psychology Today*, January 1987, 58–62; and Alfie Kohn, "Shattered Innocence," *Psychology Today*, February 1987, 54–58.

6. Wolf echoes the pioneering research of Jean Kilbourne on the dangers of advertising, which Kilbourne presented in two educational films: *Killing Us Softly: Advertising's Image of Women* (1979) and *Still Killing Us Softly* (1987). On body image, see Kilbourne, *Deadly Persuasion: Why Women and Girls Must Fight the Addictive Power of Advertising* (New York: Free Press, 1999), 128–154.

7. Naomi Wolf, *The Beauty Myth: How Images of Beauty Are Used Against Women* (New York: Random House, 1990), 270.

8. See, for example, "Critic's Notebook: Feminine Beauty as a Masculine Plot," *New York Times*, 7 May 1991.

9. Wolf, *The Beauty Myth*, 289. See also Arnold E. Andersen, *Males with Eating Disorders* (New York: Brunner/Mazel, 1990): Andersen estimates that eating disorders among men occur at about a tenth of the frequency of women.

10. Hilde Bruch, *The Golden Cage: The Enigma of Anorexia Nervosa* (Cambridge, MA: Harvard University Press, 1978), vii.

11. Adrienne Rich, "For Ellen West, Mental Patient and Suicide" (1971), first published in Kim Chernin, *The Obsession: Reflections on the Tyranny of Slenderness* (1981; repr., New York: Harper, 1994), 178–179. For the importance of the Ellen West case, see Martin Halliwell, *Therapeutic Revolutions: Medicine, Psychiatry, and American Culture, 1945–1970* (New Brunswick, NJ: Rutgers University Press, 2013), 244–245 and Gail Weiss, *Body Images: Embodiment as Intercorporeality* (New York: Routledge, 1999), 101–102.

12. Temple Grandin, *Thinking in Pictures and Other Reports from My Life with Autism* (New York: Doubleday, 1995), 215.

13. Hilde Bruch, "Approaches to Anorexia Nervosa," in *Anorexia and Obesity*, ed. Christopher V. Rowland Jr. (Boston: Little, Brown, 1970). See also Hilde Bruch, *Eating Disorders: Obesity, Anorexia Nervosa, and the Person Within* (New York: Basic, 1973).

14. "Clinton Calls Fashion Ads' 'Heroin Chic' Deplorable,'" *New York Times*, 22 May 1997. See also Sarah Grogan, *Body Image: Understanding Body Dissatisfaction in Men, Women, and Children* (London: Routledge, 1999), 15–16.

15. Jean Baudrillard, "The Anorexic Ruins," in *Looking Back on the End of the World*, ed. Dietmark Kampfer and Christoph Wulf (New York: Semiotext(e), 1989), 30.

16. Morag MacSween, *Anorexic Bodies: A Feminist and Sociological Perspective on Anorexia Nervosa* (London: Routledge, 1993), 113.

17. Slavoj Žižek, *The Sublime Object of Ideology* (London: Verso, 1989), 75.

18. *DSM-IV* distinguished body dysmorphic disorder (an imagined physical anomaly or exaggerated concern about a physical anomaly) from anorexia nervosa, although the manual acknowledges that anorexics typically experience distortions of "body weight and shape." *Diagnostic and Statistical Manual of Mental Disorders*, 4th ed. (Washington, DC: American Psychiatric Association, 1994), 466, 540.

19. Susan Bordo, *Unbearable Weight: Feminism, Western Culture, and the Body* (Berkeley: University of California Press, 1993), 55. Bordo's "Anorexia Nervosa: Psychopathology as the Crystallization of Culture" was originally published in *Philosophical Forum* 17 (Winter 1985) and is reproduced in *Unbearable Weight*, 139–164.

20. Ibid., 141. Research on body image and anorexia has grown significantly since the millennium, integrating details from Internet sites with information from print and broadcasting media, but in this chapter I limit my discussion to primary and secondary literature published up to 2000. For an overview of scholarship up to 2010, see Thomas F. Cash and Linda Smolak, *Body Image: A Handbook of Science, Practice, and Prevention*, 2nd ed. (New York: Guilford Press, 2011), 4–6.

21. Katharine A. Phillips, *The Broken Mirror: Understanding and Treating Body Dysmorphic Disorder* (New York: Oxford University Press, 1996), 221. Phillips has run a neuroscientific program on body dysmorphic disorder at Rhode Island Hospital and Brown University since the mid-1990s. See also Lisa J. Fabian and J. Kevin Thompson, "Body Image and Eating Disturbance in Young Females," *International Journal of Eating Disorders* 8, no. 1 (1989): 63–74; James C. Rosen, "Body Image Disturbance in Eating Disorders," in *Body Images: Development, Deviance, and Change* ed. Thomas F. Cash and Thomas Pruzinsky

(New York: Guilford Press, 1990), 190–216; L. K. George Hsu and Theresa A. Sobkiewicz, "Body Image Disturbance: Time to Abandon the Concept for Eating Disorders?," *International Journal of Eating Disorders* 10 (January 1991): 15–30.

22. Bordo, *Unbearable Weight*, 56.

23. Nixon made this comment at The White House on 1 May 1973 when introducing The Carpenters to his guests: for commentary, see Randy L. Schmidt, *Little Girl Blue: The Life of Karen Carpenter* (Chicago: Chicago Review Press, 2010), 101.

24. Paula Saukko, *The Anorexic Self: A Personal, Political Analysis of a Diagnostic Discourse* (Albany: State University of New York Press, 2008), 58.

25. Charlie Tuna, "Karen Carpenter: Nothing to Hide Behind" (1976) and Richard Carpenter, "Karen Was Wasting Away . . ." (1988), in *Yesterday Once More: The Carpenters Reader*, ed. Randy L. Schmidt, rev. ed. (Chicago: Chicago Review Press, 2012), 189, 262. Of the newspaper coverage that marked the death of Karen Carpenter, the most insightful is Robert Hilburn and Dennis Hunt's "Behind Carpenter's Girl-Next-Door Image," *Los Angeles Times*, 7 February 1983. Two retrospective pieces by Rob Hoerburger revisited Carpenter's cultural image and the factors that led to her death: "Revisionist Thinking on the Carpenters," *New York Times*, 3 November 1991; and "Karen Carpenter's Second Life," *New York Times*, 6 October 1996.

26. "Doctors Cite Emetic Abuse," *New York Times*, 22 March 1985. See also Schmidt, *Little Girl Blue*, 252, 259–260.

27. "She Can't Seem to Break Her Destructive Eating Habits," *Boston Globe*, 15 April 1983.

28. "Self-Starvation in America," *Chicago Tribune*, 14 February 1983.

29. Joan Jacobs Brumberg, *Fasting Girls: The History of Anorexia Nervosa* (1988; repr., New York: Vintage, 2000), 8. See also Joan Jacobs Brumberg, "Anorexia Nervosa in Context," in *The Sociology of Health and Illness: Critical Perspectives*, ed. Peter Conrad, 7th ed. (1997; repr., New York: Worth 2005), 107–121.

30. Eric Lott, "Perfect Is Dead: Karen Carpenter, Theodor Adorno, and the Radio, or if Hooks Could Kill," in *Pop: When the World Falls Apart*, ed. Eric Weisbard (Durham, NC: Duke University Press, 2012), 74–79.

31. Music critic Robert Hilburn wrote the phrase "audio wallpaper" and then changed his mind about Carpenter after her death. See "A Lesson in Art of Emotion," *Los Angeles Times*, 13 February 1983.

32. Todd Haynes, Far from Heaven, Safe, *and* Superstar*: The Karen Carpenter Story: Three Screenplays* (New York: Grove, 2003), ix.

33. Ibid., 185.

34. Ibid., 186.

35. Ibid., 189.

36. Ibid., 190.

37. Ibid., 193–194.

38. Terence J. Sandbek, *The Deadly Diet: Recovering from Anorexia and Bulimia* (Oakland, CA: New Harbinger, 1986), 21–44.

39. See Cherry Boone O'Neill, *Starving for Attention* (New York: Dell, 1982).

40. Haynes, Far from Heaven, Safe, *and* Superstar, 219.

41. Julia Leyda, *Todd Haynes Interviews* (Jackson: University of Mississippi Press, 2014), 6.

42. Mary Desjardins, "The Incredible Shrinking Star: Todd Haynes and the Case History of Karen Carpenter," *Camera* 19, no. 3 (2004): 32.

43. Ibid., 43. Haynes claimed that his co-writer Cynthia Schneider had an important role in making the film yet comments that "the pressures and the kinds of neurotic motivations that would result in eating disorders are the same pressures and neurotic feelings that I've experienced but taken out in other ways": Leyda, *Todd Haynes Interviews*, 7.

44. Mitchell Morris, *The Persistence of Sentiment: Display and Feeling in Popular Music of the 1970s* (Berkeley: University of California Press, 2013), 119.

45. Jane Fonda, *Jane Fonda's Workout Book* (New York: Simon and Schuster, 1981), 20.

46. "Jane Fonda: Finding Her Golden Pond," *Cosmopolitan*, 26 January 1985, 168–171, 205. Fonda discusses her insecurity during the 1960s, noting that bulimia did not really have a name until the publication of a 1979 essay, Gerald Russell. "Bulimia Nervosa: An Ominous Variant of Anorexia Nervosa," *Psychological Medicine* 9, no. 3 (1979): 429–448.

47. "Jane Fonda: Finding Her Golden Pond," 170. Fonda features in an important book on the phenomenology of self-starvation: Maud Ellman, *The Hunger Artists: Starving, Writing and Imprisonment* (Cambridge, MA: Harvard University Press, 1993), 9–10.

48. "First Lady Down to Size 2," *Los Angeles Times*, 30 September 1983; "President's Advisers Harbor Worries about First Lady's Health," *Washington Post*, 10 October 1983.

49. Davis, *The Way I See It*, 136.

50. For the case of Tracey Gold, see Elizabeth Sporkin, "A Terrible Hunger," *People*, 17 February 1992, 92–95.

51. Marilyn Lawrence, ed., *Fed Up and Hungry: Women, Oppression and Food* (New York: Peter Bedrick, 1987), 3.

52. Wolf, *The Beauty Myth*, 202.

53. Ibid., 203.

54. Ibid., 207.

55. Bruch, *The Golden Cage*, vii.

56. Deborah Hautzig, *Second Star to the Right* (1981; repr., New York: Puffin, 1999), 114.

57. Ibid., 6.

58. For the formulaic nature of some anorexia narratives, see Brumberg, *Fasting Girls*, 19–20.

59. Bruch, *The Golden Cage*, 3.

60. Hautzig, *Second Star to the Right*, 12.

61. See Christine Pollice, Walter H. Kaye, Catherine G. Greeno, and Theodore E. Weltzin, "Relationship of Depression, Anxiety, and Obsessionality to State of Illness in Anorexia Nervosa," *International Journal of Eating Disorders* 21 (May 1997): 367–376.

62. Steven Levenkron, *Treating and Overcoming Anorexia Nervosa* (New York: Scribner, 1982), 4.

63. Levenkron made this remark at the Center for the Study of Anorexia and Bulimia in 1983; see Bordo, *Unbearable Weight*, 60. See also Levenkron, *Treating and Overcoming Anorexia Nervosa*, 4.

64. Ibid., 2–3.

65. Lori Gottlieb, *Stick Figure: A Diary of My Former Self* (New York: Berkeley Books, 2000), 237.

66. Christopher Lasch, *The Culture of Narcissism: American Life in an Age of Diminishing Expectations* (New York: Norton, 1979), 95.

67. Gottlieb, *Stick Figure*, 225.

68. Ibid., 131.

69. Marya Hornbacher, *Wasted: A Memoir of Anorexia and Bulimia* (New York: Harper, 1998), 3.

70. Ibid., 4.

71. Sue Vice, "The Well-Rounded Anorexic Text," in *American Bodies: Cultural Histories of the Physique*, ed. Tim Armstrong (Sheffield: Sheffield Academic Press, 1996), 196–203.

72. Hornbacher, *Wasted*, 4.

73. Ibid., 15.

74. The two *Mork and Mindy* episodes about the birth of the Orkan "child" Mearth (who emerges as an elderly man and lives his life backward) aired in October 1981.

75. Hornbacher, *Wasted*, 24–25.

76. The trope of performance is taken much further theoretically in Patrick Anderson's *So Much Wasted: Hunger, Performance, and the Morbidity of Resistance* (Durham, NC: Duke University Press, 2010).

77. Hornbacher, *Wasted*, 29–30.

78. Ibid., 129.

79. Ibid., 159, 158.

80. Ibid., 144.

81. For the relationship between psychic numbing and lying, see Dorothy Rowe, *Why We Lie* (London: Fourth Estate, 2011), 73.

82. Susanna Kaysen, *Girl, Interrupted* (London: Virago, 1993), 45.

83. See, for example, Susan C. Wooley, "Sexual Abuse and Eating Disorders: The Concealed Debate," in *Feminist Perspectives on Eating Disorders*, ed. Patricia Fallon, Melanie A. Katzman, and Susan C. Wooley (New York: Guilford Press, 1994), 171–211.

84. Kaysen, *Girl, Interrupted*, 38.

85. Angelina Jolie's role as Lisa is telling because as a young actress she battled with the pressure to remain thin. See "A Chic Heroine, but Not a Pretty Story," *New York Times*, 25 January 1998.

86. Hornbacher, *Wasted*, 2.

87. Ibid., 196.

88. Ibid., 61.

89. See Marion Nestle and Michael F. Jacobson, "Halting the Obesity Epidemic: A Public Health Policy Approach," *Public Health Report* 115 (January–February 2000): 12–24.

90. Abigail C. Saguy and Kjerstin Gruys, "Morality and Health: News Media Constructions of Overweight and Eating Disorders," *Social Problems* 57 (May 2010): 231–250. For eating disorders among different racial groups, see Denise E. Wilfley, George B. Schreiber, Kathleen M. Pike, Ruth H. Striegel-Moore, David J. Wright, and Judith Rodin, "Eating Disturbance and Body Image: A Comparison of a Community Sample of Adult Black and White Women," *International Journal of Eating Disorders* 20 (December 1996): 377–387.

91. On the intersection of race, class, and eating disorders, see Becky W. Thompson, "'A Way Outa No Way': Eating Problems among African American, Latina, and White Women," in *Race, Class, and Gender: Common Bonds, Different Voices*, ed. Esther Ngan-Ling Chow, Doris Wilkinson, and Maxine Baca Zinn (London: Sage, 1996), 52–69.

92. See Susie Orbach, *Hunger Strike: The Anorectic's Struggle as a Metaphor for Our Age* (New York: Norton, 1986). The issue of balance had been explored three years earlier by Susan Squire in *The Slender Balance: Causes and Cures for Bulimia, Anorexia and the Weight-Loss/Weight-Gain Seesaw* (New York: Putnam, 1983).

93. See Mary Belenky, *Women's Ways of Knowing: The Development of Self, Voice and Mind* (New York: Basic Books, 1986) and Nancy Goldberger, *Knowledge, Difference, and Power: Essays Inspired by Women's Ways of Knowing* (New York: Basic Books, 1996).

94. Carol Gilligan, *In a Different Voice: Psychological Theory and Women's Development* (1982; repr., Cambridge, MA: Harvard University Press, 1993), 173–174.

95. Wolf, *The Beauty Myth*, 275.

96. For data that documents cases of eating disorders among nonwhites, see Bridget Dolan, "Cross-Cultural Aspects of Anorexia Nervosa and Bulimia: A Review," *International Journal of Eating Disorders* 10, no. 1 (1991): 67–79; Jane E. Smith and Jonathan Krejci, "Minorities Join the Majority: Eating Disturbances among Hispanic and Native American Youth," *International Journal of Eating Disorders* 10, no. 2 (1991): 179–186; Linda Smolak, Michael P. Levine, and Ruth Striegel-Moore, eds., *The Developmental Psychopathology of Eating Disorders* (Mahwah, NJ: Lawrence Erlbaum, 1996), 259–284. For work that challenges the correlation between middle-class status and anorexia, see Maisie C. E. Gard and Chris P. Freeman, "The Dismantling of a Myth: A Review of Eating Disorders and Socioeconomic Status," *International Journal of Eating Disorders* 20, no. 1 (1996): 1–12.

97. Hornbacher, *Wasted*, 204.

98. Ibid., 203.

99. Ibid., 212–213.

100. "Jane Fonda: Finding Her Golden Pond," 170.

101. Hornbacher, *Wasted*, 298, 300. Kelly Osgood criticizes *Wasted* for glamorizing anorexia and for mixing a how-to manual with a critique of the disorder. See Kelly Osgood, *How to Disappear Completely: On Modern Anorexia* (New York: Overlook Press, 2013).

102. See David M. Garner, Paul E. Garfinkel, Donald Schwartz, and Michael Thompson, "Cultural Expectations of Thinness in Women," *Psychological Reports* 47 (1980): 483–491; Claire V. Wiseman, James J. Gray, James E. Mosimann, and Anthony H. Ahrens, "Cultural Expectations of Thinness in Women: An Update," *International Journal of Eating Disorders* 11 (January 1992): 85–89; Dale L. Cusumano and J. Kevin Thompson, "Body Image and Body Shape Ideals in Magazines: Exposure, Awareness, and Internalization," *Sex Roles* 37, no. 9–10 (1997): 701–721.

103. Grogan, *Body Image*, 97–101.

104. Emily Fox-Kales, *Body Shots: Hollywood and the Culture of Eating Disorders* (Albany: State University of New York Press, 2011), 5.

105. Ibid., 7.

106. Lawrence, *Fed Up and Hungry*, 7.

107. Bordo, *Unbearable Weight*, 198.

108. See Eugenia Kaw, "Medicalization of Racial Features: Asian-American Women and Cosmetic Surgery," *Medical Anthropology Quarterly* 7, no. 1 (1993): 74–89, reprinted in Rose Weitz, ed., *The Politics of Women's Bodies: Sexuality, Appearance, and Behavior* (Oxford: Oxford University Press, 1998), 167–183.

109. "Feeling Fat in a Thin Society," *Glamour*, February 1984, 198–201, 251–252; "If You Could Change Your Breasts," *Self*, May 1996, 186–189, 210–211.

110. Gloria Steinem, *Revolution from Within: A Book of Self-Esteem* (New York: Little, Brown 1992), 222.

111. On the politics and health implications of cosmetic surgery, see Kathy Davis, *Reshaping the Female Body: The Dilemma of Cosmetic Surgery* (New York: Routledge, 1994) and Deborah A. Sullivan, *Cosmetic Surgery: The Cutting Edge of Commercial Medicine in America* (New Brunswick, NJ: Rutgers University Press, 2001).

112. James E. Mitchell, Richard L. Pyle, and Elke D. Eckert, "Diet Pill Usage in Patients with Bulimia Nervosa," *International Journal of Eating Disorders* 10 (March 1991): 233–237. See also James E. Mitchell, "A Clinician's Guide to the Eating Disorders' Medicine Cabinet," *International Journal of Eating Disorders* 7, no. 2 (1998): 211–223.

113. See Robert Langreth, "Critics Claim Diet Clinics Misuse Obesity Drugs," *Wall Street Journal*, 31 March 1997; and Howard Brody, *Hooked: Ethics, the Medical Profession, and the Pharmaceutical Industry* (Lanham, MD: Rowman & Littlefield, 2007), 269–275.

114. See "Diet to Death," *Boston Herald*, 6 May 1997; "2 Top Diet Drugs Are Recalled amid Reports of Heart Defects," *New York Times*, 16 September 1997; "Now That Two Popular Weight-Loss Drugs Are Off the Market, What's Left for Dieters?," *Washington Post*, 16 September 1997. Meridia was withdrawn in 2010.

115. On this point, see Julie Hepworth, *The Social Construction of Anorexia Nervosa* (London: Sage, 1999), 99–130.

116. Weiss, *Body Images*, 97, 102.

117. Hornbacher, *Wasted*, 306.

CHAPTER 7 — DISORDERS OF MOOD AND IDENTITY

1. Edward Jay Epstein, "Good News from Mr. Bad News," *New York*, 9 August 1976.

2. Temple Grandin, *The Way I See It: A Personal Look at Autism and Asperger's*, rev. ed. (Arlington, TX: Future Horizons, 2011), 206; Max Fink, *Electroshock: Healing Mental Illness* (New York: Oxford University Press, 1999), 35–36.

3. Peter D. Kramer, *Listening to Prozac* (1993; repr., London: Fourth Estate, 1994), 57.

4. Ibid., 64. On the marketing of Prozac, see Gary Greenberg, *Manufacturing Depression* (London: Bloomsbury, 2010), 274–276.

5. On enhancement technology, see Carl Elliott and Tod Chambers, eds., *Prozac as a Way of Life* (Chapel Hill: University of North Carolina Press, 2004). On identity transformation, see Carl Elliot, *Better than Well: American Medicine Meets the American Dream* (New York: Norton, 2003), 50–51.

6. Prozac was the fourth best-selling drug in 2000. See Peter Breggin, *Toxic Psychiatry* (New York: St Martin's Press, 1991); Peter Breggin, *Talking Back to Prozac* (New York: St Martin's, 1994). *Time* labeled Breggin "Prozac's Worst Enemy" in its 10 October 1994 issue. For overmedicated children, see "The Way We Live Now: Generation Rx," *New York Times Magazine*, 12 March 2000.

7. Lauren Slater, *Prozac Diary* (New York: Penguin, 1998), 162.

8. "The Promise of Prozac," *Newsweek*, 26 March 1990. Prozac prescriptions had risen to 9.9 million by 1997. See "Lusting after Prozac," *New York Times*, 11 October 1998; Bradley Lewis, *Moving beyond Prozac, DSM, and the New Psychiatry* (Ann Arbor: University of Michigan Press, 2006), 122.

9. Elizabeth Wurtzel, *Prozac Nation: Young and Depressed in America* (1994; repr., London: Quarter, 1995), 297.

10. These texts include David Healy, *Let Them Eat Prozac* (New York: New York University Press, 2004); Joanna Moncrieff, *The Myth of the Chemical Cure: A Critique of Psychiatric Drug Treatment* (London: Palgrave, 2008); and Irving Kirsch, *The Emperor's New Drugs: Exploding the Antidepressant Myth* (London: Bodley Head, 2009).

11. Slater, *Prozac Diary*, 81.

12. See Judith Guest, *Ordinary People* (New York: Ballantine Books, 1976); Raymond Carver, *What We Talk about When We Talk about Love* (New York: Knopf, 1981); and Richard Ford, *The Sportswriter* (New York: Vintage, 1986).

13. *Diagnostic and Statistical Manual of Mental Disorders*, 4th ed. (Washington, DC: American Psychiatric Association, 1994), 320, 328.

14. Patients with degenerative dementia are often excluded from *DSM* categorizations because it is a brain disease rather than a psychiatric disorder.

15. See Roy W. Menninger and John C. Nemiah, *American Psychiatry after World War II, 1944–1994* (Washington, DC: American Psychiatric Press, 2000), 603–604. The *DSM-IV* casebook tried to observe cultural difference: *DSM-IV Casebook*, 419–478.

16. Stephen M. Stahl, *Depression and Bipolar Disorder: Stahl's Essential Psychopharmacology*, 3rd ed. (Cambridge: Cambridge University Press, 2008), 9, 13.

17. Hannah S. Decker, *The Making of DSM-III: A Diagnostic Manual's Conquest of American Psychiatry* (Oxford: Oxford University Press, 2013), 170.

18. "Washington Town Full of Prozac," *New York Times*, 30 January 1994.

19. For the therapeutic effects of lithium carbonate, see Joe Mendels, "Lithium in the Treatment of Depression," *American Journal of Psychiatry* 133 (April 1976): 373–378.

20. A profile of Ruth Hayes, who had suffered violent mood swings for twenty years before successfully starting on lithium with Fieve, appeared as "Saved by Lithium" in "Drugs for the Mind: Psychiatry's Newest Weapon," *Newsweek*, 12 November 1978, 102.

21. Patty Duke and Kenneth Turan, *Call Me Anna: The Autobiography of Patty Duke* (New York: Bantam, 1987), 290.

22. On Nixon and Eagleton, see Ronald R. Fieve, *Moodswing*, rev. ed. (1975; repr.; New York: Bantam, 1997), 165–166, 176–179. Emily Martin credits theater director Josh Logan's 1976 autobiography, *Josh: My Up and Down, In and Out Life*, with exploring the creativity of manic depression: Emily Martin, *Bipolar Expeditions: Mania and Depression in American Culture* (Princeton, NJ: Princeton University Press, 2007), 22.

23. See Kay Redfield Jamison, *Touched with Fire: Manic-Depressive Illness and the Artistic Temperament* (New York: Free Press, 1993); Patty Duke and Gloria Hochman, *A Brilliant Madness: Living with Manic Depressive Illness* (New York: Bantam, 1992).

24. Fieve, *Moodswing*, 42.

25. Jamison prefers "manic depression" to "bipolar" because she thinks it captures both the "nature and seriousness" of her condition: Kay Redfield Jamison, *An Unquiet Mind: A Memoir of Moods and Madness* (London: Picador, 1996), 182.

26. Ibid., 4.

27. Kate Millett decided to come off lithium in 1980 because of the drug's side effects and the stigma associated with it. See Millett, *The Looney-Bin Trip* (New York: Simon and Schuster, 1990), 12.

28. Jamison, *An Unquiet Mind*, 13.

29. Ibid., 34.

30. Jamison tried to tackle the fear of professional disclosure when she moved from UCLA to Johns Hopkins University in 1986: ibid., 204–207.

31. Wurtzel, *Prozac Nation*, 260.

32. Jamison, *An Unquiet Mind*, 89, 214–215.

33. Ibid., 93, 123.

34. Wurtzel, *Prozac Nation*, 305.

35. Ibid., 263.

36. On the discursive construction of depression, see Dwight Fee, "The Project of Pathology: Reflexivity and Depression in Elizabeth Wurtzel's *Prozac Nation*," in *Pathology and the Postmodern: Mental Illness as Discourse and Experience*, ed. Dwight Fee (London: Sage, 2000), 74–98.

37. Carrie Fisher, another Hollywood casualty, attributed her long-term codeine addiction to bipolar disorder. Fisher was diagnosed in the mid-1980s and subsequently received electroshock treatment; ABC *Primetime* interview, 21 December 2000.

38. Duke and Turan, *Call Me Anna*, 311.

39. *DSM-IV*, 629.

40. Ibid., 630.

41. Philip Manfield, *Split Self/Split Object: Understanding and Treating Borderline, Narcissistic, and Schizoid Disorders* (Northvale, NJ: Aronson, 1992), xviii.

42. The fifth edition of *DSM* in 2013 dropped the multiaxial system but retained the diagnostics for borderline and narcissistic personality disorders (there was much discussion about the ongoing validity of the latter disorder during the planning stage of *DSM-5*).

43. *DSM-IV*, 650.

44. Ibid., 651.

45. For the Personality Disorders Advisory Group, see Decker, *The Making of DSM-III*, 167–169.

46. Theodore Millon, "The Borderline Construct," in *Borderline Personality Disorder: Clinical and Empirical Perspectives*, ed. John F. Clarkin, Elsa Marzioli, and Heather Munroe-Blum (New York: Guilford, 1992), 4.

47. Ibid., 5.

48. Millon, "The Borderline Construct," 17. See also Louis Sass, "The Borderline Personality," *New York Times Magazine*, 22 August 1982; Michael H. Stone, "Borderline Personality Disorder," in *New Psychiatric Syndromes: DSM III and Beyond*, ed. Salman Akhtar (New York: Aronson, 1983), 19.

49. See Robert Jay Lifton, *The Protean Self: Human Resilience in the Age of Fragmentation* (New York: HarperCollins, 1993), 30, 232.

50. The film was based on a 1990 thriller *SWF Seeks Same* by John Lutz.

51. See Susan Faludi, *Backlash: The Undeclared War against Women* (New York: Crown, 1991), 145–152.

52. *Malicious* also recycles *Play Misty for Me* when the obsessive stalker masquerades as the roommate of the protagonist's girlfriend.

53. See, for example, "Frustrated by the Odds, Single Women over 30 Seek Answers in Therapy," *Los Angeles Times*, 6 November 1986.

54. Susanna Kaysen, *Girl, Interrupted* (London: Virago, 1993), 105, 145.

55. Ibid., 151, 154.

56. Ibid., 154, 157–158. For self-harm and impulsivity linked to borderline personality disorder, see Nancy Nyquist Potter, *Mapping the Edges of the In-Between* (Oxford: Oxford University Press, 2009), 70–71, 92–94. Armando Favazza's 1987 book *Bodies under Siege: Self-mutilation in Culture and Psychiatry*, updated in 1996, is a key text for understanding self-harm and body modification.

57. In early 2000, shortly after the cinema release of *Girl, Interrupted*, Angelina Jolie spent three days as an inpatient at UCLA's neuropsychiatric hospital. She admitted herself to the facility after experiencing a psychotic episode on a road trip, but it is interesting that she describes herself as having lost her "speech almost completely." Jolie spoke about this experience on CNN's *Larry King Live* on 4 August 2001.

58. Slater, *Prozac Diary*, 50. For mythic resonances, see Nathan Schwartz-Salant, *The Borderline Personality: Vision and Healing* (Wilmette, IL: Chiron, 1989).

59. *Borderline Syndrome: A Personality Disorder of Our Time*, dir. John Peter Spellos (New York: Filmmakers Library, 1989). The film includes an interview with John Gunderson of McLean Hospital, who chaired the personality disorder work group for *DSM-IV*.

60. For Cobain's suicidal tendencies and substance abuse, see Charles R. Cross, *Heavier than Heaven: A Biography of Kurt Cobain* (2001; repr., New York: Hyperion, 2014). For a more speculative account, see Christopher Sandford, *Kurt Cobain* (New York: Da Capo, 1995).

61. See Joan Lachkar, *The Narcissistic/Borderline Couple: New Approaches to Marital Therapy*, rev. ed. (1992; repr., New York: Routledge, 2004).

62. See Maya Pines, "New Focus on Narcissism Offers Analysts Insight into Grandiosity and Emptiness," *New York Times*, 16 March 1982.

63. *DSM-IV*, 658.

64. Erich Fromm, *The Art of Loving* (New York: Harper, 1956), 57.

65. Erich Fromm, *Escape from Freedom* (New York: Rinehart & Co., 1941), 115.

66. Ibid., 116. "The Survival Mentality" is the second chapter of Christopher Lasch's *The Minimal Self: Psychic Survival in Troubled Times* (New York: Norton, 1984), 60–99.

67. Alice Miller, *The Drama of the Gifted Child: The Search for the True Self*, trans. Ruth Ward (1979; repr., New York: Basic Books, 1981), xvi.

68. Therapists at the time were reluctant to abandon the idea of a "true self." See, for example, Alexander Lowen. *Narcissism: Denial of the True Self* (New York: Macmillan, 1983).

69. Heinz Kohut, *The Analysis of the Self: A Systematic Approach to the Psychoanalytic Treatment of Narcissistic Personality Disorders* (Chicago: University of Chicago Press, 1971), xiv.

70. Ibid., 3, 9. In the late 1980s, forensic psychologist J. Reid Meloy discussed the differences between narcissistic personality disorder and its "more severe and aggressive variant, the psychopathic personality"; J. Reid Meloy, *The Psychopathic Mind: Origins, Dynamics, and Treatment* (Northvale, NJ: Aronson, 1988), 52.

71. Kohut, *The Analysis of the Self*, 4.

72. Ibid., 11.

73. Ibid., 9.

74. Don DeLillo, *Americana* (1971; repr., New York: Penguin, 1989), 11.

75. Kohut, *The Analysis of the Self*, 192. Otto Kernberg distinguished between emptiness and loneliness, which is often bound up with a sense of guilt, conflict, and self-punishment: Otto F. Kernberg, *Borderline Conditions and Pathological Narcissism* (1975; repr., New York: Rowman & Littlefield, 2004), 214–215.

76. DeLillo, *Americana*, 11.

77. Ibid., 130, 58.

78. For Bell's relationship with her mother and the role of images in *Americana*, see David Cowart, "For Whom Bell Tolls: *Americana*," *Contemporary Literature* 37, no. 4 (1996): 602–619.

79. DeLillo, *Americana*, 341.

80. Ibid., 205, 347. See Mark Osteen, *American Magic and Dread: Don DeLillo's Dialogue with Culture* (Philadelphia: University of Pennsylvania Press, 2000), 28–30.

81. Georgina Colby, *Bret Easton Ellis: Underwriting the Contemporary* (New York: Palgrave, 2006), 59. Angela Woods makes a similar point in her reading of the actor Victor Ward in Ellis's 2000 novel *Glamorama* as "a self evacuated of psychic depth": Angela Woods, *The Sublime Object of Psychiatry: Schizophrenia in Clinical and Cultural Theory* (Oxford: Oxford University Press, 2011), 219.

82. Brett Easton Ellis, *American Psycho* (New York: Vintage, 1991), 304.

83. Kernberg, *Borderline Conditions and Pathological Narcissism*, 232.

84. Ibid., 233.

85. Annesley, *Blank Fictions*, 18; Colby, *Bret Easton Ellis*, 59.

86. Kernberg, *Borderline Conditions and Pathological Narcissism*, 233.

87. Bateman's violent behavior may be more attributable to the pressures of advertising and consumerism than to a problematic maternal relationship. See James Annesley, *Blank Fictions: Consumerism, Culture, and the Contemporary American Novel* (London: Pluto, 1998), 20.

88. Kernberg, *Borderline Conditions*, 268.

89. Kramer, *Listening to Prozac*, 312.

90. Manuel Babbitt was executed in 1999 for homicide, but not before he was awarded the Purple Heart in prison for his valor during two tours of duty in Vietnam: "Vietnam Veteran Executed for 1980 Murder," *New York Times*, 5 May 1999. The hard-hitting 2015

animated film *Last Day of Freedom* retells Babbitt's story from the perspective of his brother.

91. For Hinckley's personality disorder, see Donald Capps, "John W. Hinckley, Jr.: A Case of Narcissistic Personality Disorder," *Pastoral Psychology* 62, no. 3 (2013): 247–269.

92. Cited in Gerald Posner, *Case Closed: Lee Harvey Oswald and the Assassination of JFK* (London: Warner, 1993), 12.

93. Don DeLillo, *Libra* (New York: Penguin, 1988), 166.

94. Norman Mailer, *Oswald's Tale: An American Mystery* (1995; repr., New York: Random House, 2007), 365.

95. The playwright Harding Lemay's introduction to Bremer's diary portrays an impressionable young man growing up in the shadow of the Vietnam War: Arthur H. Bremer, *An Assassin's Diary* (New York: Harper's, 1973).

96. For the differing diagnostic views brought to the trial, see "Excerpts from Psychiatric Evaluation of Hinckley by the Mental Hospital," *New York Times*, 10 August 1982.

97. See James W. Clarke, *On Being Mad or Merely Angry: John W. Hinckley, Jr., and Other Dangerous People* (Princeton, NJ: Princeton University Press, 1990). In 1986, a woman from Maine, Joanne Harris, wrote to President Reagan asking him to "reduce youth suicides, addiction, abuses, mental illness, future criminals, potential John Hinckleys dramatically" and urging Mrs. Reagan to address developmental issues. She received a standard reply but tried again with Barbara Bush in 1988: Joanne Harris to Ronald Reagan, 19 May 1986 and Joanne Harris to Barbara Bush, 11 November 1988, OA/ID 28719, HE 1–5 [Health: Disease: Physically Handicapped], George H. W. Bush Vice Presidential Records, Mrs. Bush's Office, George Bush Presidential Library, College Station, Texas.

98. Hinckley was released in September 2016 on what the judge called "full-time convalescent leave."

99. See Steven N. Gold, "Fight Club: A Depiction of Contemporary Society as Dissociogenic," *Journal of Trauma and Dissociation* 5 (July 2004): 13; Heike Schwarz, *Beware of the Other Side(s): Multiple Personality Disorder and Dissociative Identity Disorder in American Fiction* (Berlin: Transcript-Verlag, 2013), 321–322.

100. David Eldridge, "The Generic American Psycho," *Journal of American Studies* 42 (April 2008): 27.

101. Jeff Baker, "Bret Easton Ellis Talks about Writing Novels, Making Movies," *California Chronicle*, July 2010; Jaime Clarke, "Interview with Bret Easton Ellis," *Mississippi Review* 27 (Spring–Summer 1999): 74.

102. Ellis, *American Psycho*, 5. For the parodic view of "media-fueled misconceptions" of AIDS in the novel, see Colby, *Bret Easton Ellis*, 69–72.

103. Ibid., 115, 179. See also Martin Weinreich, "'Into the Void': The Hyperrealism of Simulation in Bret Easton Ellis's 'American Psycho,'" *Amerikastudien/American Studies* 49, no. 1 (2004): 71–72.

104. Chuck Palahniuk, *Fight Club* (London: Vintage, 1997), 32.

105. Ibid., 51, 63.

106. Ibid., 59–60, 71.

107. Ibid., 97.

108. Ibid., 168.

109. Jamison, *An Unquiet Mind*, 120.

110. Ibid., 120.

111. See Flora Rheta Schreiber, *Sybil* (1973; repr., New York: Grand Central, 2009). For context for the Sybil case, see Debbie Nathan, *Sybil Exposed: The Extraordinary Story behind the Famous Multiple Personality Case* (New York: Free Press, 2012); Lisa Appignanesi, *Mad, Bad and Sad: A History of Women and the Mind Doctors from 1800 to the Present* (London: Virago, 2008), 486–492. Cornelia Wilbur continued to write about abuse: see, for example, "Multiple Personality and Child Abuse: An Overview," *Psychiatric Clinics of North America* 7, no. 1 (1984): 3–7.

112. Miller, *The Drama of the Gifted Child*, x.

113. Joanne Woodward switched from playing a split-personality patient in the 1957 film *Three Faces of Eve* to the role of the healer figure in the 1976 adaptation of *Sybil*. For discussion of *Three Faces of Eve* and the clinical study on which it is based, see Martin Halliwell, *Therapeutic Revolutions: Medicine, Psychiatry, and American Culture, 1945–1970* (New Brunswick, NJ: Rutgers University Press, 2013), 74, 223, 248.

114. Ibid., 26. For these physical manifestations, see "Multiple Personalities Yielding Clues on Mind-Body Connection," *Chicago Tribune*, 9 June 1985.

115. Nicholas P. Spanos, *Multiple Identities and False Memories: A Sociocognitive Perspective* (Washington, DC: American Psychological Association, 1996), 7.

116. One example of this arose in 1979 at the legal defense of the Ohioan robber and rapist William Milligan. Although the insanity defense at Milligan's trial seemed to be opportunist (citing physical abuse by his stepfather), during his incarceration it was confirmed that Milligan had twenty-four distinct alters, half of whom (the ones he called "The Undesirables") led him astray. See Daniel Keyes, *The Minds of Billy Milligan* (New York: Random House, 1981).

117. Ian Hacking, *Rewriting the Soul: Multiple Personality and the Sciences of Memory* (Princeton, NJ: Princeton University Press, 1995), 96–97; Jennifer Radden, *Divided Minds and Successive Selves: Ethical Issues in Disorders of Identity and Personality* (Cambridge, MA: MIT Press, 1996), 46–57.

118. The first international conference on multiple personality disorder was held in Chicago in 1983. By the end of the 1980s, 1 to 3 percent of the population was thought to have the disorder. See Frank W. Putnam, *Diagnosis and Treatment of Multiple Personality Disorder* (New York: Guilford, 1989); Colin A. Ross, *Multiple Personality Disorder: Diagnosis, Clinical Features, and Treatment* (New York: Wiley, 1989).

119. This episode of *The Oprah Winfrey Show* aired on 21 May 1990, and coincided with a two-part ABC mini-series, *Voices Within: The Lives of Truddi Chase* which reduced Chase's unprecedented number of alters to twenty-two. The *New York Times Magazine* luridly

called them "myriad characters [that] are seething inside the same skull": John Leonard, "All of Me," *New York Times Magazine*, 21 May 1990. This number might stem from the fact that the "Eve" of *The Three Faces of Eve* had recently published an account of the fusion of her twenty-two identities (not three, as originally identified): see Chris Costner Sizemore, *A Mind of My Own* (New York: Morrow, 1989). For the link to PTSD, see Alfie Kohn, "Shattered Innocence," *Psychology Today*, February 1987, 54–58.

120. Truddi Chase, *When Rabbit Howls* (1987; repr., New York: Berkeley, 1990), 22–24.

121. For alternative mothers in *Sybil* and *The Flock*, see Rosaria Champagne, "True Crimes of Motherhood: Mother-Daughter Incest, Multiple Personality Disorder, and the True Crime Novel," in *Feminist Nightmares, Women at Odds: Feminism and the Problems of Sisterhood*, ed. Susan Weisser and Jennifer Fleischner (New York: New York University Press, 1994), 142–158.

122. Joan Frances Casey with Lynn Wilson, *The Flock: The Autobiography of a Multiple Personality* (1991; repr., London: Abacus, 1993), 20. On *The Flock* and *When Rabbit Howls*, see Schwarz, *Beware of the Other Side(s)*, 173–184. For a more recent disclosure of multiple personality disorder, see Robert B. Oxnam, *A Fractured Mind* (New York: Hyperion, 2005).

123. Casey and Wilson. *The Flock*, 160.

124. Ibid., 156.

125. Ibid., 280–281.

126. St. Paul therapist Diane Humenansky's license was permanently suspended in 1997 after ten patients sued her for misdiagnosis and for planting false memories of abuse. See Joan Acocella, *Creating Hysteria: Women and Multiple Personality Disorder* (San Francisco: Jossey-Bass, 1999), 1–25. Richard Schwartz reframed the language of personalities with his Internal Family Systems Theory in the 1990s: see Richard Schwartz, *Internal Family Systems Therapy* (New York: Guilford, 1995).

127. Slater, *Prozac Diary*, 9. Slater had earlier discussed her life as a patient in her collection *Welcome to My Country* (New York: Random House, 1996).

128. Slater, *Prozac Diary*, 45.

129. Ibid., 47.

130. For the health risks of serotonin boosters such as Prozac, see Joseph Glenmullen, *Prozac Backlash* (New York: Simon and Schuster, 2000).

131. See, for example, Lauren Slater, *Love Works Like This: Moving from One Kind of Life to Another* (New York: Random House, 2002).

132. Slater, *Prozac Diary*, 184.

133. See Ian Hacking, "Making Up People," in *Reconstructing Individualism: Autonomy, Individuality, and the Self in Western Thought*, ed. Thomas C. Heller, David Wellbery, and Morton Sosna (Stanford, CA: Stanford University Press, 1986), 222–237; Paul Roth, "Ways of Pastmaking," *History of the Human Sciences* 15 (November 2002): 125–143.

134. Lindsey Grubbs, "Lauren Slater and the Experts: Malingering, Masquerade, and the Disciplinary Control of Diagnosis," *Literature and Medicine* 33 (Spring 2015): 30.

CHAPTER 8 — MENTAL HEALTH AT THE MILLENNIUM

1. George H. W. Bush, "Statement on Signing the ADAMHA Reorganization Act," 10 July 1992, in *Public Papers of the Presidents of the United States: George Bush, 1992*, Book 1 (Washington, DC: U.S. Government Printing Office, 1993), 207, 210.

2. "Magic Johnson Quits Panel on AIDS," *New York Times*, 26 September 1992. There is evidence that Johnson did not really engage with the commission beyond the first two months of his appointment. See Daniel Casse to Ede Holiday, 13 July 1992, OA/ID 07133, AIDS Commission, Bush Presidential Records, White House Office of Cabinet Affairs–Daniel Cass Files, George Bush Presidential Library, College Station, Texas. Johnson's successor on the AIDS Commission, artist Mary Fisher, later called Bush's response to AIDS "personally sympathetic but publicly lame." See the 2012 foreword to Mary Fisher, *My Name Is Mary: A Memoir* (New York: Scribner's, 1995). Both Johnson and Fisher were HIV positive (Fisher had contracted AIDS from her second husband at the turn of the 1990s).

3. Earvin Johnson Jr. to George Bush, 14 January 1992, OA/ID 07133, AIDS Commission, White House Office of Cabinet Affairs–Daniel Cass Files, George Bush Presidential Library.

4. Bush, "Remarks on Signing the Americans with Disabilities Act of 1990," 26 July 1990, in *Public Papers of the Presidents of the United States: George Bush, 1990*, Book 2 (Washington, DC: U.S. Government Printing Office, 1991), 1068. Randy Shilts was deeply critical of the inaction of the Reagan administration in *And the Band Played On: Politics, People, and the AIDS Epidemic* (New York: Penguin, 1987). In contrast, Bush took seriously the 1988 report of the President's Commission on the HIV Epidemic.

5. George H. W. Bush, "Statement on Congressional Action on the Americans with Disabilities Act," 13 July 1990, in *Public Papers of the Presidents of the United States: George Bush, 1990*, Book 1 (Washington, DC: U.S. Government Printing Office, 1991), 207, 210. For mental health and the ADA, see William Eaton, ed., *Public Mental Health* (Oxford: Oxford University Press, 2012), 356, 366; and Leonard S. Rubenstein, "People with Psychiatric Disabilities," in *Implementing the Americans with Disabilities Act*, ed. Jane West (Oxford: Blackwell, 1996), 339–364.

6. George H. W. Bush, "Statement on Signing the ADAMHA Reorganization Act," 207–210. See also George H. W. Bush, "Remarks at the National Institute of Health Clinical Center, Rockville, Maryland, NIH Clinical Center, 12//22/89," OA/ID 04939, Office of Policy Development–James Pinkerton Chronological File, George Bush Presidential Library.

7. George Bush, "Proclamation 6158: Decade of the Brain, 1990–1999," July 1990, *The American Presidency Project*, accessed 28 December 2016, www.presidency.ucsb.edu/ws/?pid=1869. On the "brain revolution," see Jeffry Lieberman with Ogi Ogas, *Shrinks: The Untold Story of Psychiatry* (New York: Little, Brown, 2015).

8. For example, the 1992 issue of *Our Bodies, Ourselves* begins with a discussion of healthism and cites Robert Crawford's foundational 1980 essay "Healthism and the Medicalization of Everyday Life" (as discussed in the introduction). See Boston Women's

Health Book Collective, *The New Our Bodies, Ourselves: A Book by and for Women* (New York: Simon & Schuster, 1992), 3.

9. George H. W. Bush, "Remarks at the Swearing-in Ceremony for Louis W. Sullivan as Secretary of Health and Human Services," 10 March 1989, in *Public Papers of the Presidents of the United States* (Washington, DC: U.S. Government Printing Office, 1990), Book 1, 207–210. For criticisms of Sullivan, see "HHS Secretary Sullivan's Unofficial Portfolio," *Washington Post*, 18 August 1990. For Sullivan's work in and beyond the Bush administration, see Louis Wade Sullivan, *Breaking Ground: My Life in Medicine* (Athens: University of Georgia Press, 2014).

10. See George H. W. Bush, "Address before a Joint Session of Congress on the State of the Union," 31 January 1990, in *Public Papers of the Presidents, George Bush*, 1990, Book 1, 129–134; Daniel R. Heimbach to Ede Holiday, 25 July 1990, OA/ID 04810, Health (File J)–National Health Reform, Bush Presidential Records, Domestic Policy Council Files, George Bush Presidential Library. For Bush's healthcare plan, see *The President's Comprehensive Health Reform Program* (Washington, DC: U.S. Government Printing Office, 1992).

11. Arthur J. Barsky, "The Paradox of Health," *New England Journal of Medicine* 318 (February 1988): 414–418.

12. See Aaron T. Beck, *The Diagnosis and Management of Depression* (Philadelphia: University of Pennsylvania Press, 1967); Aaron T. Beck, *Depression: Causes and Treatment* (Philadelphia: University of Pennsylvania Press, 1972).

13. Kurt Kroenke, R. L. Spitzer, and J. B. Williams, "The PHQ-9: Validity of a Brief Depression Severity Measure," *Journal of General Internal Medicine* 16 (September 2001): 606–613.

14. On 24 June 1993, Rosalynn Carter and Tipper Gore spoke at a conference organized by the Mental Health Program of the Carter Center in Washington, DC.

15. See *Healthy People 2000*, accessed 11 December 2016, www.cdc.gov/nchs/data/hp2000/mentalhlth/objtbls.pdf.

16. See the National Comorbidity Study, 1992, accessed 22 December 2016, www.hcp.med.harvard.edu/ncs.

17. Mrs. Gore spoke at Howard University to open the White House Conference on Mental Health on 7 June 1999: Master Tape 10101–10104, Audio Visual Archive, William J. Clinton Presidential Library, Little Rock, Arkansas. For a video version of her remarks, see "White House Conference on Mental Health (1999)," YouTube video, accessed 2 February 2017, https://www.youtube.com/watch?v=WixpTOGXhIc. Tipper Gore gave a number of related public speeches in the period 1997–1999, four of which are collected on the archived Clinton White House website: clinton5.nara.gov/WH/EOP/VP_Wife/mental_health.html, accessed 11 December 2016.

18. *The World Health Organization 1999 Report: Making a Difference* (Geneva: World Health Organization, 1999), accessed 11 December 2016, www.who.int/whr/1999/en/whr99_en.pdf and U.S. Department of Health and Human Services, *Mental Health: A Report of the Surgeon General* (Washington, DC: Department of Health and Human

Services, National Institutes of Health, 1999), profiles.nlm.nih.gov/ps/access/NNBBHS.pdf, accessed 5 January 2017.

19. Clinton spoke eloquently about the "managed competition" model of health insurance during the second presidential debate held in Richmond, Virginia in October 1992; see Oct 15, 1992–2nd Presidential Debate Bush, Clinton & Perot, YouTube video, accessed 7 February 2017, https://www.youtube.com/watch?v=4-m5bW-13us. In response, President Bush blamed malpractice cases for breaking the system.

20. Bill Clinton, "Address Accepting the Presidential Nomination at the Democratic National Convention," 16 July 1992, *The American Presidency Project*, accessed 28 December 2016, www.presidency.ucsb.edu/ws/?pid=25958.

21. See George H. W. Bush, "Address before a Joint Session of Congress on the State of the Union," 28 January 1992; and George H. W. Bush, "Radio Address to the Nation on Health Care Reform," 3 July 1992, in *Public Papers of the Presidents, George Bush, 1992*, Book 1, 156–163, 205–209. For media reaction to Bush's stance on healthcare reform, see Lori Cox Han, *A Presidency Upstaged: The Public Leadership of George H. W. Bush* (College Station: Texas A&M University Press, 2011), 186–194.

22. Bill Clinton, "Remarks on Signing the Health Insurance Portability and Accountability Act of 1996," 21 August 1996, in *Public Papers of the Presidents, William J. Clinton, 1996*, Book 2, 1319. In this speech, Clinton cited his chairing of the healthcare panel in Memphis as a formative moment in his commitment to healthcare reform.

23. For example, at a Democratic Leadership Council luncheon on 11 December 1996, Clinton mentioned a woman from New Hampshire with Down syndrome who had given him a badge that morning with the word "Down" crossed out, replaced by the word "Up." This led him to comment: "You must believe in the potential of the American people. We cannot afford to patronize each other with cynicism": *Public Papers of the Presidents, William J. Clinton, 1996*, Book 2, 2191.

24. Ibid.

25. "Remarks by the President in Lunch with Columnists," 21 September 1993, Box 2, Health Care–BC Interviews, 2006–0885-F, Segment 1, Health Care Task Force Records, William J. Clinton Presidential Library. See also Arthur King, Thomas Hyclak, and Samuel McMahon, eds., *North American Health Care Policy in the 1990s* (New York: Wiley, 1993), 199.

26. "First Lady Hillary Rodham Clinton's Remarks to Magazine Publishers of America," Orlando, Florida, 12 October 1993, Box 23, HC–HRC Magazine Speech, 2006–0885-F, Segment 1, Health Care Task Force Records, William J. Clinton Presidential Library. For Hillary Clinton's influential role as chair of the task force, see Jeff Gerth and Don Van Natta Jr., *Her Way: The Hopes and Ambitions of Hillary Rodham Clinton* (New York: Back Bay, 2007), 117–131 and Carl Bernstein, *A Woman in Charge* (New York: Vintage, 2008), 284–294.

27. "The Clinton Health Plan Is Alive on Arrival," *New York Times*, 3 October 1993.

28. Richard M. Nixon, *Beyond Peace* (New York: Random House, 1994), 209.

29. Ibid., 210.

30. Colin Gordon, *Dead on Arrival: The Politics of Health Care in Twentieth-Century America* (Princeton, N.J.: Princeton University Press, 2003), 41, 43.

31. Alex Waddan, *Clinton's Legacy: A New Democrat in Governance* (London: Palgrave, 2002), 90. For the aftermath of the failed Health Security Act, see Paul Starr, *Remedy and Reaction: The Peculiar American Struggle over Health Care Reform* (New Haven, CT: Yale University Press, 2011), 129–146.

32. On the Health Security Act, see, for example, Daniel Yankelovich, "The Debate that Wasn't: The Public and the Clinton Plan," *Health Affairs* 15 (Spring 1994): 7–23; Haynes Johnson and David S. Broder, *The System: The American Way of Politics at Breaking Point* (Boston: Little, Brown, 1996); Theda Skocpol, *Boomerang: Health Care Reform and the Turn Against Government* (New York: Norton, 1996); and Jacob S. Hacker, *The Road to Nowhere: The Genesis of President Clinton's Plan for Health Security* (Princeton, NJ: Princeton University Press, 1997).

33. "Mental Health Fact Sheet," Box 6, OA/ID 3017, Ira Magaziner, Behavioral Health Care Tomorrow, Health Care Task Force Records, William J. Clinton Presidential Library.

34. "Coverage for Mental Illness, Drug Abuse Urged," *Washington Post*, 8 March 1994.

35. For Donna Shalala on managed competition see, for example, "Clinton Plan: Tough Sell Yet to Come," *USA Today*, 14 April 1993.

36. See Richard A. Hogarty, *Massachusetts Politics and Public Policy: Studies in Power and Leadership* (Amherst: University of Massachusetts Press, 2002), 89–90, 102–105; "Report on the Working Group on Mental Health," Box 6, OA/ID 4959, Ira Magaziner: Conference on Health Care Reform, 5 April 1999 (1), Health Care Task Force Records, William J. Clinton Presidential Library. A scathing critique of Magaziner's health plans appeared in the liberal magazine *The New Republic* a year later. See Jacob Weisberg, "Dies Ira," *The New Republic*, 24 January 1994, 18–24.

37. Charles B. Nemeroff, "The Neurobiology of Depression," *Scientific American* 278, no. 6 (1998): 42–49.

38. "Schizophrenia and Psychiatry's Limits," *Wall Street Journal*, 9 March 1994. See also Tipper Gore, "The High Social Cost of Mental Illness," *Wall Street Journal*, 12 January 1994.

39. See "Administration Rethinking Mental-Health Coverage," *New York Times*, 10 June 1993; "Mental Health Coverage Being Drafted," *Washington Post*, 4 July 1993.

40. "Dukakis Releases Medical Details to Stop Rumors on Mental Health," *New York Times*, 4 August 1988.

41. The information about Dukakis's brother came to light in Charles Kenney and Robert L. Turner's *Dukakis: An American Odyssey* (Boston: Houghton Mifflin, 1988). Kitty Dukakis addressed her addiction in her 1990 autobiography *Now You Know* and later became an advocate of electroconvulsive treatment.

42. Martha Manning, *Undercurrents: A Life beneath the Surface* (New York: HarperCollins, 1994); Tracy Thompson, *The Beast: A Journey through Depression* (New York: Penguin, 1995). See also Henry H. Kim, ed., *Depression* (San Diego, CA: Greenhaven, 1999).

43. Styron noted in 1953 (when he was 28) that his life felt like "a long gray depression interrupted by moments of high hilarity": William Styron, *Selected Letters of William Styron*, ed. Rose Styron with R. Blakeslee Gilpin (New York: Random House, 2013), 184.

44. William Styron, *Darkness Visible: A Memoir of Madness* (1990; repr., London: Vintage, 2004), 84, 64. Styron's article "Darkness Visible" was published in *Vanity Fair*, December 1989, 212–215, 278–286.

45. Betty Friedan discussed the sense of powerlessness that often accompanies depression in the middle-aged and elderly in Frieden, *The Fountain of Age* (New York: Simon Schuster, 1993), 61–62.

46. Styron, *Darkness Visible*, 72.

47. Hopelessness was thought at the time to be the chief precipitating factor in suicide. See Herbert Hendin, *Suicide in America* (1984; repr. New York: Norton, 1995), 15.

48. Philip Roth, *The Facts: A Novelist's Autobiography* (1988; repr., London: Vintage, 2007), 5.

49. Styron, *Darkness Visible*, 36, 12.

50. Ibid., 5.

51. Ibid., 44, 47.

52. Ibid., 84.

53. Styron's interview with Diane Sawyer was broadcast on 30 August 1990, followed the next day by the ABC documentary *Depression: Beyond the Darkness*. Sawyer re-aired the interview footage with Styron a week after Kurt Cobain's suicide in April 1994.

54. Styron, *Selected Letters*, 637. For the theme of authenticity in *Darkness Visible*, see Abigail Cheever, "Prozac Americans: Depression, Identity, and Selfhood," *Twentieth Century Literature* 46 (Autumn 2000): 346–368.

55. Styron, *Selected Letters*, 636, 639. This letter to biographer Gavin Cologne-Brookes, dated 11 February 2002, is Styron's final full published letter, even though he lived for four more years. Cologne-Brookes notes the paradox of *Darkness Visible*: Styron uses "beautiful prose" to describe "depression's messy reality": Gavin Cologne-Brookes, *Rereading William Styron* (Baton Rouge: Louisiana State University Press, 2014), 59.

56. As a student at Amherst, Wallace published a short story on depression: "The Planet Trillaphon as It Stands in Relation to the Bad Thing," *Amherst Review* 12 (1984): 26–33. I am grateful to Adam Kelly for his insights on Wallace's work.

57. David Foster Wallace, *Infinite Jest* (1996; repr., New York: Back Bay, 2006), 695–696.

58. See Lewis H. Lapham, "Omens," *Harper's*, January 1998, 9–11; and Ronald J. Glasser, "The Doctor Is Not In," *Harper's*, March 1998, 35–41.

59. D. T. Max, *Every Love Story Is a Ghost Story* (New York: Granta, 2012), 202–203, 241.

60. David Foster Wallace, "The Depressed Person," *Harper's*, January 1998, 57.

61. Ibid., 61.

62. Ibid., 64.

63. Ibid.

64. David Foster Wallace, *Brief Interviews with Hideous Men* (Boston: Little, Brown, 1999), 283.

65. Wallace hung himself in September 2008, a year after he decided to stop taking the antidepressant phenelzine (sold as Nardil).

66. Andrew Solomon, *The Noonday Demon: An Anatomy of Depression* (2001; repr., London: Vintage, 2015), 17.

67. Ibid., 12, 14.

68. Wallace, *Infinite Jest*, 696.

69. Solomon, *The Noonday Demon*, 17.

70. Andrew Solomon, "Anatomy of Melancholy," *New Yorker*, 12 January 1998, 46.

71. Andrew Solomon, "A Death of One's Own," *New Yorker*, 28 May 1995, 54–60, 62–69. See Andrew Solomon, *A Stone Boat: A Novel* (New York: Scribner, 1994).

72. Solomon, "Anatomy of Melancholy," 46, 48.

73. Ibid., 48.

74. Ibid., 58, 61.

75. Wallace, *Infinite Jest*, 694; Solomon, "Anatomy of Melancholy," 61.

76. See Emmy Gut, *Productive and Unproductive Depression: Success or Failure of a Vital Process* (New York: Basic Books, 1989).

77. Solomon, *The Noonday Demon*, 19.

78. Ibid., 21.

79. Dana Crowley Jack, *Silencing the Self: Women and Depression* (Cambridge, MA: Harvard University Press, 1991), 30–37. For stress, alcoholism, substance abuse, and suicide among young women, see "Women's Health: Report of the Public Health Service Task Force on Women's Health Issues," *Public Health Reports* 100 (January–February 1985): 98–101.

80. Boston Women's Health Book Collective, *The New Our Bodies, Ourselves*, 57.

81. Ibid., 476, 485–487. Journalist Tracy Thompson explored postpartum depression in *The Beast* and actress Brooke Shields's 2005 autobiographical account *Down Came the Rain* helped raise awareness of the condition.

82. See Cheryl T. Beck, "Predictors of Postpartum Depression: An Update," *Nursing Research and Practice* 50 (September–October 2001): 275–285.

83. See Sandra Morgen, *Into Our Own Hands: The Women's Health Movement in the United States, 1969–1990* (New Brunswick, NJ: Rutgers University Press, 2002), 85–90.

84. Rosalynn Carter and Susan K. Golant, *Helping Yourself Help Others: A Book for Caregivers* (New York: Random House, 1994), 46. Eighty percent of the caregivers who took part in a Georgia-based CARE-NET survey of 1990 (covering 175 informal caregivers drawn from a sample of 543) were women, of which more than half feared burnout.

85. The National Mental Health Association gave Rosalynn Carter its Into the Light award on 25 September 1997, in Alexandria, Virginia.

86. Rosalynn Carter and Susan K. Golant, *Helping Someone with Mental Illness: A Compassionate Guide for Family, Friends, and Caregivers* (New York: Random House, 1998), 144.

87. Ibid., 146.

88. Ibid., 152.

89. Rod Steiger and Joan Rivers both feature in Kathy Cronkite's *On the Edge of Darkness: Conversations about Conquering Depression* (New York: Delta, 1994). For an example of Rod Steiger discussing his depressive episodes, see his interview with Matias Bombal at the Reno Film Festival, October 2000, https://www.youtube.com/watch?v=MmzCFM9_U80.

90. "Joan Rivers Offers Some Stand-Up Therapy," *New York Times*, 29 January 1995; and Joan Rivers, *Bouncing Back* (New York: Harper, 1997).

91. See "Rod Steiger: The Climb out of the Depths of Despair," *Los Angeles Times*, 14 October 1979.

92. Emily Martin, *Flexible Bodies: Tracking Immunity in American Culture from the Days of Polio to the Age of AIDS* (Boston: Beacon, 1994), 127–142.

93. Todd Haynes, *Far from Heaven, Safe, and Superstar: The Karen Carpenter Story* (New York: Grove, 2003), 103, 180.

94. Rob White compares the self-help ethos of Wrenwood to self-styled guru Louise L. Hay's philosophy in her 1984 book *You Can Heal Your Life* and her bogus suggestion that the cause of AIDS is a feeling of hopelessness and denial of the self: Rob White, *Todd Haynes* (Champaign: University of Illinois Press, 2013), 52.

95. Ibid., 56.

96. Morgen, *Into Our Own Hands*, 235.

97. "'You Have to Get Help': Frightening Experience Now a Tool to Help Others," *USA Today*, 7 May 1999. See also "Tipper Gore Says She Took Treatment for Depression," *New York Times*, 7 May 1999; "Tipper Gore Details Depression Treatment," *Washington Post*, 8 May 1999; "Mrs. Gore's Depression," *New York Times*, 11 May 1999.

98. "Tipper Gore Keeps Cautious Watch at Door She Opened," *New York Times*, 7 June 1999.

99. See "Tipper Steps Out," *Newsweek*, 24 May 1999, 48–51.

100. JoAnn Bren Guernsey, *Tipper Gore: Voice for the Voiceless* (Minneapolis, MN: Lerner, 1994), 26, 40, 43.

101. "Equal Coverage of Physical and Mental Ills Is White House Goal for Federal Employees," *New York Times*, 25 May 1999.

102. "White House Conference on Mental Health: Working for a Healthier America" briefing paper, 6 June 1999, Box 18, 2011-0688-S, Health Reform: Mental Health Conference [June 7, 1999], Domestic Policy Council–Neera Tanden, William J. Clinton

Library. The initial brief for the conference is held in the Gore Vice Presidential Records: "Draft Proposal: White House Conference on Mental Health," Box 12, OA/ID 01017, Health: Mental Health [1], Records of the Office of Domestic Policy–David W. Beier Files, National Archives and Records Administration, Washington DC.

103. Tipper Gore, "From Discovery to Recovery," speech at the meeting of the National Alliance for the Mentally Ill, Washington, DC 16 July 1998, accessed 11 December 2016, clinton5.nara.gov/WH/EOP/VP_Wife/speeches/19980716.html.

104. "A Policeman Who Rescued 4 in Bombing Kills Himself," *New York Times*, 11 May 1996. For the impact of Columbine, see "Horror that Burned into Littleton Minds," *The Washington Post*, May 15, 1999.

105. Bill Clinton, "Remarks at the White House Conference on Mental Health," 7 June 1999, in *Public Papers of the Presidents of the United States: William J. Clinton, 1999*, Book 1 (Washington, DC: U.S. Government Printing Office, 2001), 895.

106. Ibid.

107. Ibid.

108. For the phrase "science and services," see Nelba Chavez, Steven E. Hyman, and Bernard S. Arons, "Foreword," in U.S. Department of Health and Human Services, *Mental Health: A Report of the Surgeon General* (Washington, DC: Department of Health and Human Services, National Institutes of Health, 1999).

109. Al and Tipper Gore, *Joined at the Heart: The Transformation of the American Family* (New York: Henry Holt, 2002), 296.

110. Ibid., 297–298.

111. "What It Would Really Take," *Time*, 7 June 1999, 54–56. In 1992, Senator Gore associated mental illness with "spiritual loss" and the growth of a materialistic culture: see Al Gore, *Earth in the Balance* (Boston: Houghton Mifflin, 1992), 221.

112. See Charles Barber, *Comfortably Numb: How Psychiatry Is Medicating a Nation* (New York: Pantheon, 2008), 224; Sherry Turkle, *Life on the Screen: Identity in the Age of the Internet* (1995; repr., New York: Simon & Schuster, 2011), 255–269.

113. See Alexander Cockburn and Jeffrey St. Clair, *Al Gore: A User's Manual* (London: Verso, 2000).

114. See "They Threaten, Seethe and Unhinge, Then Kill in Quantity," *New York Times*, 9 April 2000.

115. National Council of La Raza, Center for Health Promotion Fact Sheet, November 1993 and internal memos on Native American Mental Health, May 1999, Box 43, 206–0197-F Segment 3, Records on President Clinton's Indian Native American Policy, Mary Smith Files, William J. Clinton Presidential Library. Hillary Clinton convened a session on Hispanic Children and Youth at the White House on 2 August 1999; see "The White House Convening on Hispanic Children and Youth," *La Prensa San Diego*, 13 August 1999, accessed 3 February 2017, http://laprensa-sandiego.org/archieve/august13/white.htm.

116. "Remarks to the Community at Pine Ridge Indian Reservation," 7 July 1999, *Public Papers of the Presidents: William J. Clinton, 1999*, Book 1, 1149–1153.

117. Paul B. Simms, "Regional Health Councils: An Alternative Approach to Health Reform," 2–3 May 1993, Box 6, Ira Magaziner, Regional Health Councils, 2006–0885-F, Health Care Task Force Records, William J. Clinton Presidential Library. For broader context, see the first section of Arlene Rubin Stiffman and Larry E. Davis, ed., *Ethnic Issues in Adolescent Mental Health* (London: Sage, 1990).

118. "U.S. AIDS Cases Reported through December 1992," *HIV/AIDS Surveillance Report*, 5, no. 1 (1993): 1–23. At the close of the Sixth International AIDS Conference in June 1990, while being heckled by AIDS activists, Louis Sullivan spoke about the need to develop "culturally relevant and sensitive programs" for poor and minority communities affected by AIDS. "Remarks by Louise W. Sullivan, M.D., Sixth International Conference on AIDS", OA/ID 049807, Health (File A)–AIDS [1], Domestic Policy Council Files, George Bush Presidential Library. For Sullivan's speech and the demonstration, see "Sixth International AIDS Conference," accessed 7 January 2017, https://www.c-span.org/video/?12863-1/sixth-international-aids-conference. On the voices of HIV-positive African American women, see Rosanna DeMarco, "Supporting Voice in Women Living with HIV/AIDS," in *Silencing the Self across Cultures: Depression and Gender in the Social World*, ed. Dana Crowley Jack and Alisha Ali (Oxford: Oxford University Press, 2010), 343–362.

119. Joseph R. Berger and Robert M. Levy, eds., *AIDS and the Nervous System*, 2nd ed. (Philadelphia: Lippincott-Raven, 1997), 433–436. The level of clinical depression among the HIV-positive population was similar to the levels among those with Alzheimer's or Parkinson's. There had been only marginal discussion of psychological stress in relation to AIDS at the Third International Conference on AIDS held in June 1987, a conference at which Vice-President Bush gave the keynote address. "Remarks for Vice President George Bush, Third International Conference on AIDS," OA/ID 14874, 6/1/87 Third International Conference on AIDS, Washington, DC, Speechwriter Files, George H. W. Vice Presidential Records Office, George Bush Presidential Library.

120. See "The Alarming Spread of AIDS among Women," *Washington Post*, 11 December 1990.

121. *One America in the 21st Century: Forging a New Future: The President's Initiative on Race* (Washington, DC: U.S. Government Printing Office, 1997), 89.

122. Bill Clinton, "Remarks at the White House Conference on Mental Health."

123. Michael Winerip, "Bedlam on the Streets: Increasingly the Mental Ill Have Nowhere to Go. That's Their Problem and Ours," *New York Times*, 23 May 1999. See also "Real Help for the Mentally Ill," *New York Times*, 11 January 1999.

124. For a similar argument, see "Why Deinstitutionalization Turned Deadly," *Wall Street Journal*, August 4, 1998.

125. See *Outcasts on Main Street: Report on the Federal Task Force on Homelessness and Severe Mental Illness* (Rockland, MD: Department of Health and Human Services, 1995).

126. For Massachusetts initiatives, see the special issue of *New England Journal of Public Policy* 8, no. 1 (1992): 11, 16, 419–430.

127. Ralph Nader, "The Greens and the Presidency: A Voice, not an Echo," *The Nation*, 8 July 1996.

128. "The President's Radio Address," 1 January 2000, in *Public Papers of the Presidents of the United States: William J. Clinton, 2000–2001*, Book 1 (Washington, DC: U.S. Government Printing Office, 2002), 1.

129. "Gore Calls for Better Benefits for Children with Mental Ills," *New York Times*, 1 June 2000.

130. George W. Bush mentioned community health centers frequently in 2006–2007. See "Remarks at a Luncheon for Congressional Candidate Jon A. Porter in Las Vegas, Nevada," 24 April 2006, in *Public Papers of the Presidents of the United States: George W. Bush, 2006*, Book 1 (Washington, DC: National Archives and Records Administration, 2010), 798; George W. Bush, "Remarks Following a Meeting on Health Care and an Exchange with Reporters in Omaha," 5 December 2007, in *Public Papers of the Presidents of the United States: George W. Bush, 2007*, Book 2 (Washington, DC: National Archives and Records Administration, 2011), 1526.

CONCLUSION

1. Walker Percy, *Love in the Ruins* (New York: Picador, 1974), 56–58.

2. "College Youth Presentation," 17 January 1971, Box 21, Value Added Tax [1970]–Youth [1–24–72], White House Special Files–Egil Krogh, Richard Nixon Presidential Library, Yorba Linda, California. The data was provided by pollster Daniel Yankelovich.

3. Dr. Hafden Mahler to President Carter, 11 August 1978, Box 52, Addendum–International Health, Records of Peter Bourne, Jimmy Carter Presidential Library, Atlanta, Georgia. See also Mahler, "World Health Is Indivisible," address to the World Health Assembly in Geneva, 9 May 1978, published in *Health Values*, 3 (January–February 1979): 61–66.

4. David Satcher, "Foreword," in Daniel E. Dawes, *150 Years of Obamacare* (Baltimore, MD: Johns Hopkins University Press, 2016), ix.

5. *Depression: A Global Crisis* was released on Mental Health Day (10 October 2012): www.who.int/mental_health/management/depression/wfmh_paper_depression_wmhd_2012.pdf

6. Michael F. Hogan to President George W. Bush, 22 July 2003, in The President's New Freedom Commission on Mental Health, *Achieving the Promise: Transforming Mental Health Care in America* (Washington, DC: Department of Health and Human Services, 2003), n.p. Mrs. Carter noticed similarities between the 2002 New Freedom Commission and the 1977 President's Commission on Mental Health. See Rosalynn Carter, with Susan Golant and Kathryn Cade, *Within Our Reach: Ending the Mental Health Crisis* (Emmaus, PA: Rodale, 2010), xxii. For connections between the two commissions, see John K. Inglehart, "The Mental Health Maze and the Call for Transformation," *The New England Journal of Medicine* 350 (January 2004): 507–514.

7. "From Paternalism to Productivity: 'Whatever It Takes,'" Report of the President's Committee on the Employment of People with Disabilities, 8 April 1990, OA/ID 04808, Health (File E)–Handicapped, Domestic Policy Council Files, George Bush Presidential Library, College Station, Texas.

8. For a comparative study of health inequalities, see Clare Bambra, *Health Divides: Where You Live Can Kill You* (Bristol: Polity Press, 2016).

9. George W. Bush, "Remarks at the University of New Mexico in Albuquerque, New Mexico," 29 April 2002, in *Public Papers of the Presidents of the United States: George W. Bush, 2002*, Book 1 (Washington, DC: National Archives and Records Administration, 2004), 677–678. For Bill Clinton's links to Bellah, see Robert D. Linder, "Universal Pastor: President Bill Clinton's Civil Religion," *Journal of Church and State* 38 (Autumn 1996): 733–749.

10. Bush, "Remarks at the University of New Mexico," 678.

11. *Emergency Response: A Roadmap for Federal Action in America's Mental Health Crisis* (Washington, DC: Campaign for Mental Health Reform, 2005).

12. Gerald N. Grob and Howard H. Goldman, *The Dilemma of Federal Mental Health Policy: Radical Reform or Incremental Change?* (New Brunswick, NJ: Rutgers University Press, 2006), 179–180.

13. On what was called "Buffalo Creek syndrome," see James T. Titchener and Frederic T. Kapp, "Family and Character Change at Buffalo Creek," *American Journal of Psychiatry* 133 (March 1976): 295–301; Kai T. Erikson, *Everything in Its Path: Destruction of Community in the Buffalo Creek Flood* (New York: Simon and Schuster, 1976). On Hurricane Katrina, see Jean Rhodes, Christian Chan, Christina Paxson, Cecilia Rouse, and Elizabeth Fussell, "The Impact of Hurricane Katrina on the Mental and Physical Health of Low-Income Parents in New Orleans," *American Journal of Orthopsychiatry* 80 (April 2010): 237–247; Gary Rivlin, *Katrina: After the Flood* (New York: Simon and Schuster, 2015), 259–260, 367–368. The Carter Center held a symposium entitled "Mental Health in the Wake of Katrina" on 8–9 November 2006.

14. George W. Bush, "Remarks on Compassionate Conservatism in San Jose, California," 30 April 2002, in *Public Papers of the Presidents of the United States: George W. Bush, 2002*, Book 1, 693.

15. This phrase was used on the Points of Light awards certificates. On the Points of Light Foundation see the press releases of 5 January 1990 and 22 May 1990, OA/ID 07633, Washington Post, Bruce Chapman–11/2/90, National Service: A Bad Idea, Office of National Service–Miscellaneous Files, George Bush Presidential Library.

16. For the Carter quote, see *The Presidential Campaign 1976*, vol. 1, part 2 (Washington, DC: U.S. Government Printing Office, 1978), 999–1000.

17. See Theda Skocpol, *Boomerang: Health Care Reform and the Turn against Government* (New York: Norton, 1996).

18. For the statistics, see National Institute of Mental Health, "Inmate Mental Health," accessed 28 December, 2016, www.nimh.nih.gov/health/statistics/prevalence/inmate-mental-health.shtml. In 2004, George W. Bush launched a Prisoner Reentry Initiative as a form of faith-based and community support, but he did not discuss the health challenges inmates or released prisoners face. For mental health issues in prisons, see Terry Kupers, *Prison Madness* (New York: Wiley, 1999); Michelle Alexander, *The New Jim*

Crow: Mass Incarceration in the Age of Colorblindness (New York: New Press, 2011); and Joseph D. Galanek, "The Cultural Construction of Mental Illness in Prison: A Perfect Storm of Pathology," *Culture, Medicine and Psychiatry* 37 (March 2013): 195–225. See also "Even Nightmares are Classified: Interrogation's Shadow Hampers Mental Care in Guantánamo," *New York Times*, 13 November 2016.

19. Institute of Medicine, *The Future of the Public's Health in the 21st Century* (Washington, DC: National Academies Press, 2003), xv.

20. Satcher, "Foreword," xi.

21. The second White House-sponsored National Conference on Mental Health was held on 3 June 2013, three weeks after the publication of the fifth edition of *DSM*.

22. President Obama signed the Mental Health Reform Act on 15 March 2016; he signed the 21st Century Cures Act on 13 December 2016. For Donald Trump's healthcare pledges, see "Healthcare Reform to Make America Great Again," www.donaldjtrump.com/positions/healthcare-reform. Hillary Clinton's campaign healthcare plans were more detailed. On mental health, see "Hillary Clinton's Comprehensive Agenda on Mental Health," a speech to the American Legion in Cincinnati, Ohio, 31 August 2016, http://time.com/4474619/read-hillary-clinton-american-legion-speech, accessed 6 January 2017. See also "Hope for Americans with Mental Illness," *New York Times*, 5 September 2016; Hillary Clinton and Tim Kaine, *Stronger Together: A Blueprint for America's Future* (New York: Simon & Schuster, 2016), 89–95.

23. One example is the National Institute of Mental Health's "Real Men, Real Depression" multimedia campaign of 2003.

24. See Kimberlé Crenshaw's address at the "Women of the World" festival, Southbank Centre, London, 12 March 2016, "Kimberlé Crenshaw, On Intersectionality, WOW 2016 keynote," YouTube video, accessed 6 January 2017, https://www.youtube.com/watch?v=-DW4HLgYPlA.

25. Nancy J. Hirschmann and Beth Linker, eds., *Civil Disabilities: Citizenship, Membership, and Belonging* (Philadelphia: University of Pennsylvania Press, 2015), 2.

26. See James Berger, *The Disarticulate: Language, Disability, and the Narratives of Modernity* (New York: New York University Press, 2014), 186–188. For a recent critique of both the medical and social models see Jonas-Sébastien Beaudry, "Beyond (Models of) Disability," *Journal of Medicine and Philosophy* 41 (April 2016): 210–228.

27. On health citizenship, see Stuart Murray, "Afterword: Health, Care, Citizenship," in *The Edinburgh Companion to Critical Medical Humanities*, ed. Anne Whitehead and Angela Woods (Edinburgh: Edinburgh University Press, 2016), 627–632. For the mental healthcare challenges of undocumented immigrants, see Kurt C. Organista and Maria Y. Hernandez, "The Mental Health Needs of Illegalized Latinos," in *Hidden Lives and Human Rights in the United States*, vol. 2, ed. Lois Ann Lorentzen (Santa Barbara, CA: Praeger, 2014), 321–353.

28. Stephen Jay Gould, *The Mismeasure of Man* (New York: Norton, 1981), 24.

29. See the postscript in Elyn R. Saks, *The Center Cannot Hold: My Journey through Madness* (2007; repr., New York: Hachette, 2015), 345–347.

30. Joyce Carol Oates, *The Lost Landscape: A Writer's Coming of Age* (New York: HarperCollins, 2015), 207. Glenn and Jessie Close offer a contrasting example of sisters' stories in Jessie Close, *Resistance: Two Sisters and a Story of Mental Illness* (New York: Grand Central, 2015), written with Glenn Close and Pete Earley.

31. For concerns that *DSM-IV* was becoming an all-powerful "statute book" underpinning health insurance claims see Mary Sykes Wylie, "The Power of DSM-IV: Diagnosing for Dollars?," *Family Therapy Networker*, May/June 1995, 23–33, 65–68.

32. Satcher, "Foreword," *150 Years of Obamacare*, xii. For discussion of the deleterious effects of social isolation on mental health, see Erin York Cornwell and Linda J. Wait, "Social Disconnectedness, Perceived Isolation, and Health among Older Adults," *Journal of Health and Social Behavior* 50 (March 2009): 31–48; and Kerstin Gerst-Emerson and Jayani Jayawardhana, "Loneliness as a Public Health Issue," *American Journal of Public Health* 105 (May 2015): 1013–1019.

33. See Robert N. Bellah, Richard Madsen, William M. Sullivan, Ann Swidler, and Steven M. Tipton, *The Good Society* (New York: Knopf, 1991), 82–84; Robert N. Bellah, "Understanding Care in Contemporary America," in *The Crisis of Care: Affirming and Restoring Caring Practices in the Helping Professions*, ed. Susan S. Phillips and Patricia Benner (Washington, DC: Georgetown University Press, 1994), 21–35.

Index

About the Author

Martin Halliwell is a professor of American studies at the University of Leicester in the United Kingdom. His published work spans American cultural and intellectual history, the medical humanities, twentieth-century American literature, American film after 1945, and popular music. He is the author of nine monographs, including *Therapeutic Revolutions: Medicine, Psychiatry, and American Culture, 1945–1970* (2013), and the co-editor of three volumes, including *William James and the Transatlantic Conversation* (2014) and *Reframing 1968: American Politics, Protest, and Identity* (forthcoming). He was the chair of the British Association for American Studies from 2010–2013 and is the current chair of the English Association.